Rheumatology: An Evidence-Based Approach

Rheumatology: An Evidence-Based Approach

Editor: Jeffrey Cain

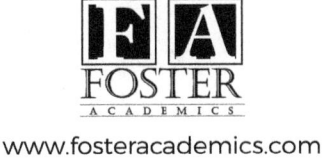

www.fosteracademics.com

www.fosteracademics.com

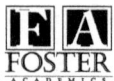

Cataloging-in-Publication Data

Rheumatology : an evidence-based approach / edited by Jeffrey Cain.
        p. cm.
Includes bibliographical references and index.
ISBN 978-1-63242-853-0
1. Rheumatology. 2. Rheumatism. 3. Joints--Diseases. 4. Connective tissues--Diseases. I. Cain, Jeffrey.
RC927 .R44 2019
616.723--dc23

© Foster Academics, 2019

Foster Academics,
118-35 Queens Blvd., Suite 400,
Forest Hills, NY 11375, USA

ISBN 978-1-63242-853-0 (Hardback)

Contents

Preface

The field of medicine concerned with the diagnosis and treatment of rheumatic diseases is known as rheumatology. It is often termed as the study and practice of medical immunology. Rheumatologists deal with diseases related to the soft tissues, musculoskeletal system, heritable connective tissue disorders, vasculitides and autoimmune diseases. Some common rheumatic diseases are osteoarthritis, tendinitis, capsulitis, palindromic rheumatism, Sjögren syndrome, dermatomyositis and systemic lupus erythematosus. The intake of analgesics and non-steroidal anti-inflammatory drugs (NSAIDs) are considered to be effective in treating rheumatic diseases. Surgical methods to treat such diseases include synovectomies and corrective interventions. This book is a compilation of chapters that discuss the most vital concepts and emerging trends in the field of rheumatology. The various advancements in this domain are glanced at and their applications as well as ramifications are looked at in detail. This book includes contributions of experts and doctors, which will provide innovative insights into rheumatology.

This book unites the global concepts and researches in an organized manner for a comprehensive understanding of the subject. It is a ripe text for all researchers, students, scientists or anyone else who is interested in acquiring a better knowledge of this dynamic field.

I extend my sincere thanks to the contributors for such eloquent research chapters. Finally, I thank my family for being a source of support and help.

Editor

Sarcoidosis and Histoplasmosis: Is One a Consequence of the Other?

Anupam Bansal[1] and Rupali Drewek[2]

[1]Atlantic University School of Medicine, Gros Islet Highway, Rodney Bay, Saint Lucia
[2]Phoenix Children's Hospital, 1919 E. Thomas Road, Phoenix, AZ 85016, USA

Correspondence should be addressed to Rupali Drewek; rdrewek@gmail.com

Academic Editor: Mario Salazar-Paramo

Sarcoidosis involves abnormal collections of inflammatory cells (granulomas) which may form as nodules in multiple organs. 90% of affected patients have respiratory tract abnormalities. We present a 61-year-old male with sarcoidosis who was admitted for respiratory distress. Fibrosing mediastinitis was seen in the chest computograph. Management was conservative and included steroids, antibiotics, and oxygen therapy. Sarcoidosis and fibrosing mediastinitis are rare. Fibrosing mediastinitis is more commonly seen with histoplasmosis. We explore the clinical similarities between histoplasmosis and sarcoidosis. We also explore the potential cause and effect relationship and workup for each disease entity.

1. Introduction

Sarcoidosis involves abnormal collections of inflammatory cells (granulomas), which may form as nodules in multiple organs. It is considered a diagnosis of exclusion and most commonly presents with respiratory symptoms. Histoplasmosis is caused by the fungus *H. capsulatum* and causes symptoms that are almost identical to those present with sarcoidosis. Clinicians rely on patient history, lab values, and radiological and pathological studies to distinguish between them. However, there are false negative tests and atypical findings which may complicate the diagnosis. Misdiagnosing one for the other and starting the incorrect treatment plan could cause significant morbidity. In this case, we present a male patient diagnosed with sarcoidosis. History was obtained by personal interview and clinic and hospital medical records. His radiographic finding of fibrosing mediastinitis is rare in sarcoidosis and more commonly seen with histoplasmosis. We review this case to make clinicians aware of the striking resemblance between these two entities and the workup that is recommended to accurately diagnose each disease.

2. Case Presentation

A 61-year-old male with past medical history significant for sarcoidosis was admitted with acute respiratory distress. He had severe baseline lung disease with the most recent forced expiratory volume in 1 second (FEV1) at 18%. Arterial blood gas analysis revealed respiratory acidosis with a pH of 7.27 and CO_2 of 57 (on 50% FiO_2). Due to his level of respiratory distress, he was intubated with ventilator support. He was treated with antibiotics, steroids, and airway clearance measures. Chest X-ray (CXR) showed extensive fibrocalcific scarring in the upper lobes and compensatory emphysema of the lower lobes (Figure 1). Cultures from the endotracheal tube were negative. Viral Direct Fluorescence Antibody (Viral DFA) was negative. Echocardiogram (ECHO) showed normal left ventricular systolic function with an ejection fraction of 60%, right ventricular enlargement, diastolic dysfunction, and normal pulmonary artery pressures. Ventilation/Perfusion Scan (V/Q Scan) was negative for pulmonary embolism.

Our patient first presented with respiratory symptoms at 28 years of age. His symptoms at that time included intermittent fatigue, shortness of breath, a "sore" tongue, and "facial

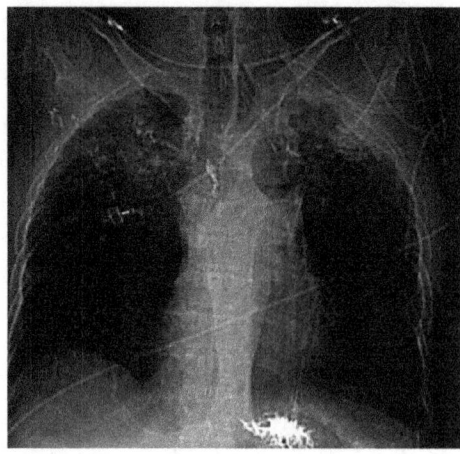

FIGURE 1: Chest X-ray (CXR) showed extensive fibrocalcific scarring in the upper lobes and compensatory emphysema of the lower lobes.

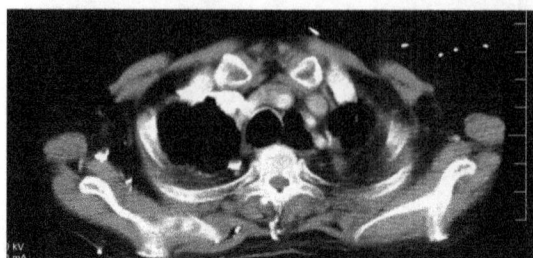

FIGURE 2: Chest computography shows the dilated esophagus above the fibrosing mediastinum.

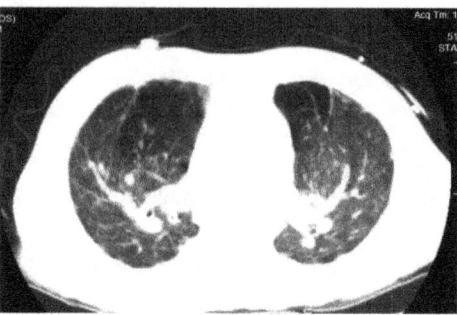

FIGURE 3: Chest computography with extensive calcification, scarring, and areas of hyperinflation.

swelling." While spirometry was normal, his CXR revealed left hilar adenopathy and calcification. Mediastinoscopy was performed, including a mediastinal lymph node biopsy where he was found to have noncaseating granulomas. The fungal cultures and AFB (acid fast bacilli) stains by bronchoscopy were negative. The patient was diagnosed with sarcoidosis and started on prednisone for several months, to which his symptoms responded favorably. For 2 decades, he was treated with inhaled steroids and intermittent courses of prednisone. In his 40s, he presented to an ENT (ear, nose, and throat) specialist with uveitis and a hoarse voice. The ENT physician felt that the cause of the hoarse voice was iatrogenic (secondary to inhaled steroids). No biopsy was performed. At the age of 55, a cavitary lesion was detected on chest CT, and sputum cultures were positive for *Aspergillus*. For this reason, oral antifungal therapy was instituted.

Initial CXRs at the age of 28 showed left hilar and left paratracheal adenopathy. There were also calcified nodules in right and left lung fields. CXRs from the age of 45 through 52 showed progressive upper lobe fibrotic changes. From the age of 52 to 62, the images were stable. The CT scan during the most recent admission was stable as compared to the one done 3 years prior. It showed extensive calcification and soft tissue within the mediastinum with retraction of the mediastinum consistent with fibrosing mediastinitis. Both upper lobes had extensive calcifications and scarring. The esophagus was dilated above the fibrosing mediastinum (Figures 2 and 3). Pulmonary lung function just before admission showed an FVC of 56% FEV1 22% with a ratio of 35%. There was no postbronchodilator response. DLCO (diffusion capacity) was 69%. TLC was 62%, FRC was 75%, and RV was 69%. These values were unchanged as compared to 5 years ago. MRI of the brain showed no evidence of neurosarcoidosis.

Socially, the patient was a nonsmoker and was not exposed to any known environmental toxins which could cause interstitial lung disease. His immunizations were up to date including BCG. He was born in India and lived in Ohio at the age of 20–30 years and in Illinois thereafter. There was no known family history of lung disease.

3. Discussion

Sarcoidosis and histoplasmosis have a striking resemblance in terms of clinical presentation. Table 1 outlines the shared clinical characteristics [1, 2]. The radiographic finding of fibrosing mediastinitis is commonly associated with histoplasmosis [3]. The fact that our patient lives in Ohio (where histoplasmosis is most common) brings up the question of whether our patient could have had a concurrent histoplasmosis infection at the time of initial presentation. This scenario would complicate management since treatment with immunosuppressants for sarcoidosis would worsen any underlying infection. Even though bronchoscopy cultures were negative for fungal infections, there is a significant rate of false negatives [4]. Wheat et al. described 11 patients diagnosed as having sarcoidosis who had laboratory evidence of histoplasmosis [4]. The diagnosis of histoplasmosis in these patients was confirmed by urine antigen, serologic tests, and/or immunodiffusion. These patients all received steroids prior to the diagnosis of histoplasmosis being confirmed. Therefore, it is difficult to say whether histoplasmosis was the primary diagnosis or was a secondary diagnosis secondary to an immunocompromised state. Baughman described 2 cases where sarcoid patients with declining respiratory status attributed their symptoms to sarcoidosis [5]. Their corticosteroid dosage was increased and their condition deteriorated even further. Ultimately, they were detected to have culture evidence of histoplasmosis. Reimann described a case of histoplasmosis in Pennsylvania which was mistakenly diagnosed as sarcoidosis [6]. Sharma described cases where diffuse histoplasmosis was found in a patient with sarcoidosis [7]. It is evident that misdiagnosis can

TABLE 1: Shared characteristics and differences between histoplasmosis and sarcoidosis.

	Histoplasmosis	Sarcoidosis
Clinical symptoms	Cough Dyspnea Adrenal involvement Erythema nodosum Splenomegaly Anorexia Fever Arthralgia Skin ulcers Uveitis/retinitis Hepatitis Parotid gland involvement Cervical myelopathy	Cough Dyspnea Adrenal involvement Erythema nodosum Splenomegaly Anorexia Fever Arthralgia Skin ulcers Uveitis/retinitis Hepatitis Parotid gland involvement Cervical myelopathy
Laboratory findings	Histology Cultures (bronchoalveolar lavage) Immunoassays	Histology: noncaseating granulomas Elevated angiotensin converting enzyme Elevated vitamin D Gammaglobulinemia Kveim
Radiographic findings	Hilar lymphadenopathy Fibrosing mediastinitis Nodules Reticulonodular opacities	Hilar lymphadenopathy Upper lobe involvement Nodules Reticulonodular opacities Granulomas along lymphatic vessels Air trapping
Treatment	Itraconazole/amphotericin Streptomycin Bacillomycin B	Prednisone

happen and an incorrect treatment plan can cause significant morbidity.

Sarcoidosis is a disease process with unknown etiology. Various genetic, environmental, and infectious processes have been hypothesized. *Mycobacterium* has been the longest hypothesized and most investigated potential etiology of sarcoidosis [8]. Other infectious etiologies proposed include *Propionibacterium acnes* and certain viruses [9]. Mycetic agents have also been proposed as potential etiologies [9]. We explored the possibility of histoplasmosis as a causal agent for development of sarcoidosis. Israel et al. investigated a case of chronic disseminated histoplasmosis and its relationship to sarcoidosis [10]. He suggested that histoplasmosis could be the primary disease and stimulate the sarcoidosis [10]. Wynbrandt and Crouser described a case in which documented pulmonary histoplasmosis allegedly evolved into sarcoidosis [11]. Interestingly, there seems to be a higher prevalence of sarcoidosis in Franklin County, Ohio (the demographic profile of which is nearly identical to that of the US) [12]. Ohio is the state where histoplasmosis is also most commonly found.

In addition to similar clinical findings, both histoplasmosis and sarcoidosis present with similar radiographic findings. Chest X-ray will show hilar lymphadenopathy, reticulonodular opacities, nodules, and air trapping. Fibrosing

mediastinitis is more commonly found with histoplasmosis. However, it is (albeit rarely) associated with sarcoidosis. Devaraj et al. reported two cases in a series of 12 patients with CT images and histology of fibrosing mediastinitis (16% of patients) [13]. There were 3 separate case reports discussing fibrosing mediastinitis in patients with sarcoidosis developing complications such as pulmonary edema, pulmonary hypertension, and pulmonary artery occlusion [14–16]. Strock recently found that certain HLA typing within histoplasmosis could carry a higher predisposition towards development of fibrosing mediastinitis [17]. This suggests that an aberrant host immune response could be contributing to its pathogenesis.

There are other clinical markers which can be used to diagnose sarcoidosis. However, these also can be misleading. ACE (angiotensin converting enzyme) levels are usually only elevated in sarcoidosis but there was a reported case where a patient had elevated ACE levels and *Histoplasma* grew from the liver biopsy specimens [7]. ACE levels can also have false positive and negative rates [18]. Noncaseating granulomas, which are the hallmark for sarcoidosis, are also seen in tissues from patients with histoplasmosis [19]. Histoplasmosis usually exhibits few angular ragged granulomas, while sarcoidosis usually contains more granulomas and has a rounded morphology [20]. A positive Kveim-Siltzbach test provides strong support for the diagnosis of sarcoidosis [21]. However, this test is rarely performed.

Laboratory methods to diagnose histoplasmosis include cultures, histology, molecular techniques, serology, and antigen detection. *Histoplasma* organisms are difficult to visualize in tissues and have often been initially overlooked [22]. In addition, the sensitivity can be low (9–34%) especially in acute or localized cases [23, 24]. Histopathological evaluation oftentimes lacks sensitivity. Urine antigen sensitivity was noted to be 93–100% [25]. In recent years, *Histoplasma capsulatum* has been identified in clinical samples by a highly sensitive molecular marker, a fragment of the Hcp 100 gene. PCR assays for the Hcp 100 gene have been validated in several studies and have shown high specificities [26–29].

In summary, chronic disseminated histoplasmosis and sarcoidosis have strikingly similar features. Diagnostic tests including radiography also have similarities. Unfortunately, applying loose criteria for the diagnosis of sarcoidosis may result in overlooking specific infectious diseases including histoplasmosis. Cultures alone cannot exclude histoplasmosis due to a significant rate of false negatives. As a result, the recommended workup to accurately differentiate between sarcoidosis and histoplasmosis should include radiography, tissue biopsies, cultures, ACE level, serology, PCR assay, and urine antigen. Future studies will be needed to investigate the link between these two diseases.

References

[1] T. E. King, *Patient Information: Sarcoidosis (Beyond the Basics)*, UpToDate, 2013.

[2] J. L. Wheat and C. A. Kaufmann, *Pathogenesis and Clinical Manifestations of Disseminated Histoplasmosis*, UpToDate, 2014.

[3] T. Peikert, T. V. Colby, D. E. Midthun et al., "Fibrosing mediastinitis: clinical presentation, therapeutic outcomes, and adaptive immune response," *Medicine*, vol. 90, no. 6, pp. 412–423, 2011.

[4] L. J. Wheat, M. L. V. French, and J. L. Wall, "Sarcoidlike manifestations of histoplasmosis," *Archives of Internal Medicine*, vol. 149, no. 11, pp. 2421–2426, 1989.

[5] R. P. Baughman and E. E. Lower, "Fungal infections as a complication of therapy for sarcoidosis," *QJM*, vol. 98, no. 6, pp. 451–456, 2005.

[6] H. A. Reimann and A. H. Price, "Histoplasmosis in Pennsylvania; confusion with sarcoidosis," *Pennsylvania Medical Journal*, vol. 52, no. 4, pp. 367–371, 1949.

[7] O. P. Sharma, "Histoplasmosis: a masquerader of sarcoidosis," *Sarcoidosis*, vol. 8, no. 1, pp. 10–13, 1991.

[8] I. Brownell, F. Ramirez-Valle, M. Sanchez, and S. Prystowsky, "Evidence for mycobacteria in sarcoidosis," *American Journal of Respiratory and Critical Care Medicine*, vol. 183, no. 5, pp. 573–581, 2011.

[9] R. P. Baughman, D. A. Culver, and M. A. Judson, "A concise review of pulmonary sarcoidosis," *American Journal of Respiratory and Critical Care Medicine*, vol. 183, no. 5, pp. 573–581, 2011.

[10] H. L. Israel, E. DeLamater, M. Sones, W. D. Willis, and A. Mirmelstein, "Chronic disseminated histoplasmosis. An investigation of its relationship to sarcoidosis," *The American Journal of Medicine*, vol. 12, no. 2, pp. 252–260, 1952.

[11] J. H. Wynbrandt and E. D. Crouser, "Transformation of pulmonary histoplasmosis to sarcoidosis: a case report," *Respiratory Medicine*, vol. 101, no. 4, pp. 863–864, 2007.

[12] B. S. Erdal, B. D. Clymer, V. O. Yildiz, M. W. Julian, and E. D. Crouser, "Unexpectedly high prevalence of sarcoidosis in a representative U.S. Metropolitan population," *Respiratory Medicine*, vol. 106, no. 6, pp. 893–899, 2012.

[13] A. Devaraj, N. Griffin, A. G. Nicholson, and S. P. G. Padley, "Computed tomography findings in fibrosing mediastinitis," *Clinical Radiology*, vol. 62, no. 8, pp. 781–786, 2007.

[14] C. R. Hamilton-Craig, R. Slaughter, K. McNeil, F. Kermeen, and D. L. Walters, "Improvement after angioplasty and stenting of pulmonary arteries due to sarcoid mediastinal fibrosis," *Heart Lung and Circulation*, vol. 18, no. 3, pp. 222–225, 2009.

[15] M. Załeska, K. Błasińska-Przerwa, K. Oniszh, B. Roszkowska-Śliz, and K. Roszkowski-Śliz, "Fibrosing mediastinitis with pulmonary hypertension as a rare complication of sarcoidosis," *Pneumonologia i Alergologia Polska*, vol. 81, no. 3, pp. 273–280, 2013.

[16] F. Yangui, J.-P. Battesti, D. Valeyre, A. B. Kheder, and P.-Y. Brillet, "Fibrosing mediastinitis as a rare mechanism of pulmonary oedema in sarcoidosis," *European Respiratory Journal*, vol. 35, no. 2, pp. 455–456, 2010.

[17] S. B. Strock, S. Gaudieri, S. Mallal et al., "Fibrosing mediastinitis complicating prior histoplasmosis is associated with human leukocyte antigen DQB1 04:02—a case control study," *BMC Infectious Diseases*, vol. 15, article 206, 2015.

[18] J. Lieberman, "Enzymes in sarcoidosis. Angiotensin-converting-enzyme (ACE)," *Clinics in Laboratory Medicine*, vol. 9, no. 4, pp. 745–755, 1989.

[19] J. V. Walker, D. Baran, Y. N. Yakub, and R. B. Freeman, "Histoplasmosis with hypercalcemia, renal failure, and papillary necrosis. Confusion with sarcoidosis," *The Journal of the American Medical Association*, vol. 237, no. 13, pp. 1350–1352, 1977.

[20] M. P. Gailey, M. E. Keeney, and C. S. Jensen, "A cytomorphometric analysis of pulmonary and mediastinal granulomas: differentiating histoplasmosis from sarcoidosis by fine-needle aspiration," *Cancer Cytopathology*, vol. 123, no. 1, pp. 51–58, 2015.

[21] W. J. Williams and D. G. James, "Kveim-Siltzbach test revisited," *Sarcoidosis*, vol. 8, no. 1, pp. 6–9, 1991.

[22] L. J. Wheat, R. B. Kohler, and R. P. Tewari, "Diagnosis of disseminated histoplasmosis by detection of *Histoplasma capsulatum* antigen in serum and urine specimens," *The New England Journal of Medicine*, vol. 314, no. 2, pp. 83–88, 1986.

[23] L. J. Wheat, "Improvements in diagnosis of histoplasmosis," *Expert Opinion on Biological Therapy*, vol. 6, no. 11, pp. 1207–1221, 2006.

[24] L. J. Wheat, "Current diagnosis of histoplasmosis," *Trends in Microbiology*, vol. 11, no. 10, pp. 488–494, 2003.

[25] C. A. Hage, J. A. Ribes, N. L. Wengenack et al., "A multicenter evaluation of tests for diagnosis of histoplasmosis," *Clinical Infectious Diseases*, vol. 53, no. 5, pp. 448–454, 2011.

[26] D. Maubon, S. Simon, and C. Aznar, "Histoplasmosis diagnosis using a polymerase chain reaction method. Application on human samples in French Guiana, South America," *Diagnostic Microbiology and Infectious Disease*, vol. 58, no. 4, pp. 441–444, 2007.

[27] A. I. Toranzo, I. N. Tiraboschi, N. Fernández et al., "Molecular diagnosis of human histoplasmosis in whole blood samples," *Revista Argentina de Microbiologia*, vol. 41, no. 1, pp. 20–26, 2009.

[28] C. Muñoz, B. L. Gómez, A. Tobón et al., "Validation and clinical application of a molecular method for identification of *Histoplasma capsulatum* in human specimens in Colombia, South America," *Clinical and Vaccine Immunology*, vol. 17, no. 1, pp. 62–67, 2010.

[29] M. J. Buitrago, C. E. Canteros, G. Frías De León et al., "Comparison of PCR protocols for detecting *Histoplasma capsulatum* DNA through a multicenter study," *Revista Iberoamericana de Micologia*, vol. 30, no. 4, pp. 256–260, 2013.

Myasthenia Gravis and Stroke in the Setting of Giant Cell Arteritis

Elli-Sophia Tripodaki,[1] Sotirios Kakavas,[1,2] Ioanna Skrapari,[1] Dimitrios Michas,[3] Giorgios Katsikas,[4] Charikleia Kouvidou,[5] Theodoros Gounaris,[1] and Euaggelia Sioula[1]

[1] *1st Department of Internal Medicine, Evangelismos General Hospital, Ypsilanti 45-47, 10676 Athens, Greece*
[2] *9 Kosma Aitolou, Herakleio, 14121 Athens, Greece*
[3] *Department of Neurology, Evangelismos General Hospital, Ypsilanti 45-47, 10676 Athens, Greece*
[4] *Department of Rheumatology, Evangelismos General Hospital, Ypsilanti 45-47, 10676 Athens, Greece*
[5] *Department of Pathology, Evangelismos General Hospital, Ypsilanti 45-47, 10676 Athens, Greece*

Correspondence should be addressed to Sotirios Kakavas; sotikaka@yahoo.com

Academic Editors: H. Alexanderson, G. O. Littlejohn, and M. Salazar-Paramo

This case report concerns the diagnosis of two independent chronic diseases in a patient hospitalized for stroke, myasthenia gravis (MG) and giant cell arteritis (GCA). MG has been found to be associated with several diseases, but there are very few cases documenting its coexistence with GCA. We report the case of a 79-year-old woman initially hospitalized for stroke. Patient's concurrent symptoms of blepharoptosis, dysphagia, and proximal muscle weakness were strongly suggestive of myasthenia gravis. The persistent low-grade fever and elevated inflammatory markers in combination with the visual deterioration that developed also raised the suspicion of GCA. Histological examination confirmed GCA, while muscle acetylcholine receptor antibodies were also present. Even though in medicine one strives to interpret a patient's symptoms with one diagnosis, when one entity cannot fully interpret the clinical and laboratory findings, clinicians must consider the possibility of a second coexisting illness.

1. Introduction

Myasthenia gravis (MG) is an immune-mediated disease that compromises the postsynaptic membrane of the neuromuscular junction and usually leads to symptoms of fatigability and decreased muscle strength. It is characterized by the production of antibodies to the n-acetylcholine receptor (AChR) as a dominating feature. Some MG patients, who do not have AChR antibodies, have antibodies to muscle-specific kinase (MuSK) or other muscle proteins such as titin, ryanodine receptor (RyR), and voltage-gated potassium receptor. MG remains a challenging medical diagnosis due to its fluctuating symptoms and similarity to other disorders. A clinical diagnosis (patient history and findings of fluctuating and fatigable weakness, particularly involving extraocular and bulbar muscles) may be confirmed by laboratory testing including (1) pharmacologic testing with edrophonium chloride that elicits unequivocal improvement in strength;

(2) electrophysiologic testing with repetitive nerve stimulation (RNS) studies and/or single-fiber electromyography (SFEMG) that demonstrates a primary postsynaptic neuromuscular junctional disorder; (3) by serological demonstration of AChR or MuSK antibodies [1].

Giant cell arteritis (GCA) also referred to as cranial arteritis or temporal arteritis is a vasculitis of predominantly large- and medium-sized arteries and is the most prevalent of the systemic vasculitis syndromes. Inflammation of the vessel wall is characterized by infiltration of T cells and macrophages, presence of eponymous giant cells, granulomatous lesions, intimal hyperplasia, and destruction of elastic fibres [2]. Symptomatic vessel inflammation usually involves cranial branches of arteries originating from the aortic arch, including the superficial temporal artery, the ophthalmic artery, and the posterior ciliary arteries [3]. The incidence of GCA increases after the age of 50 and peaks between 70 and 80 years of age, with a current prevalence of approximately

20/100000 in Central Europe. Women are affected more frequently than men (3 : 1). The disease is associated with polymyalgia rheumatica. Typical symptoms owing to temporal artery involvement in GCA include unilateral headache, jaw claudication, and visual loss due to ischaemic optic neuropathy. When arteries, however, other than the temporal artery are involved (in more than half of GCA cases), symptoms are often atypical and may involve arm claudication, signs of regional or global cerebral hypoperfusion, low grade fever, and general malaise. Diagnosis is based on typical clinical symptoms, raised serologic inflammatory markers, response to glucocorticoids, and exclusion of other diseases. The gold standard for diagnosis remains temporal artery biopsy.

MG has been found to be associated with a large number of autoimmune diseases (primary sclerosing cholangitis, autoimmune thyroiditis, systemic lupus erythematosus, rheumatoid arthritis, ankylosing spondylitis, Sjogrens) but there are very few cases documenting the coexistence of MG and GCA.

2. Case Presentation

A 79-year-old woman presented to the emergency department with left arm and leg weakness and dysarthria. She had previously experienced several weeks of generalized weakness, malaise, temporal headache, and left palpebral ptosis, without a recording of her temperature. She did not mention any episodes of jaw claudication or scalp tenderness. Her medical history was significant for arterial hypertension, cholecystectomy, and a cataract operation in the right eye.

On examination, reduced power was noted in her left arm and leg with normal speech and no facial droop. The left palpebral ptosis was noted which upon repeat questioning she insisted to be contained to the left eye lid and did not fluctuate during the day. A low-grade fever was recorded. Physical examination of both temporal arteries showed no abnormalities. Auscultation of the chest revealed a systolic murmur.

Computed tomography (CT) of brain performed upon admission revealed ischaemic leukoencephalopathy but no infarcts, whereas the repeat CT showed subacute infarcts in the right posterior parietal and occipital lobes. Ultrasound of carotids showed no significant stenosis, and ECG revealed a sinus rhythm.

Initial investigations revealed anemia (normochromatic and normocytic) and moderately elevated transaminases. Our patient's erythrocyte sedimentation rate (ESR) was 112 mm/h, and her C-reactive protein level (CRP) was 14.4 (normal < 0.5) mg/dL.

A lumbar puncture was performed which revealed an absence of cells with normal protein and glucose (the fluid culture that ensued was negative).

A transthoracic cardiac ultrasound showed a mild hypertrophy of the left ventrical, an exertion fraction of 60%, and mild mitral valve regurgitation. Vegetations were not observed.

A computed tomography of the thorax and upper and lower abdomen was performed which did not reveal any significant findings.

Thyroid function tests were within normal range. Antinuclear antibody assay was negative, as were antineutrophil cytoplasmic antibody, rheumatoid factor, PANCA, CANCA, and anti-Jo1. Complement factors C3 and C4 were elevated. Repeated blood and urine cultures were negative. The Mantoux screening test was negative.

A gastroscopy and colonoscopy were performed which were normal.

Due to the low-grade fever which persisted and the elevated inflammatory markers, despite the absence of other signs or symptoms of infection, broad spectrum antibiotics were initiated, as was antiplatelet therapy (clopidogrel). The low-grade fever and inflammatory markers persisted despite the antibiotic regime.

On the 10th day of hospitalization and although patient's left arm and leg weaknesses were improving, the unilateral blepharoptosis evolved into bilateral blepharoptosis, and she presented with acute onset dysphagia involving liquids and solids, dysarthria, and proximal muscle weakness. She also mentioned deterioration in her vision, which was objectively confirmed with reduced optical acuity and a limitation in the visual fields (completely in the right eye).

Magnetic resonance imaging (MRI) of brain confirmed the CT findings without revealing significant additional pathologic features.

Due to the reduced optical acuity and the limitation in the visual fields—although the full clinical picture of the patient could not be interpreted by a probable diagnosis of giant cell arteritis—a temporal artery biopsy as well as skin, muscle, and vessel biopsy was performed. Pending biopsy results, we found it prudent to treat the patient with high-dose intravenous methylprednisolone (1 mg/kg) without delay due to the vision deterioration. We also proceeded to an investigation of serum antibodies to muscle acetylcholine receptors (AChR-Ab) as patient's symptoms of blepharoptosis, dysphagia, and proximal muscle weakness were strongly suggestive of myasthenia gravis (MG).

Histological examination indeed confirmed giant cell arteritis, while the AChR-Ab were also positive (Figure 1). The skin muscle vessel biopsy did not reveal any pathology.

The dysphagia, dysarthria, and blepharoptosis showed immediate response to the steroid treatment. Patient's temperature readings returned to normal, and the inflammatory markers (ESR and CRP) gradually decreased, until they returned within normal range.

Upon the result of AChR-Ab, oral pyridostigmine was added to the patient's treatment (60 mg three times daily).

Patient was discharged with high-dose oral steroids (prednisolone 55 mg daily), oral pyridostigmine (60 mg three times daily), and antiplatelet therapy.

Upon reexamination in two weeks time, due to a slight deterioration in patient's status (blepharoptosis, dysphagia and dysphagia were exasperated), the pyridostigmine dose was increased (60 mg 4 times daily).

Four weeks after she was discharged from our department, the patient presented to the emergency room with

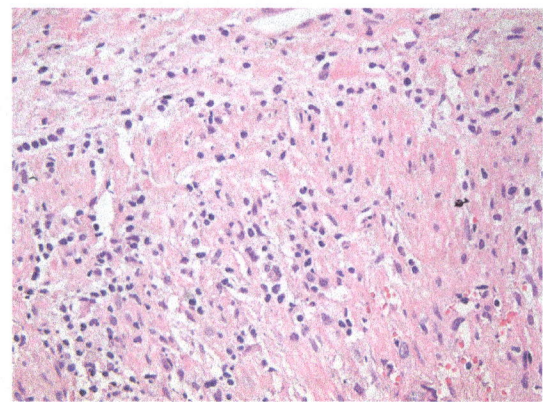

FIGURE 1: Destruction of the wall by an inflammatory infiltrate containing multinucleated giant cells associated with the internal elastic lamina of the artery (Hematoxylin-Eosin ×40).

dyspnea and palpitations. Upon physical examination, except for tachypnea and tachycardia, an edema of her right leg was noted. ECG showed a sinus tachycardia. She had respiratory alkalosis and elevated D-dimers levels. She underwent a triplex ultrasound which revealed deep vein thrombosis of the right leg, while C/T angiography demonstrated a massive pulmonary embolism. Deep vein thrombosis was probably the result of the limited mobility of the patient due to myasthenia, as the evaluation for thrombophilia was unrevealing.

We continue to reassess the patient monthly in cooperation with our hospital's rheumatologists and neurologists. After the initial two-month-high dose steroid regimen, they will gradually be tapered, depending on the patient's condition.

3. Discussion

This case presents clinical interest because it involves the diagnosis of two independent chronic diseases in a patient hospitalized for stroke. Several clinical observations support the idea that a general derangement of the immune system regulation plays an important role in the pathophysiology of MG. MG has been reported to be associated with a number of autoimmune disorders including more frequently rheumatoid arthritis [4], Graves' disease [4, 5], and systemic lupus erythematosus [6] but also Type I diabetes [5]. Moreover, similar genetic associations, overlapping with other autoimmune conditions, including the HLA-B8, DR3 haplotypes and the R620W variants of PTPN22 have been demonstrated in the case of MG [7]. Finally, patients with MG demonstrate a therapeutic response to various immunomodulating therapies, immunosuppressants, and thymectomy [8].

These observations suggest that common mechanisms may exist which predispose MG patients for additional autoimmune disorders. In our patient, MG was found to overlap with GCA which to our knowledge is extremely rare. An extensive review of the literature revealed very few cases of the coexistence of MG and vasculitis. In a case series of 25 patients with GCA, only one also had MG [9]. In a more recently published study by Liozon et al. [10], only one case of MG is reported in a series of 250 patients with GCA during a study period of 27 years. We also found one case report describing the concurrence of MG with polyarteritis nodosa [11], as well as a case of myasthenia gravis in the setting of microscopic polyangiitis [12].

In our patient, as was presented in the brief history, there was a time coincidence of the clinical manifestation of the two diseases. The persistent fever, headache, and especially the decrease in optical acuity demanded that the diagnostic followup includes GCA. Nevertheless, solely this diagnosis was not adequate to interpret the entire clinical picture.

The blepharoptosis was unilateral in the beginning, which is quite unusual in MG [13]. This is why the suspicion of MG intensified when during her hospitalization bilateral blepharoptosis, dysphagia, and proximal muscle weakness were added to the clinical picture.

It is usual in medicine to strive to interpret a patient's symptoms with one diagnosis. In some cases though when patient's clinical and laboratory findings cannot all be comprehended by one entity, it is imperative that the diagnostic followup investigates the possibility of a second coexisting illness.

It is worth noting that our patient presented to the ER and was initially hospitalized due to symptoms of left pyramidal syndrome which were found to be caused by an ischemic brain infarct. We speculate that the stress of the stroke led to an exasperation of the symptoms of MG in our patient. We consider the stroke to be associated with the history of arterial hypertension. It is important to add that there are very few cases of concomitant stroke and GCA in the literature. This can be explained by the fact that the inflammatory response in GCA is directed towards the elastic fibres in the media and adventia, which are sharply reduced within about 5 mm of the artery entering the dura. GCA is reportedly the cause of first-ever stroke in only 0.11% of patients. 50%–75% of strokes associated with GCA occur in the vertebrobasilar circulation (compared with 15%–20% of strokes in patients without GCA) [14]. Stroke associated with extracranial involvement in GCA occurs in 3 to 7% of GCA patients, which was not the case in our patient as carotid artery and vertebrobasilar circulation triplex revealed no abnormal findings [15].

4. Conclusion

Myasthenia gravis has been associated with a number of autoimmune disorders; we report a rare case of its coexistence with giant cell arteritis. The diagnosis of GCA can prove to be very challenging especially in the case of the coexistence of a second newly diagnosed disease such as MG. Moreover, clinicians should keep in mind that MG may occur in the setting of other autoimmune diseases. It is of special significance to note how vigilant clinicians must be in rapidly considering the possibility of MG but mainly GCA, especially when it presents with visual disturbances. The early recognition of symptoms and rapid initiation of treatment are critical not only in relieving the patient's symptoms but also in preventing the potentially catastrophic progression of the illness.

References

[1] V. C. Juel and J. M. Massey, "Myasthenia gravis," *Orphanet Journal of Rare Diseases*, vol. 2, no. 1, article 44, 2007.

[2] C. Salvarani, F. Cantini, and G. G. Hunder, "Polymyalgia rheumatica and giant-cell arteritis," *The Lancet*, vol. 372, no. 9634, pp. 234–245, 2008.

[3] I. M. Wilkinson and R. W. Russell, "Arteries of the head and neck in giant cell arteritis. A pathological study to show the pattern of arterial involvement," *Archives of Neurology*, vol. 27, no. 5, pp. 378–391, 1972.

[4] P. Brogger Christensen, T. S. Jensen, I. Tsiropoulos et al., "Associated autoimmune diseases in myasthenia gravis. A population-based study," *Acta Neurologica Scandinavica*, vol. 91, no. 3, pp. 192–195, 1995.

[5] C. Toth, D. McDonald, J. Oger, and K. Brownell, "Acetylcholine receptor antibodies in myasthenia gravis are associated with greater risk of diabetes and thyroid disease," *Acta Neurologica Scandinavica*, vol. 114, no. 2, pp. 124–132, 2006.

[6] G. Vaiopoulos, P. P. Sfikakis, V. Kapsimali et al., "The association of systemic lupus erythematosus and myasthenia gravis," *Postgraduate Medical Journal*, vol. 70, no. 828, pp. 741–745, 1994.

[7] R. Ramanujam, F. Piehl, R. Pirskanen, P. K. Gregersen, and L. Hammarström, "Concomitant autoimmunity in myasthenia gravis—lack of association with IgA deficiency," *Journal of Neuroimmunology*, vol. 236, no. 1-2, pp. 118–122, 2011.

[8] J. Y. Kim, K. D. Park, and D. P. Richman, "Treatment of myasthenia gravis based on its immunopathogenesis," *The Journal of Clinical Neurology*, vol. 7, pp. 173–183, 2011.

[9] B. Dare and E. Byrne, "Giant cell arteritis. A five-year review of biopsy-proven cases in a teaching hospital," *Medical Journal of Australia*, vol. 1, no. 8, pp. 372–373, 1980.

[10] E. Liozon, V. Loustaud-Ratti, P. Soria et al., "Disease associations in 250 patients with temporal (giant cell) arteritis," *Presse Medicale*, vol. 33, no. 19, pp. 1304–1312, 2004.

[11] F. El Sayed, R. Dhaybi, A. Ammoury, M. Chababi, and J. Bazex, "Myasthenia gravis with cutaneous polyarteritis nodosa," *Clinical and Experimental Dermatology*, vol. 31, no. 2, pp. 215–217, 2006.

[12] M. V. Holmes and D. Sen, "Microscopic polyangiitis and myasthenia gravis: the battle of Occam and Hickam," *Clinical Rheumatology*, vol. 26, no. 11, pp. 1981–1983, 2007.

[13] D. Grob, N. Brunner, T. Namba, and M. Pagala, "Lifetime course of myasthenia gravis," *Muscle and Nerve*, vol. 37, no. 2, pp. 141–149, 2008.

[14] M. Wiszniewska, G. Devuyst, and J. Bogousslavsky, "Giant cell arteritis as a cause of first-ever stroke," *Cerebrovascular Diseases*, vol. 24, no. 2-3, pp. 226–230, 2007.

[15] M. A. Gonzalez-Gay, T. R. Vazquez-Rodriguez, I. Gomez-Acebo et al., "Strokes at time of disease diagnosis in a series of 287 patients with biopsy-proven giant cell arteritis," *Medicine*, vol. 88, no. 4, pp. 227–235, 2009.

3

Association of Sweet's Syndrome and Systemic Lupus Erythematosus

J. L. Barton, L. Pincus, J. Yazdany, N. Richman, T. H. McCalmont, L. Gensler, M. Dall'Era, and K. H. Fye

Division of Rheumatology, Department of Medicine, University of California, San Francisco, CA 94143, USA

Correspondence should be addressed to J. L. Barton, jennifer.barton@ucsfmedctr.org

Academic Editors: A. Chalmers and J. C. Nossent

Sweet's syndrome is an acute febrile neutrophilic dermatosis which usually presents as an idiopathic disorder but can also be drug induced, associated with hematopoetic malignancies and myelodysplastic disorders, and more, infrequently, observed in autoimmune disorders. Sweet's syndrome has been reported in three cases of neonatal lupus, three cases of hydralazine-induced lupus in adults, and in nine pediatric and adult systemic lupus erythematosus (SLE) patients. We describe three additional adult cases of Sweet's associated with SLE and provide a focused review on nondrug-induced, nonneonatal SLE and Sweet's. In two of three new cases, as in the majority of prior cases, the skin rash of Sweet's paralleled underlying SLE disease activity. The pathogenesis of Sweet's remains elusive, but evidence suggests that cytokine dysregulation may be central to the clinical and pathological changes in this condition, as well as in SLE. Further research is needed to define the exact relationship between the two conditions.

1. Introduction

Sweet's syndrome represents an acute neutrophilic dermatitis, often with associated fever [1], first described by Sweet in 1964 [2]. Although the syndrome often presents in idiopathic fashion, it can also be induced by medications and has been associated with hematopoietic malignancies and myelodysplastic disorders. It has also been observed in association with certain autoimmune disorders, such as Sjogren's syndrome. Nine patients with both Sweet's syndrome and systemic lupus erythematosus (SLE) have been previously reported [3–10]. Because the diagnosis of Sweet's syndrome can be challenging, particularly when associated with other connective tissue disorders such as SLE, a set of diagnostic criteria were proposed initially by Su and Liu [11] and then revised by Von den Driesch [12]. The diagnosis is based upon the presence of two major and two of the four minor criteria. The two major criteria are (1) abrupt onset of painful erythematous plaques or nodules and (2) histopathologic evidence of a dense neutrophilic infiltrate. The minor criteria include (1) fever >38 degrees centigrade; (2) presence of a malignancy or connective tissue disease; (3) dramatic response to corticosteroids or potassium iodide therapy; (4) an elevated erythrocyte sedimentation rate or leukocytosis.

We herein report our experience with Sweet's syndrome among adult patients in the Lupus Clinic at the University of California, San Francisco, along with a review of the literature.

2. Case 1

A 26-year-old previously healthy Japanese female presented with nine days of myalgias, subjective fevers, and soaking night sweats. Four days prior, she developed multiple zerythematous nodules on her face, chest, abdomen, and upper and lower extremities bilaterally. She complained of sore throat, nonproductive cough, painless oral ulcers, hand swelling, Raynaud's phenomenon, erythroderma, and abdominal bloating. She denied illicit or prescribed drug use, drug allergies, alcohol, or tobacco. She emigrated from Japan at age eight and received a BCG vaccination as a child. She reported recent travel to Europe and was sexually active with one partner.

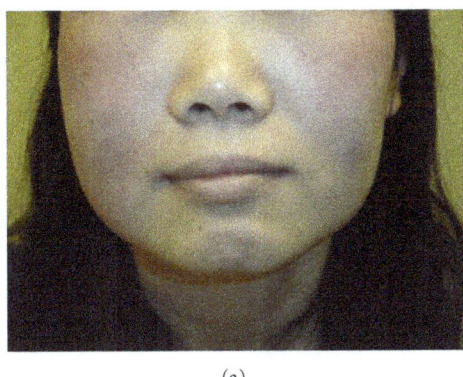
(a)

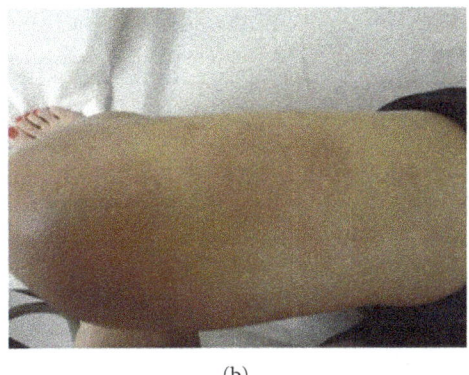
(b)

Figure 1: Multiple 2-3 cm tender, erythematous, subcutaneous nodules were present over (a) the face and (b) lower extremities.

On physical examination, the patient was normotensive and afebrile. There was a tender right submandibular node and diffuse swelling of the hands without synovitis. Multiple 2-3 cm tender, erythematous, subcutaneous nodules were present over the face, chest, abdomen, and upper and lower extremities bilaterally (Figures 1(a) and 1(b)). She subsequently developed a fever of 39.5 Celsius. Initial laboratory tests included a hematocrit of 30.9%, an LDH of 329 iu/L, a positive Coombs antibody assay, an erythrocyte sedimentation rate of 58 mm/hr Westergren, a c-reactive protein of 182 mg/L (normal <6.3 mg/L), and a prolonged partial thromboplastin time of 38.7 sec (normal 20.9–33.6). Histochemical staining of the skin biopsy did not reveal organisms. A CT scan of the chest revealed interlobular septal and bronchial wall thickening of multiple lobes and patchy ground glass opacities suggestive of pulmonary edema or atypical or viral pneumonia. Further laboratory testing revealed an antinuclear antibody titer >640, speckled with positive anti-Smith and anti-Sm/RNP antibody assays. Complement levels and urinalysis were normal. A tuberculin skin test was positive to 14 mm at 48 hours. A quantiferon gold assay was indeterminate. A skin biopsy from her left thigh showed a relatively sparse interstitial inflammatory infiltrate composed of neutrophils, lymphocytes, and histiocytes. In addition, there were some foci of leukocytoclastic vasculitis. Neutrophils were also found in the subcutaneous tissue.

The patient was treated with prednisone 40 mg and hydroxychloroquine 400 mg daily with a dramatic response. Dapsone was later added in an effort to taper the prednisone. She was also treated for latent tuberculosis with four months of rifampin.

3. Case 2

A 23-year-old Asian-American female with a history of SLE presented to the emergency department with a five-day history of diffuse myalgias, fatigue, dizziness, and three days of erythematous papules and plaques which began on the left side of the face and then spread to the upper trunk, arms and legs. On presentation, temperature was 38.9 Celsius. Routine blood tests, chest radiograph, rapid strep, blood cultures, and throat swabs for gonorrhea and Chlamydia were negative. An erythrocyte sedimentation rate was 54 mm/hr Westergren. The patient was instructed to follow up in the lupus clinic. Manifestations of SLE diagnosed at age 20 included malar rash, arthritis, pericarditis, Raynaud's, Coombs positive autoimmune hemolytic anemia, antinuclear antibody titer >640 speckled, and elevated titers of anti-dsDNA antibodies. She was a nursing student, denied tobacco, alcohol, or illicit drug use, and was sexually active with one partner. Medications included hydroxychloroquine 400 mg, prednisone 3 mg, and calcium with vitamin D.

The following day in clinic, the patient complained of painful erythematous papules and plaques as well as intermittent discomfort over the left chest which worsened with deep inspiration, palpitations, and Raynaud's phenomenon. She denied hair loss, arthralgias, dyspnea, oral ulcerations, or new medications. Physical examination revealed an afebrile, normotensive female with tachycardia (pulse 114), cobblestone appearance and erythema of bilateral tonsils with slight exudate, and shotty cervical lymphadenopathy. Cardiac and chest exam were normal. Skin exam revealed large erythematous, tender, and indurated papules and plaques over the face with smaller lesions scattered over the upper chest, back, upper legs, and arms.

Repeat laboratories and skin biopsy were performed. Hemoglobin dropped from 13.7 g/dL to 10.9 g/dL over two days. A skin biopsy of the right upper arm revealed an extensive interstitial infiltrate of neutrophils and histiocytes accompanied by leukocytoclastic debris, suggestive of Sweet's syndrome. A skin biopsy over the chin 17 months later showed neutrophilic dermatitis with leukocytoclasis. Treatment with higher dose prednisone and azathioprine resulted in a good response. However, as indicated by the repeat biopsy, the rash recurred as prednisone was tapered.

4. Case 3

A 23-year-old Asian male with a history of SLE diagnosed at age 16 presented for followup with his nephrologist. He complained of persistent right facial swelling for 12 months. The swelling was limited to the skin over the right parotid gland and was associated with intermittent pruritic vesicles. Manifestations of SLE included a discoid rash and lupus nephritis. Abnormal serologies included antinuclear antibody titer >640 diffuse and elevated titers of anti-dsDNA antibodies. Medications included prednisone 5 mg, enalapril 5 mg, and tacrolimus 2 mg twice daily. The patient was an engineer, used tobacco and alcohol occasionally, and was not sexually active. On examination, the patient was normotensive and afebrile. He had slight warmth and erythema over the right parotid gland without tenderness. Laboratory data revealed an elevated anti-dsDNA antibody titer of 271 iu/mL (250 iu/mL one month prior). Complete blood count, complement levels, creatinine, urinalysis, and c-reactive protein were all normal. A fine needle aspiration of the parotid gland revealed a mixed population of lymphocytes with scattered lymphoepithelial islands, diagnostic of lymphoepithelial sialadenitis. Skin biopsy of the right cheek showed a diffuse infiltrate of neutrophils and leukocytoclastic debris consistent with Sweet's syndrome (Figures 2(a) and 2(b)). The patient was started on hydroxychloroquine 400 mg and prednisone with an excellent response.

5. Discussion

While Sweet's syndrome can occur in idiopathic fashion, it can also be drug induced, associated with malignancy [13], or connective tissue diseases. Concurrent Sweet's disease and SLE are exceedingly rare. Only two other papers reported Sweet's syndrome as an initial presentation in adult SLE [6, 8]. Our Case 1 is the third. Three cases of Sweet's syndrome-like nonbullous neutrophilic dermatosis and neonatal lupus have been reported [14, 15], as well as three cases of hydralazine-induced SLE and Sweet's [16–18], but will not be discussed here. In addition, cases with some features of SLE that did not meet full criteria for SLE were excluded from this paper.

The skin lesions in Sweet's syndrome typically start as erythematosus papules, plaques, and nodules. The lesions can take on a pseudovesicular or pseudopustular appearance, and sometimes fully formed vesicles or pustules develop. The lesions are usually painful, and typical sites include the head, neck, and upper extremities, although lesions can be found anywhere. Lesions usually develop abruptly, resolve over 1–3 months, and can recur in 30% of patients [19]. One of the two major criteria as outlined by Von den Driesch is a typical cutaneous rash [12]. Indeed, all three patients described herein had a rash compatible with Sweet's syndrome. Both Cases 1 and 2 had lesions on the face, upper trunk, arms, and legs. Patient 3 had erythematosus swelling on his right face with vesicles within it for 12 months. Although the time course of this patient's lesion was atypical for Sweet's, the vesicles waxed and waned, suggesting resolution and recurrence, as can be seen.

The prototypical histopathologic findings in Sweet's syndrome include a diffuse dermal infiltrate of neutrophils accompanied by leukocytoclasis with overlying papillary dermal edema and, in some cases, extending into the subcutaneous septa. Although older studies reported that leukocytoclastic vasculitis is not seen [20], more recent reports have convincingly demonstrated that leukocytoclastic vasculitis

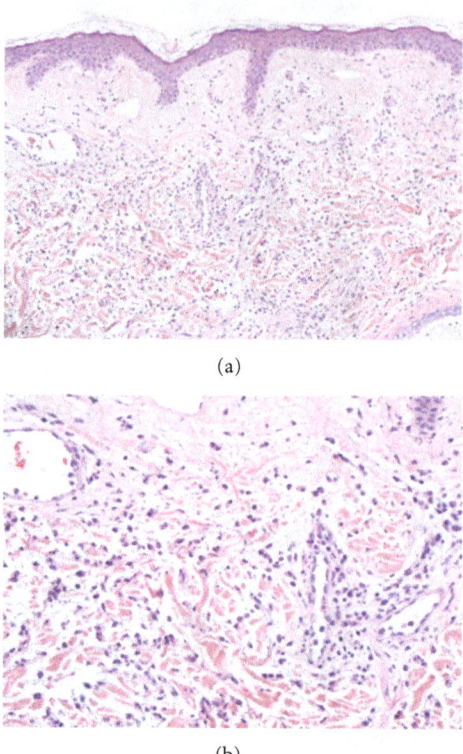

(a)

(b)

Figure 2: (a) Low magnification showing a diffuse dermal infiltrate of neutrophils accompanied by leukocytoclastic debris. (b) High magnification highlighting the neutrophils.

can occasionally be found [21]. The skin biopsies from all patients described herein were compatible with Sweet's syndrome as they exhibited a dermal neutrophilic infiltrate accompanied by leukocytoclasis (Table 1). In Cases 2 and 3, the neutrophilic infiltrate was diffuse and extensive, although in Case 1 it was relatively sparse. Additional histopathologic findings in Case 1 included extension of the neutrophilic infiltrate into subcutaneous septa and accompanying leukocytoclastic vasculitis.

As posited by Gleason and colleagues [9], infiltrates that are less dense than what is typically observed in Sweet's disease may be classified as "neutrophilic dermatosis of LE (lupus erythematosus)." In fact, our Case 1 probably best fits into this classification. It seems most plausible that Sweet's syndrome and neutrophilic dermatosis of LE are related and on a spectrum. It is important for rheumatologists and dermatologists to recognize the possibility, as suggested by Gleason, that what appears to be a distinct entity (Sweet's syndrome) may in fact be a variant of cutaneous LE and may represent the first manifestation of the systemic disease, as in Case 1.

These new cases, combined with nine others in the literature, raise several important questions. Does Sweet's syndrome occur as an independent process, or is it merely a manifestation of the underlying autoimmune disease and an underrecognized variant of cutaneous LE? In two out of three new cases, the rash consistent with Sweet's syndrome

TABLE 1: Demographic and clinical characteristics of SLE patients at time of presentation with Sweet's.

Patient	Gender	Age	Race/ethnicity	Clinical manifestations of SLE at time of Sweet's presentation	Serologies	Histopathology	Treatment	Response
1	Female	26	Asian	Oral ulcers, Raynaud's, hemolytic anemia	ANA, anti-Sm, anti-Sm/RNP	Sparse interstitial neutrophilic dermatitis	Prednisone 40 mg, hydroxychloroquine	Responsive to treatment
2	Female	23	Asian	Malar rash, pericarditis, arthritis, hemolytic anemia	ANA, anti-dsDNA, anti-La,	Neutrophilic dermatitis	Prednisone	Responsive to treatment
3	Male	23	Asian		ANA, dsDNA	Neutrophilic dermatitis	Hydroxychloroquine, prednisone	Responsive to treatment
Goette 1985 [7]	Male	67	NA	Arthritis, malar, and discoid rashes, leukopenia, thrombocytopenia	ANA	Prominent dermal edema, extensive infiltration with intact and karyorrhectic PMNs	Prednisone 30–40 mg, quinacrine hydrochloride 100 mg	Responsive to treatment
Choi and Chung, 1999 [5]	Female	13	Asian	Malar rash, oral ulcers, leukopenia, thrombocytopenia, nephritis	ANA, anti-Sm, anti-dsDNA	Neutrophilic dermatosis	Pulse methylprednisolone	Responsive to treatment
Burnham and Cron, 2005 [10]	Female	14	African American	Arthritis, oral ulcer, leukopenia	ANA, anti-dsDNA, anti-Ro, anti-La, anti-SM/RNP	Marked edema of papillary dermis with early subepidermal bullae, PMNs and karyorrhexis	NA	NA
Hou et al., 2005 [8]	Female	38	Asian	Arthritis, proteinuria >0.5 mg/day,	ANA, anti-Ro, anti-La	Neutrophilic dermatosis	Prednisolone 20 mg	Responsive to treatment
Gleason et al., 2006 [9]	Female	16	NA	Arthritis, serositis, leukopenia	ANA, anti-dsDNA	Neutrophilic dermatosis	Hydroxychloroquine, prednisone	Responsive to treatment
Gleason et al., 2006 [9]	Female	35	NA	Arthritis, hematuria (lupus nephritis on prior biopsy)	ANA, anti-dsDNA, anti-Ro	Neutrophilic dermatosis	Corticosteroids, dapsone, azathioprine	Responsive to treatment
Camarillo et al., 2008 [3]	Female	9	NA	Lymphopenia, (mesangial glomerulonephritis prior)	ANA, anti-dsDNA, anti-RNP	Interstitial dermal infiltrate of histiocytelike cells, lymphocytes and segmented neutrophils and leukocytoclastic debris	Methylprednisolone, dapsone	Responsive to treatment
Fernandes et al., 2009 [6]	Male	25	NA	Leukopenia, proteinuria, malar rash	ANA, anti-Sm/RNP, anti-dsDNA	Neutrophilic dermatitis	Prednisone	Responsive to treatment
Gollol-Raju et al., 2009 [4]	Female	23	NA	Malar rash (lupus nephritis previously)	ANA	Acute inflammatory cells with overlying keratin debris, abundant neutrophilic dust	Corticosteroids	Responsive to treatment

paralleled underlying SLE activity. In Case 1, the patient had concomitant oral ulcerations, hand swelling, and a Coombs positive hemolytic anemia. In Case 2, the patient had serositis and a Coombs positive hemolytic anemia. The nine other cases in the literature reflect a similar pattern of Sweet's presenting along with manifestations of active SLE.

Although the pathogenesis of Sweet's syndrome remains elusive, evidence suggests that cytokine dysregulation may be central to the clinical and pathological changes. Studies have implicated a variety of cytokines, including IL-1, IL-3, IL-6, and IL-8 and G-CSF, GM-CSF and interferon gamma [22, 23]. Some of these cytokines, such as IL-6, may also play a role in SLE through a variety of mechanisms, including B cell stimulation and induction of acute phase reactants [24]. Similarly, interferon gamma may be involved in the pathogenesis of SLE. In one series of experiments, NZB mice treated with interferon developed hemolytic anemia earlier and had a significant increase in renal immune complex deposition and renal failure [25]. This preliminary evidence suggests that cytokine dysregulation plays a role in both conditions. It may be that in certain patients during a SLE flare, some cytokines implicated in eliciting Sweet's syndrome are released, resulting in clinical manifestations on the spectrum of Sweet's syndrome and Sweet's syndrome-like neutrophilic dermatitis.

Like other cases in the literature, our patients responded dramatically to corticosteroids, which are the mainstay of therapy for Sweet's syndrome. Other immunosuppressive treatments, including cyclosporine, have also been used successfully. Additional treatments include potassium iodide, dapsone, colchicine, indomethacin, and clofazimine.

In summary, Sweet's syndrome is a neutrophilic dermatoses that may be more commonly associated with SLE than previously suspected because of the role of cytokine dysregulation in the pathogenesis of both conditions. Sweet's disease observed in the setting of lupus may also be classified as "neutrophilic dermatosis of LE" and may be the first manifestation of SLE. Further research is needed to define the exact relationship between the two conditions and to enhance awareness among both rheumatologists and dermatologists.

Dedication

The authors would like to dedicate this paper to the memory of their senior author and beloved teacher, Dr. Kenneth H. Fye, who died on March 28, 2010.

Acknowledgments

Dr. J. L. Barton's work was supported by a Physician Scientist Development Award from the American College of Rheumatology Research and Education Foundation. Drs. J. L. Barton, J. Yazdany, N. Richman, L. Gensler, M. Dall'Era and K. H. Fye's work was supported by the Rosalind Russell Medical Research Center for Arthritis, University of California, San Francisco. Dr. J. Yazdany also received support from the Arthritis Foundation Arthritis Investigator Award, and Dr. N. Richman received support from NIH T32 AR007304.

References

[1] J. S. Storer, L. T. Nesbitt, W. K. Galen, and V. A. DeLeo, "Sweet's syndrome," *International Journal of Dermatology*, vol. 22, no. 1, pp. 8–12, 1983.

[2] R. D. Sweet, "An acute febrile neutrophilic dermatosis," *British Journal of Dermatology*, vol. 76, pp. 349–356, 1964.

[3] D. Camarillo, T. H. McCalmont, I. J. Frieden, and A. E. Gilliam, "Two pediatric cases of nonbullous histiocytoid neutrophilic dermatitis presenting as a cutaneous manifestation of lupus erythematosus," *Archives of Dermatology*, vol. 144, no. 11, pp. 1495–1498, 2008.

[4] N. Gollol-Raju, M. Bravin, and D. Crittenden, "Sweet's syndrome and systemic lupus erythematosus," *Lupus*, vol. 18, no. 4, pp. 377–378, 2009.

[5] J. W. Choi and K. Y. Chung, "Sweet's syndrome with systemic lupus erythematosus and herpes zoster," *British Journal of Dermatology*, vol. 140, no. 6, pp. 1174–1175, 1999.

[6] N. F. Fernandes, L. Castelo-Soccio, E. J. Kim, and V. P. Werth, "Sweet syndrome associated with new-onset systemic lupus erythematosus in a 25-year-old man," *Archives of Dermatology*, vol. 145, no. 5, pp. 608–609, 2009.

[7] D. K. Goette, "Sweet's syndrome in subacute cutaneous lupus erythematosus," *Archives of Dermatology*, vol. 121, no. 6, pp. 789–791, 1985.

[8] T. Y. Hou, D. M. Chang, H. W. Gao, C. H. Chen, H. C. Chen, and J. H. Lai, "Sweet's syndrome as an initial presentation in systemic lupus erythematosus: a case report and review of the literature," *Lupus*, vol. 14, no. 5, pp. 399–402, 2005.

[9] B. C. Gleason, A. Zembowicz, and S. R. Granter, "Nonbullous neutrophilic dermatosis: an uncommon dermatologic manifestation in patients with lupus erythematosus," *Journal of Cutaneous Pathology*, vol. 33, no. 11, pp. 721–725, 2006.

[10] J. M. Burnham and R. Q. Cron, "Sweet syndrome as an initial presentation in a child with systemic lupus erythematosus," *Lupus*, vol. 14, no. 12, pp. 974–975, 2005.

[11] W. P. D. Su and H. N. H. Liu, "Diagnostic criteria for Sweet's syndrome," *Cutis*, vol. 37, no. 3, pp. 167–174, 1986.

[12] P. Von den Driesch, "Sweet's syndrome (acute febrile neutrophilic dermatosis)," *Journal of the American Academy of Dermatology*, vol. 31, no. 4, pp. 535–560, 1994.

[13] R. Kaiser, K. Connolly, C. Linker, J. Maldonado, and K. Fye, "Stem cell transplant for myelodysplastic syndrome-associated histiocytoid Sweet's syndrome in a patient with arthritis and myalgias," *Arthritis Care and Research*, vol. 59, no. 12, pp. 1832–1834, 2008.

[14] K. L. Barr, F. O'Connell, S. Wesson, and V. Vincek, "Nonbullous neutrophilic dermatosis: sweet's syndrome, neonatal lupus erythematosus, or both?" *Modern Rheumatology*, vol. 19, no. 2, pp. 212–215, 2009.

[15] E. K. Satter and W. A. High, "Non-bullous neutrophilic dermatosis within neonatal lupus erythematosus," *Journal of Cutaneous Pathology*, vol. 34, no. 12, pp. 958–960, 2007.

[16] R. Ramsey-Goldman, T. Franz, F. X. Solano, and T. A. Medsger, "Hydralazine induced lupus and Sweet's syndrome report and review of the literature," *Journal of Rheumatology*, vol. 17, no. 5, pp. 682–684, 1990.

[17] W. Sequeira, R. B. Polisky, and D. P. Alrenga, "Neutrophilic dermatosis (Sweet's syndrome). Association with a hydralazine-induced lupus syndrome," *American Journal of Medicine*, vol. 81, no. 3, pp. 558–560, 1986.

[18] O. Servitje, M. Ribera, X. Juanola, and J. Rodriguez-Moreno, "Acute neutrophilic dermatosis associated with hydralazine-induced lupus," *Archives of Dermatology*, vol. 123, no. 11, pp. 1435–1436, 1987.

[19] J. Bolognia, J. L. Jorizzo, and R. P. Rapini, *Dermatology*, Mosby, London, UK, 2nd edition, 2008.

[20] G. C. Goldman and S. L. Moschella, "Acute febrile neutrophilic dermatosis (Sweet's syndrome)," *Archives of Dermatology*, vol. 103, no. 6, pp. 654–660, 1971.

[21] J. C. Malone, S. P. Slone, L. A. Wills-Frank et al., "Vascular inflammation (vasculitis) in Sweet syndrome: a clinicopathologic study of 28 biopsy specimens from 21 patients," *Archives of Dermatology*, vol. 138, no. 3, pp. 345–349, 2002.

[22] H. Elinav, A. Maly, Y. Ilan, A. Rubinow, Y. Naparstek, and H. Amital, "The coexistence of Sweet's syndrome and Still's disease—is it merely a coincidence?" *Journal of the American Academy of Dermatology*, vol. 50, no. 5, pp. S90–S92, 2004.

[23] A. S. M. Giasuddin, A. H. A. M. El-Orfi, M. M. Ziu, and N. Y. El-Barnawi, "Sweet's syndrome: is the pathogenesis mediated by helper T cell type 1 cytokines?" *Journal of the American Academy of Dermatology*, vol. 39, no. 6, pp. 940–943, 1998.

[24] P. Youinou and C. Jamin, "The weight of interleukin-6 in B cell-related autoimmune disorders," *Journal of Autoimmunity*, vol. 32, no. 3-4, pp. 206–210, 2009.

[25] H. Heremans, A. Billiau, and A. Colombatti, "Interferon treatment of NZB mice: accelerated progression of autoimmune disease," *Infection and Immunity*, vol. 21, no. 3, pp. 925–930, 1978.

4

Refractory Rheumatic Disorder: Atypical Postpregnancy Osteoporosis

Cindy Mourgues, Sandrine Malochet-Guinamand, and Martin Soubrier

CHU Gabriel Montpied, Service de Rhumatologie, 58 rue Montalembert, 63000 Clermont-Ferrand, France

Correspondence should be addressed to Cindy Mourgues; nubecorsica@yahoo.fr

Academic Editor: Mehmet Soy

This is a case report on a young patient with severe osteoporosis that was initially revealed when she presented with polyarthralgia during her second pregnancy. Postpartum, the pain increased and her X-ray did not show any abnormalities. A bone scintigraphy was performed. It indicated an inflammatory rheumatic disorder. Six months after partum, an investigation of right coxalgia revealed a spontaneous basicervical fracture. Given the persistent polyarthralgia, the patient underwent a new scintigraphy, which revealed areas of what looked to be old rib and L1 fractures. A subsequent full body magnetic resonance imaging (MRI) scan revealed signal abnormalities that could indicate multiple lower limb bone fractures. Despite exhaustive biological, radiological, and histological testing, no secondary cause for the osteoporosis was found. The patient was started on teriparatide. We finally concluded that, despite the atypical presentation, the patient was suffering from postpregnancy osteoporosis. It is possible that the frequency of occurrence of this still poorly understood disease is underestimated.

1. Introduction

Described for the first time in 1955 by Nordin et al., postpregnancy osteoporosis typically occurs in primiparous women of a mean age of 28 years during their third trimester of pregnancy or in the immediate postpartum period [1]. To date, about a hundred case reports and four case series have been published. Postpregnancy osteoporosis is a rare condition and the cause is poorly understood. It can occur in women who have a low prepregnancy bone density. The rare occurrence of relapse in subsequent pregnancies is an original phenomenon with this condition. The frequency of occurrence is probably underestimated [2]. Joint pain during pregnancy is generally due to mechanical factors and the loosening of muscles and ligaments. We are reporting a case that was complicated by a femoral head fracture after the patient had been initially diagnosed with inflammatory rheumatic disorder.

2. Case Report

A 27-year-old female patient was hospitalized for a work-up of a spontaneous right femoral head fracture in March 2013.

The patient had a history of moderate tobacco use of less than ten pack-years. The patient has two children (4 years and 6 months of age) whom she nursed 5 months and 1 month, respectively. She also had four miscarriages, one of which occurred in her fourth month of pregnancy. Her BMI is $30 \, kg/m^2$, but her weight has drastically fluctuated in a span of less than five years.

Progressively, starting at the beginning of her 2nd pregnancy, she began experiencing daytime and nighttime arthromyalgia anteriorly and bilaterally in her legs. The pain migrated upwards from her knees to her lower thighs. Two months after partum, given the persistence of her pain, she underwent bone scintigraphy. The test revealed abnormal uptake indicating inflammation at each Chopart joint, the left talar dome, the internal left knee, the right femoropatellar joint, and finally the upper left coxofemoral joint (Figure 1). The standard X-rays were normal. One month after these tests, the patient complained of right-sided thoracic pain. Radiological testing was negative. Six months after partum, the patient's coxalgia had worsened, leading her to undergo new standard X-rays that demonstrated a fracture of the right femoral head complicated by a spontaneous basicervical

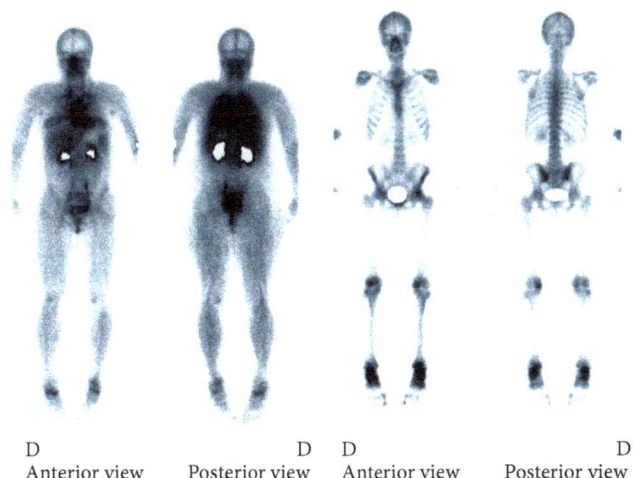

D
Anterior view   D
Posterior view   D
Anterior view   D
Posterior view

FIGURE 1: Bone scintigraphy performed two months after partum. Excessive uptake by both tali, bilaterally by the femoral condyles and by the left cotyle.

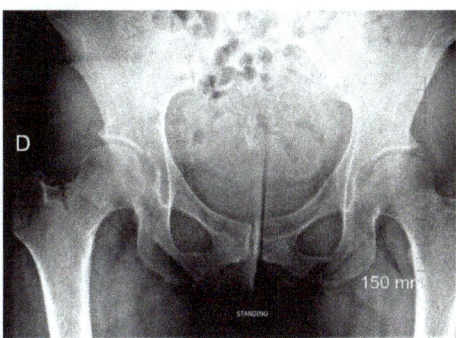

FIGURE 2: Pelvic X-ray, anteroposterior view. Basicervical fracture of the right femur.

fracture (Figure 2) treated with osteosynthesis. The bone biopsy performed during the surgery did not reveal any abnormal cells. There was no family history of bone disease. Laboratory testing one month after the femoral fracture revealed normal plasma and urinary calcium and phosphorous levels as well as normal parathyroid hormone levels. Her vitamin D was 10.8 ng/L (N > 30 ng/L). She had no signs of inflammatory syndrome and her blood protein electrophoresis levels were normal. Her biological examinations ruled out hyperthyroidism, premature ovarian insufficiency, and Cushing's syndrome. Her iron and tryptase levels were normal. Her antitransglutaminase antibody levels were normal. The only abnormal laboratory results were chronically elevated alkaline phosphatase levels of over 150 U/L (N: 5–135 U/L). Bone density testing revealed osteoporosis at two sites with a z-score of −3.1 SD at the spine and −2.7 SD at the femoral head. Endoscopy ruled out coeliac disease and inflammatory bowel disease. The patient also underwent a CT scan of her chest, abdomen, and pelvis as well as a PET scan. No tumours or lymphadenopathies were detected. However, the CT scan did reveal several old fractures, mainly of the right ribs, although no trauma was mentioned during the history. A new bone scintigraphy revealed intense uptake in several left medial ribs indicating fractures, as well as in L1 even though the patient had never experienced lumbar pain symptoms. Two months following her femoral fracture, given the onset of new pain, especially in the left lower limb, another full-body MRI was performed. The examination revealed signal abnormalities indicative of bone oedema that could mean fractures of the left talus, the internal tibial plateau of the left knee and the left greater trochanter, requiring immobilization. Given the unusual nature of this fracture-inducing osteoporosis, the patient underwent a bone biopsy after double tetracycline labelling. It revealed trabecular and cortical osteoporosis with active, highly intense hyperabsorption, especially subperiosteally, by very small osteoclasts (Figure 3) and normal or accelerated formation indicating

coupled hyperremodelling. There was no primary mineralization disorder. Unfortunately, the bone biopsy provided very little information on the trabecular bone due to the poor biopsy quality. In contrast, there were no abnormal cells found or any argument for an overload or mastocytosis. Given the exhaustive negative aetiological work-up, we diagnosed the patient with postpregnancy osteoporosis. Due to the severity of the symptoms and the successive fractures, teriparatide treatment was initiated. Despite this, the patient experienced a new rib fracture without any apparent trauma after six months of treatment.

3. Discussion

We are reporting on a case of fracture-inducing postpregnancy osteoporosis that was initially thought to be an inflammatory rheumatic disorder and became complicated by a femoral head fracture. Our case report is unusual compared with other cases found in the literature due to the type of fractures involved and the fact that onset followed a second pregnancy. The most frequently described fractures occur after an initial pregnancy and are vertebral [3]. However, observations of vertebral fractures have been reported with postpregnancy osteoporosis arising only after a second pregnancy [4]. Postpartum sacral, foot, and rib fractures have also been described [5]. Femoral fractures are generally described as transient osteoporosis or hip algodystrophy that can also become bilateral. Some femoral head fractures have also been described well after the postpartum period [6]. Our patient had no signs indicating algodystrophy on her pelvic X-ray and the presentation was indeed consistent with multiple osteoporotic fractures. Nevertheless, it is interesting to observe that transient hip osteoporosis can also be accompanied by low bone density, thereby complicating the understanding of the pathophysiology of these different postpregnancy rheumatological conditions [6].

The pathophysiology of postpartum osteoporosis is not well understood. Disturbances in phosphorous and calcium metabolism, a decline in bone density during pregnancy, bone remodelling changes, and a possible genetic predisposition given observations of family members are all etiological hypotheses traditionally described in the literature. Standard biological testing often reveals normal phosphorous

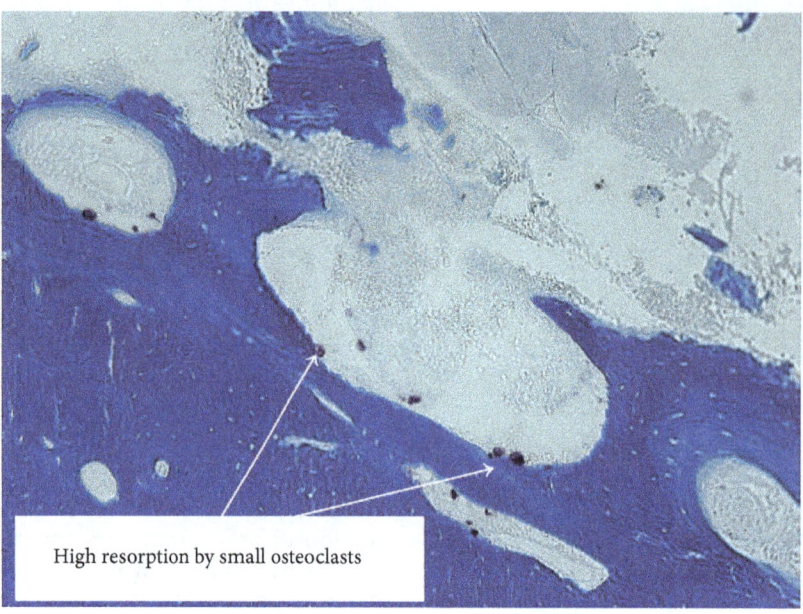

High resorption by small osteoclasts

FIGURE 3: Bone biopsy of the iliac wing with double tetracycline labelling. Active, highly intense resorption via very small osteoclasts, especially in the periosteal region.

and calcium levels except for hypercalciuria. Alkaline phosphatases are often physiologically elevated during pregnancy. Pregnancy is also often accompanied by Parathormone Relative Peptide (PTHrp) hypersecretion. PTHrp is a peptide synthesized by numerous nontumoural tissues, including the mammary glands. It plays a key role in maintaining calcium balance in pregnant and nursing woman. It promotes bone catabolism to mobilize calcium for the foetus, especially during nursing, leading to an estimated maternal bone loss of about one percent per month. When breastfeeding, calcium comes only from bone catabolism and not from food intake [7]. There are reports in the literature of postpregnancy osteoporosis associated with hypercalcemia due to persistently elevated PTHrp in a 31-year-old patient despite stopping nursing [8]. The role of PTHrp in postpregnancy osteoporosis has not been thoroughly reviewed. Its level was not determined in the case we are reporting here.

In our observation, the bone biopsy data did not help establish an aetiologic diagnosis. The literature has little histomorphometric data on postpregnancy osteoporosis, and what data are available are disparate. There are many methodological differences and the biopsies were performed at variable times ranging from several months to several years after pregnancy, or even during pregnancy. At times, osteoporosis was confirmed solely based on trabecular bone analysis and at other times based on cortical bone analysis. Bone remodelling seemed normal or exaggerated. In the majority of cases, bone mineralization was normal [9]. The bone biopsy of our patient demonstrated hyperactive subperiosteal resorption that has never been described in postpregnancy osteoporosis. This observation could indicate hyperparathyroidism, but the osteoclastic morphology was unusual and the parathyroid hormone levels were normal.

The treatment most frequently used to treat postpregnancy osteoporosis is bisphosphonates [10].

More recently, teriparatide was offered due to the fear of bone remodelling with bisphosphonates, the passage of these molecules into the placenta, and the potential impact on future pregnancies. Three patients who suffered vertebral fractures six months after partum received teriparatide treatment for six months. They experienced a 14.5 to 25% gain in lumbar spine bone mass, a 9.5% to 16.7% gain in femoral head bone mass, and a 13.4 to 17.9% gain in total hip bone mass, without experiencing any new fractures [11]. In the literature, other treatments have been offered, such as strontium ranelate [12] and even vitamin K2 or menatetrenone, which increases the carboxylation of osteocalcin [13].

Our patient received teriparatide treatment given the delay in consolidation of her femoral fracture and the severity of her fracture-related symptoms.

In our case fractures occurred during postpartum period but musculoskeletal pain has started before. We do not have any idea of the bone density of our patient before and during her pregnancy. Prevalence of osteoporosis during pregnancy is unknown because the main diagnostic methods involve radiation, which is usually avoided in pregnant women [14]. Thus, diagnosis is made often at a later stage. Our patient's observed osteoporotic risk factors were smoking and breastfeeding, although considering the latter as a risk factor is controversial. The risk of osteoporosis due to breastfeeding seems to vary with parity, duration of breastfeeding, and maternal age [15]. The aetiological investigation for secondary osteoporosis revealed only hypovitaminosis D. This condition can induce widespread pain. Kuru et al. found in their study that patients with hypovitaminosis D have a significantly higher pain scores for all scales (P value range 0.002) among

83 patients with chronic widespread pain [16]. However, to our knowledge there are no data about pain and hypovitaminosis D during pregnancy. Otherwise in our case, pain was well explained by occurrence of multiple fractures.

4. Conclusion

This is a report of a case involving a patient suffering from multiple fractures, the painful symptoms of which initially led us to believe that she was experiencing an inflammatory rheumatic disorder. Exhaustive testing revealed bone fragility but did not reveal a secondary cause of the osteoporosis. Despite the atypical manifestations, we diagnosed the patient with postpregnancy osteoporosis.

Postpregnancy osteoporosis is a rare condition whose pathophysiology is still poorly understood. There is no consensus on the optimal treatment for this condition.

References

[1] P. le Goff and A. Saraux, "Ostéoporose de la grossesse," *Revue du Rhumatisme*, vol. 68, no. 8, pp. 729–733, 2001.

[2] M.-A. Timsit, "Déminéralisation osseuse et ostéoporose de la grossesse," *Revue du Rhumatisme*, vol. 72, no. 8, pp. 725–732, 2005.

[3] D. Baszko-Błaszyk, W. Horst-Sikorska, and J. Sowiński, "Pregnancy-associated osteoporosis manifesting for the first time during second pregnancy," *Ginekologia Polska*, vol. 76, no. 1, pp. 67–69, 2005.

[4] C. Ozturk, F. C. Atamaz, H. Akkurt, and Y. Akkoc, "Pregnancy-associated osteoporosis presenting severe vertebral fractures," *Journal of Obstetrics and Gynaecology Research*, vol. 40, no. 1, pp. 288–292, 2014.

[5] M.-A. Timsit, "Grossesse et douleurs rhumatologiques lombaires basses et de la ceinture pelvienne," *Gynécologie Obstétrique & Fertilité*, vol. 32, no. 5, pp. 420–426, 2004.

[6] S. Steib-Furno, L. Mathieu, T. Pham et al., "Pregnancy-related hip diseases: incidence and diagnoses," *Joint Bone Spine*, vol. 74, no. 4, pp. 373–378, 2007.

[7] M.-C. de Vernejoul, "Métabolisme phosphocalcique lors de la grossesse et de la lactation," *Revue du Rhumatisme*, vol. 72, no. 8, pp. 695–697, 2005.

[8] I. R. Reid, D. J. Wattie, M. C. Evans, and A. A. Budayr, "Post-pregnancy osteoporosis associated with hypercalcaemia," *Clinical Endocrinology*, vol. 37, no. 3, pp. 298–303, 1992.

[9] D. W. Purdie, J. E. Aaron, and P. L. Selby, "Bone histology and mineral homeostasis in human pregnancy," *British Journal of Obstetrics and Gynaecology*, vol. 95, no. 9, pp. 849–854, 1988.

[10] L. Hellmeyer, M. Kühnert, V. Ziller, S. Schmidt, and P. Hadji, "The use of i. v. bisphosphonate in pregnancy-associated osteoporosis—case study," *The Experimental and Clinical Endocrinology and Diabetes*, vol. 115, no. 2, pp. 139–142, 2007.

[11] K. Lampropoulou-Adamidou, G. Trovas, I. P. Stathopoulos, and N. A. Papaioannou, "Case report: teriparatide treatment in a case of severe pregnancy -and lactation- associated osteoporosis," *Hormones (Athens)*, vol. 11, no. 4, pp. 495–500, 2012.

[12] M. D. Tanriover, S. G. Oz, T. Sozen, A. Kilicarslan, and G. S. Guven, "Pregnancy- and lactation-associated osteoporosis with severe vertebral deformities: can strontium ranelate be a new alternative for the treatment?" *The Spine Journal*, vol. 9, no. 4, pp. e20–e24, 2009.

[13] H. Tsuchie, N. Miyakoshi, M. Hongo, Y. Kasukawa, Y. Ishikawa, and Y. Shimada, "Amelioration of pregnancy-associated osteoporosis after treatment with vitamin K_2: a report of four patients," *Upsala Journal of Medical Sciences*, vol. 117, no. 3, pp. 336–341, 2012.

[14] L. Sanz-Salvador, M. Á. García-Pérez, J. J. Tarín, and A. Cano, "Endocrinology in pregnancy: bone metabolic changes during pregnancy: a period of vulnerability to osteoporosis and fracture," *European Journal of Endocrinology*, vol. 172, no. 26, pp. R53–R65, 2015.

[15] D. O. Okyay, E. Okyay, E. Dogan, S. Kurtulmus, F. Acet, and C. E. Taner, "Prolonged breast-feeding is an independent risk factor for postmenopausal osteoporosis," *Maturitas*, vol. 74, no. 3, pp. 270–275, 2013.

[16] P. Kuru, G. Akyuz, I. Yagci, and E. Giray, "Hypovitaminosis D in widespread pain: its effect on pain perception, quality of life and nerve conduction studies," *Rheumatology International*, vol. 35, no. 2, pp. 315–322, 2015.

5

High-Dose Subcutaneous Immunoglobulins for the Treatment of Severe Treatment-Resistant Polymyositis

Cherin Patrick,[1] Delain Jean-Christophe,[2] Crave Jean-Charles,[2] and Cartry Odile[3]

[1] Department of Internal Medicine, Pitié-Salpetrière Hospital Group, 47-83 Boulevard de l'Hôpital, 75013 Paris, France
[2] Octapharma, 92100 Boulogne-Billancourt, France
[3] Clinique Mutualiste Catalane, 66000 Perpignan, France

Correspondence should be addressed to Cherin Patrick; patrick.cherin@psl.aphp.fr

Academic Editor: Masataka Kuwana

Polymyositis is a rare debilitating condition characterized by chronic inflammation and muscle weakness. Standard treatments include corticosteroids and immunosuppressants; however, resistance to these regimens may develop. Intravenous immunoglobulins (IVIg) are thus recommended for patients with drug-resistant polymyositis. The patient presented a resistant polymyositis with severe muscle weakness, increasing dysphagia, and significant loss in weight. Subcutaneous immunoglobulins (SCIg) were initiated after failure of steroids and immunosuppressive drugs. SCIg was given twice per week (2 then 1.3 g/kg/month). Clinical recovery was observed within 2 months after the SCIg initiation. After several injections, the patient showed a progressive improvement in muscle strength. Serum creatine kinase activity decreased to normal levels, and dysphagia was resolved. The SC injections were generally well tolerated and good patient satisfaction was reported. This promising observation suggests that SCIg may be useful in active and refractory polymyositis.

1. Introduction

Polymyositis is a chronic inflammatory disorder affecting mainly the proximal skeletal muscles. This disease is associated with increased mortality and morbidity, particularly relating to life-threatening muscle weakness and visceral involvement [1–3]. Due to its low prevalence of approximately 6-7 cases per 100 000 subjects, few randomized trials have been conducted in polymyositis to define the optimal therapy [4].

To date, standard treatments include corticosteroid therapy, as a first-choice treatment, and then immunosuppressive therapy in the case of steroid-related side effects or inefficacy [5]. Intravenous immunoglobulin (IVIg) therapy is recommended in patients with polymyositis refractory to corticosteroids and immunosuppressive agents, despite the lack of randomized controlled studies [6–8]. Given the intravenous route of administration and related hospitalizations, this therapy shows an economic burden and a significant impact on patient's quality of life. Therefore, subcutaneous self-administered injections were developed as an alternative therapy to intravenous injections, but granted indications are still limited.

We report here a case of steroid/immunosuppressant resistant polymyositis, with esophageal involvement, that was successfully treated with subcutaneous immunoglobulins (SCIg).

2. Case Presentation

A Caucasian woman was referred to us with 6-year history of polymyositis, started at 43 years old. She presented severe proximal muscular weakness in the upper and lower limbs without involvement of wrist or finger flexors and increasing difficulty with standing. She had also developed dysphagia, which consequently caused weight loss of 4 kg during the last 6 months. Laboratory results revealed elevated serum creatine kinase (CK) activity (397 IU/L, normal <211 UI/L).

Polymyositis was diagnosed in 2006 while she was pregnant. The diagnosis of polymyositis was confirmed by a muscle biopsy, according to the International Consensus

Criteria [9]. Muscle biopsy showed endomysial inflammatory infiltrates (CD8 T-Cells) surrounding and invading the non-necrotic muscle fibers and a ubiquitous expression of MHC-1 by the noninvaded muscle cells. Rimmed vacuoles, ragged red fibers, and cytochrome oxidase-negative fibers suggesting inclusion body myositis were not observed.

According to the international criteria for polymyositis, the patterns of weakness were bilateral, symmetrical, and only proximal, with involvement of neck flexors. Electromyography showed increased insertional and spontaneous activity in the form of fibrillation potentials, positive sharp waves, and the presence of short duration, small amplitude, and polyphasic motor unit action potentials (MUAPs). Myositis-specific antibodies were negative. Muscle MRI was not performed as it was considered not useful for the diagnosis [9].

Intravenous immunoglobulin (IVIg, 2 g/kg/month) associated with bolus corticosteroids was therefore initiated; a significant improvement was then noticed. This treatment was followed by a maintenance therapy, during 2007, including corticosteroids and immunosuppressive treatment with either methotrexate or azathioprine, without IVIg. In September 2008, the patient showed a severe relapse despite treatments; consequently she received a course of rituximab which consisted of 4 infusions (375 mg/m^2 each) given weekly. In January 2009, immunosuppression with cyclosporine was started. Due to worsening of clinical results, plasma exchange (16 courses) was introduced in June 2010, in association with IVIg (2 g/kg/month), corticosteroids (20 mg daily), and immunosuppressive therapy with tacrolimus (4 mg, twice daily). Six months later, plasma exchange and IVIg were discontinued due to catheter-related bacteremia, and lower doses of tacrolimus were consequently given for one month (3 mg, twice daily). Meanwhile, she was admitted to an intensive outpatient physiotherapy program (4 sessions per week). In February 2011, corticosteroid treatment was reduced to 10 mg daily and tacrolimus was unchanged (4 mg, twice daily). In September 2012, she experienced worsening dysphagia with weight loss (4 kg between December and June 2012, from 48 to 44 kg). Plasma exchange was then reintroduced (12 courses), combined with IVIg (2 g/kg/month).

The patient was referred to us in November 2012. Plasma exchange and tacrolimus were discontinued and anti-interleukin-1 (anti-IL-1) was introduced to existing treatments including IVIg (2 g/kg/month) and corticosteroids (10 mg daily). Anti-IL-1 showed no clinical benefit. Due to difficult venous access, frequent hospitalizations, and the clinical benefit of immunoglobulins, SCIg (Gammanorm, 60 mL twice per week or 2 g/kg/month) was initiated in February 2013 after discussion with the patient. All other medications were stopped. At that time, the patient had severe muscle weakness; she was unable to walk or stand unaided. She was experiencing severe dysphagia which led to further loss of weight (4 kg, from 44 to 40 kg). Muscle weakness score was 55/88 (normal strength: 88 points) [6] and myositis activity scale was 49/75 (maximum disability: 75 points) [7]. CK activity was 397 UI/L. The patient was motivated for this subcutaneous treatment that was expected to prevent hospital readmissions and potential complications related to the intravenous therapy, such as her previous catheter-related

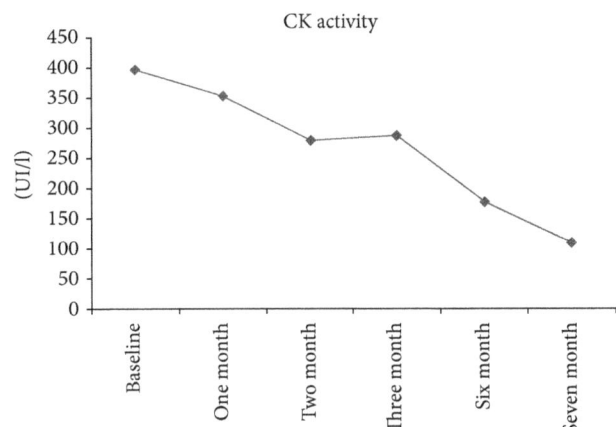

FIGURE 1: Changes in creatine kinase (CK) activity over time after SCIg initiation. Improvement in CK values was observed from the first month after the initiation of SCIg, up to 7 months.

bacteremia. Before the initiation of SCIg, a second muscle biopsy confirmed the active polymyositis.

Shortly after the first SCIg injection, the patient experienced a headache. This event was considered as related to the treatment. Therefore, SCIg was reduced to 40 mL (1.3 g/kg/month) twice per week. Two months later, her CK activity was decreased to 279 UI/L but yet no benefit was observed on the clinical status. After several courses, she showed an increasing improvement in clinical and biological parameters (Figure 1). Meanwhile, she stayed one month in an inpatient physiotherapy rehabilitation department, followed by an outpatient physical therapy program. In September 2013, CK activity was normal (177 UI/L). She was able to walk unaided and dysphagia was resolved. Neurological examination showed only mild weakness in the lower limbs. Muscle weakness score (72/88) and myositis activity scale (26/75) had improved markedly. The Life Quality Index (LQI) reflected high quality of life due to immunoglobulin treatment; score was 99% (Figure 2). No side effects were reported; particularly no local pain or rash was observed. The patient was satisfied with the SCIg injections since it was administered at home. She also reported satisfaction in achieving clinical improvement and in enjoying meals again. She showed an increase in her body weight (from 40 Kg to 45 Kg). To meet the patient's demand, the SCIg treatment was reduced to one injection (40 mL) per week. However, one month later the CK activity increased to 285 UI/L and then to 417 UI/L a couple of weeks later, with slight physical relapses. Subsequently, the previous regimen was resumed.

3. Discussion

This case shows that SCIg was safe and effective in a patient with polymyositis, presenting increasing dysphagia and subsequent weight loss, despite several lines of treatment. The patient age at disease onset, the pattern of weakness, and the two muscle biopsies confirm the definite polymyositis diagnostic.

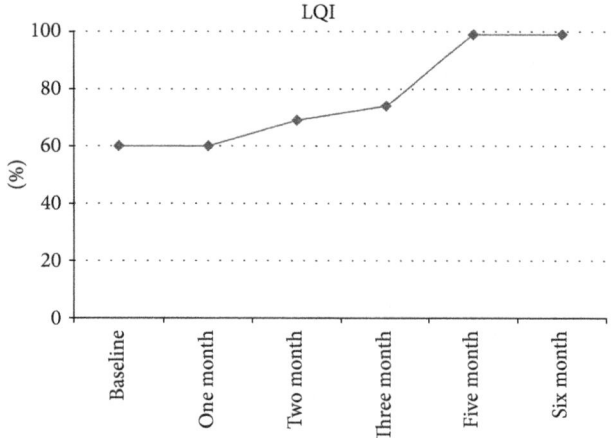

FIGURE 2: Changes in the Life Quality Index (LQI) over time after IgSC initiation. The Life Quality Index (LQI) was used to assess the treatment satisfaction. This scale comprises 18 items ranging from 1 to 7. The sum of scores is then adjusted to obtain a total score of 100 points. Improvement in LQI was observed starting from two months after the initiation of SCIg and reaching the maximum values after five months.

Significant improvement in muscle strength was observed after several courses of SCIg (1.3 g/kg/month; 40 mL twice weekly). The treatment with SCIg successfully treated dysphagia and reduced physical disability, thus preventing parenteral nutrition and allowing for normal daily activities. A slight relapse was observed when the SCIg was reduced to 0.7 g/kg/month (or 40 mL once weekly). This observation suggests that continuous higher dosage of SCIg may be advisable particularly in this case.

The clinical benefit of IVIg was recently reported in autoimmune-mediated disorders affecting nerves and muscles, including multifocal motor neuropathy, Guillain-Barré syndrome, and chronic inflammatory demyelinating polyneuropathy [10]. The subcutaneous administration of Ig has been initiated in these diseases [11–14]; few studies have reported the safety and efficacy of SCIg [15, 16].

In polymyositis and dermatomyositis, Danieli et al. described the benefit of SCIg in 7 patients with resistant disease [17]. SCIg was administered at usual IVIg monthly dose, fractioned into equal doses given weekly (in average 0.2 g/kg/week). After a median follow-up of 14 months, patients showed a favorable clinical response and improved quality of life [17]. SCIg was well tolerated in patients with PM/DM disease; no particular safety concerns were raised [17, 18].

The SCIg treatment did not result in severe adverse events. Our patient experienced a headache only after the first injection. This adverse event was considered in relation to the treatment and resolved with dosage reduction (from 2 g/kg/month, 60 mL twice weekly to 1.3 g/kg/month, 40 mL twice weekly). In general, local adverse events such as redness and swelling at the injection site are frequent with SCIg treatment [15, 16, 19]. Given the SC route of administration and the reduced doses given on a weekly schedule, systemic reactions and thromboembolic events seem to be less frequent in SCIg, compared with IVIg [20]. According to the few published reports, SCIg injections were well tolerated in patients PM/DM [17, 18]; no major adverse events were reported. No patients reported severe, local, or systemic reactions. Mild local reactions including swelling, redness, and burning sensation were reported in few patients at the infusion site that disappeared within 2 days [17, 18]. No other adverse events were reported with SCIg therapy.

Further advantages of SCIg include the home-based setting and the ease of handling infusions, which prevent hospitalizations, reduce costs, and contribute to patient autonomy [21]. Switching from IVIg to SCIg was associated with the increased quality of life and significant improvement in treatment satisfaction [22]. Consistently, our patient reported higher satisfaction and less emotional distress with the subcutaneous self-administered treatment.

In conclusion, the SCIg dose should be tapered to achieve long-lasting clinical benefit whilst preventing adverse events. This promising observation suggests that SCIg may be useful in active and refractory polymyositis, although further investigations are required to confirm these findings.

Acknowledgments

The authors would like to thank the staff of Bastide for providing monthly reports about the patient, Dominique François (Octapharma, France) for her help, and Abir Tadmouri (ClinSearch) for providing writing assistance.

References

[1] I. Marie, E. Hachulla, P.-Y. Hatron et al., "Polymyositis and dermatomyositis: short term and longterm outcome, and predictive factors of prognosis," Journal of Rheumatology, vol. 28, no. 10, pp. 2230–2237, 2001.

[2] I. Marie, P. Y. Hatron, S. Dominique, P. Cherin, L. Mouthon, and J. Menard, "Short-term and long-term outcomes of interstitial lung disease in polymyositis and dermatomyositis: a series of 107 patients," Arthritis and Rheumatism, vol. 63, no. 11, pp. 3439–3447, 2011.

[3] I. Marie, L. Lahaxe, O. Benveniste et al., "Long-term outcome of patients with polymyositis/ dermatomyositis and anti-PM-Scl antibody," British Journal of Dermatology, vol. 162, no. 2, pp. 337–344, 2010.

[4] T. A. Medsger Jr., W. N. Dawson Jr., and A. T. Masi, "The epidemiology of polymyositis," The American Journal of Medicine, vol. 48, no. 6, pp. 715–723, 1970.

[5] I. Marie and L. Mouthon, "Therapy of polymyositis and dermatomyositis," Autoimmunity Reviews, vol. 11, no. 1, pp. 6–13, 2011.

[6] P. Cherin, S. Herson, B. Wechsler et al., "Efficacy of intravenous gammaglobulin therapy in chronic refractory polymyositis and dermatomyositis: an open study with 20 adult patients," The American Journal of Medicine, vol. 91, no. 2, pp. 162–168, 1991.

[7] P. Cherin, S. Pelletier, A. Teixeira et al., "Results and long-term followup of intravenous immunoglobulin infusions in chronic, refractory polymyositis: an open study with thirty-five adult patients," *Arthritis & Rheumatism*, vol. 46, no. 2, pp. 467–474, 2002.

[8] I. Elovaara, S. Apostolski, P. Van Doorn et al., "EFNS guidelines for the use of intravenous immunoglobulin in treatment of neurological diseases: EFNS task force on the use of intravenous immunoglobulin in treatment of neurological diseases," *European Journal of Neurology*, vol. 15, no. 9, pp. 893–908, 2008.

[9] J. E. Hoogendijk, A. A. Amato, B. R. Lecky et al., "119th ENMC international workshop: Trial design in adult idiopathic inflammatory myopathies, with the exception of inclusion body myositis, 10-12 October 2003, Naarden, The Netherlands," *Neuromuscular Disorders*, vol. 14, no. 5, pp. 337–345, 2004.

[10] R. Gold, M. Stangel, and M. C. Dalakas, "Drug Insight: The use of intravenous immunoglobulin in neurology—therapeutic considerations and practical issues," *Nature Clinical Practice Neurology*, vol. 3, no. 1, pp. 36–44, 2007.

[11] P. Dacci, N. Riva, M. Scarlato et al., "Subcutaneous immunoglobulin therapy for the treatment of multifocal motor neuropathy: a case report," *Neurological Sciences*, vol. 31, no. 6, pp. 829–831, 2010.

[12] T. Harbo, H. Andersen, and J. Jakobsen, "Long-term therapy with high doses of subcutaneous immunoglobulin in multifocal motor neuropathy," *Neurology*, vol. 75, no. 15, pp. 1377–1380, 2010.

[13] D.-H. Lee, R. A. Linker, W. Paulus, C. Schneider-Gold, A. Chan, and R. Gold, "Subcutaneous immunoglobulin infusion: a new therapeutic option in chronic inflammatory demyelinating polyneuropathy," *Muscle & Nerve*, vol. 37, no. 3, pp. 406–409, 2008.

[14] K. Pars, N. Garde, T. Skripuletz, R. Pul, R. Dengler, and M. Stangel, "Subcutaneous immunoglobulin treatment of inclusion-body myositis stabilizes dysphagia," *Muscle and Nerve*, 2013.

[15] F. Eftimov, M. Vermeulen, R. J. de Haan, L. H. van den Berg, and I. N. van Schaik, "Subcutaneous immunoglobulin therapy for multifocal motor neuropathy," *Journal of the Peripheral Nervous System*, vol. 14, no. 2, pp. 93–100, 2009.

[16] L. H. Markvardsen, J.-C. Debost, T. Harbo et al., "Subcutaneous immunoglobulin in responders to intravenous therapy with chronic inflammatory demyelinating polyradiculoneuropathy," *European Journal of Neurology*, vol. 20, no. 5, pp. 836–842, 2013.

[17] M. G. Danieli, L. Pettinari, R. Moretti, F. Logullo, and A. Gabrielli, "Subcutaneous immunoglobulin in polymyositis and dermatomyositis: a novel application," *Autoimmunity Reviews*, vol. 10, no. 3, pp. 144–149, 2011.

[18] M. G. Danieli, R. Moretti, S. Gambini, L. Paolini, and A. Gabrielli, "Open-label study on treatment with 20% subcutaneous IgG administration in polymyositis and dermatomyositis," *Clinical Rheumatology*, vol. 33, no. 4, pp. 531–536, 2014.

[19] H. D. Ochs, S. Gupta, P. Kiessling, U. Nicolay, and M. Berger, "Safety and efficacy of self-administered subcutaneous immunoglobulin in patients with primary immunodeficiency diseases," *Journal of Clinical Immunology*, vol. 26, no. 3, pp. 265–273, 2006.

[20] I. Quinti, A. Soresina, C. Agostini et al., "Prospective study on CVID patients with adverse reactions to intravenous or subcutaneous IgG administration," *Journal of Clinical Immunology*, vol. 28, no. 3, pp. 263–267, 2008.

[21] C. Lazzaro, L. Lopiano, and D. Cocito, "Subcutaneous vs intravenous administration of immunoglobulin in chronic inflammatory demyelinating polyne uropathy: an Italian cost-minimization analysis," *Neurological Sciences*, vol. 35, no. 7, pp. 1023–1034, 2014.

[22] J. M. Kittner, B. Grimbacher, W. Wulff, B. Jäger, and R. E. Schmidt, "Patients' attitude to subcutaneous immunoglobulin substitution as home therapy," *Journal of Clinical Immunology*, vol. 26, no. 4, pp. 400–405, 2006.

6

Successful Treatment of Long-Term Severe Progressive Interstitial Pneumonia with Low-Dose Corticosteroid and Azathioprine in a Patient with Diffuse Systemic Sclerosis

Takuya Kotani, Tohru Takeuchi, Shigeki Makino, and Toshiaki Hanafusa

First Department of Internal Medicine, Osaka Medical College, 2-7 Daigaku-Machi, Takatsuki, Osaka 569-8686, Japan

Correspondence should be addressed to Tohru Takeuchi, t-takeuchi@poh.osaka-med.ac.jp

Academic Editors: H. Alexanderson, R. Aminov, J. V. Dunne, K. P. Makaritsis, P. E. Prete, and G. J. Tsay

For progressive interstitial pneumonia (progressive IP) that accompanies diffuse systemic sclerosis (diffuse SSc), no treatment guidelines have yet been established, and it is a complication with a poor prognosis. We herein report a case in which combination therapy of a low-dose corticosteroid and low-dose azathioprine was performed for progressive SSc-IP in a 64-year-old female whose respiratory function was severely damaged for a long period of time and for whom improvement was achieved. The beneficial effect has continued for 3 years with no side effects being observed during the course.

1. Introduction

Systemic scleroderma (SSc) is a systemic autoimmune disorder of the gastrointestinal tract, lungs, and kidneys, and so forth, which has dermal sclerosis as a major characteristic. SSc has IP as a complication at a frequency of 44 to 75% [1, 2]. SSc-IP normally progresses slowly, but in diffuse SSc-IP, there are cases in which progression is rapid and also cases in which the respiratory function is damaged for a long period of time [3]. No treatment guideline has been established for progressive SSc-IP. Treatment methods that have been attempted most frequently are oral cyclophosphamide (CY) and intravenous pulse CY (IVCY). Although improvement in respiratory function has been obtained by these methods for a short period of time of 1 to 2 years, they are not easy to be applied for longer periods of time due to serious side effects [4, 5].

Azathioprine (AZA) inhibits purine nucleotide synthesis and exerts an immunosuppressive effect. A report exists in which respiratory function stabilized upon switching treatments to AZA as a maintenance therapy after IVCY was performed monthly for 6 months for SSc-IP in addition to a low-dose corticosteroid [6]. Moreover, a report exists in which combination therapy of a steroid and AZP improved the survival rate of idiopathic interstitial pneumonia [7].

Because AZA has fewer serious side-effects than CY, there is a possibility that it can also be used for SSc-IP for a long period of time.

In this paper, we describe a case in which continuous improvement of IP was observed with combination therapy of a low-dose corticosteroid and AZA for a case of SSc-IP in which the pulmonary damage had inveterately progressed for a long period of 12 years.

2. Case Report

A 52-year-old female was admitted to our hospital for dry cough and exertional dyspnea (Hugh-Jones classification (H-J) class II) on July 1994. High-resolution computed tomography (HRCT) of the chest showed a reticular shadow on the dorsal side of both lower lungs, ground-glass opacity (GGO), and traction bronchiectasis (TBE), and she was diagnosed as having IP. Around January 2000, Raynaud's phenomenon and, in the distal portion of the limbs, dermal sclerosis appeared. The dermal sclerosis diffusely progressed throughout the entire body thereafter, and she was consequently diagnosed as having IP followed by SSc. The clinical course thereafter is shown in Figure 1 and the chest HRCT findings in July 2003 are shown in

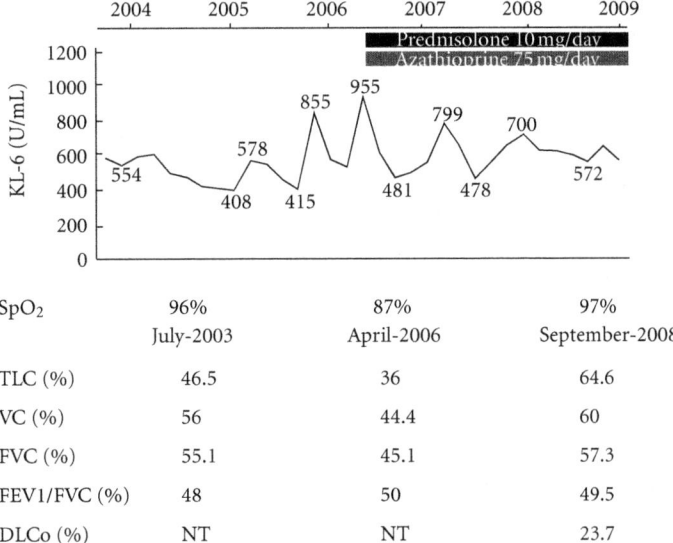

FIGURE 1: Clinical course. TLC: total lung capacity, VC: vital capacity, FVC: forced vital capacity, FEV1/FVC: forced expiratory volume in 1s/forced vital capacity, DLCo: carbon monoxide diffusing capacity, and NT: not tested.

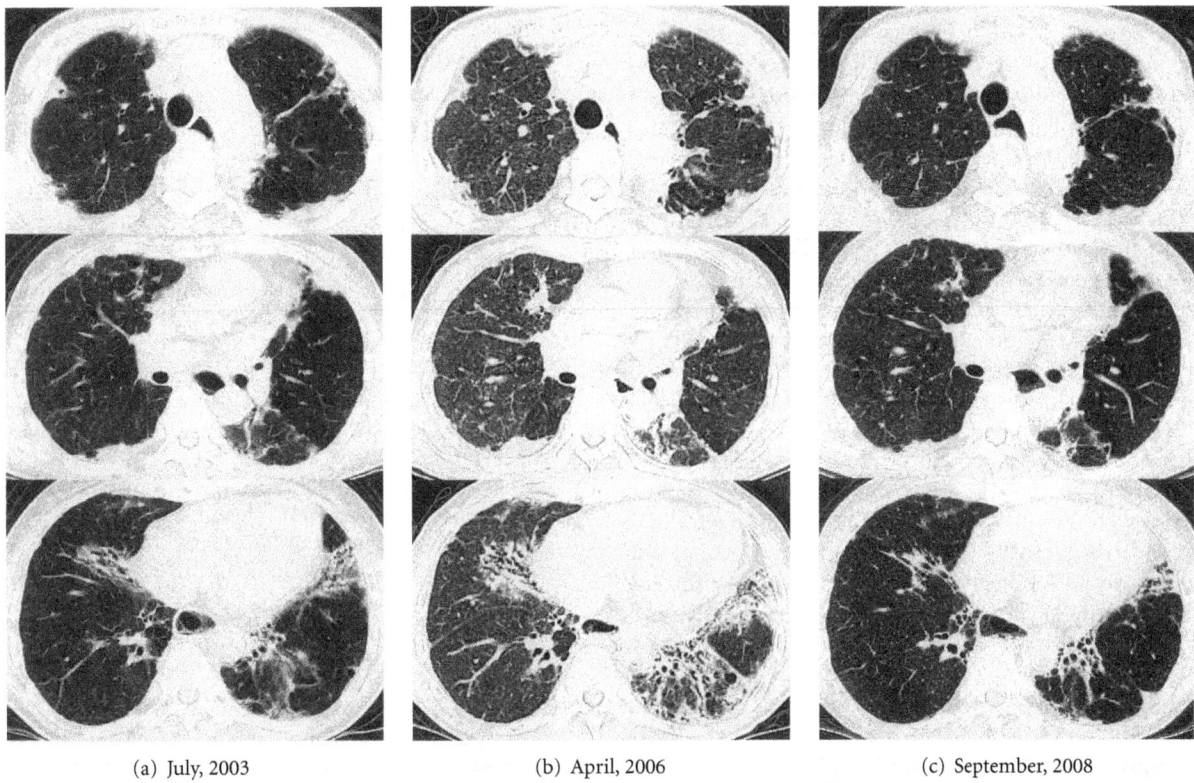

	(a) July, 2003	(b) April, 2006	(c) September, 2008

FIGURE 2: Course of chest HRCT. (a) Consolidations, ground-glass opacities (GGO), and traction bronchiectasis (TBE) were noted on chest HRCT at July, 2003. (b) Consolidations, GGO, and TBE increased on admission in April, 2006, compared with that in April, 2003. (c) Consolidations, GGO, and TBE improved with 10 mg/day of prednisolone and 75 mg/day of azathioprine at September, 2008.

Figure 2(a). In July 2003, the SpO_2 was 96% (room air), the KL-6 was 554 U/mL. In a respiratory function test, the TLC% was found to be 46.5% and the FVC% was 55.1%. From October 2005, exertional dyspnea had exacerbated from H-J class II to IV, the SpO_2 decreased to 87% (room air), and she was admitted to our hospital on April 3, 2006. On physical examination, fine crackles were observed in both lower lungs, and dermal sclerosis was diffusely observed in the facial surface and all limbs. In the laboratory findings, the WBC was 7240/μL (neutrocyte 69.2%) and the CRP was 3.20 mg/dL. The KL-6 was 955 U/mL. The antinuclear antibody was positive (speckled pattern), but the other various disease-specific autoantibodies were negative including anti-Scl-70 antibody. In a respiratory function test, the TLC% decreased to 36.0% and the FVC% to 45.1%. In the chest X-ray, both lower lungs shrank, the reticular shadow increased, and the chest HRCT showed increase in the area of the consolidation, GGO, and TBE (Figure 2(b)). SSc-IP was determined to have exacerbated, and on April 11, 2006, combination therapy of 10 mg/day of prednisolone (PSL) and 75 mg/day of AZA was initiated. The IP gradually improved, and in September 2008, the dyspnea improved to H-J class I and the SpO_2 increased to 97%. The KL-6 decreased to 572 U/mL, and in a respiratory function test, the FVC% showed improvement to 57.3%. Upon chest HRCT, decrease of the GGO, consolidation, and TBE were observed (Figure 2(c)). During the course, no obvious side effects due to the concomitant therapy of PSL and AZA were observed.

3. Discussion

For progressive SSc-IP, the treatment methods most often used are oral CY and IVCY, and it has been reported that respiratory function improves or stabilizes during a follow-up period of 1 to 2 years [4]. However, upon long-term followup, the presence of relapse cases after treatment, an unimproved survival rate, and serious side effects such as hematuria, infertility, bone marrow suppression, malignancy, and infection are problems, in addition to CY not being easy to use for SSc-IP for a long period of time [5].

AZA inhibits purine nucleotide synthesis and exerts an immunosuppressive effect mainly centering on T cells. A report exists indicating the involvement of $CD8^+$ T cells with formation of the clinical state of SSc-IP [8] and there is a possibility that AZA is effective for SSc-IP.

In the case reported herein, progressive SSc-IP over a long period of approximately 12 years improved with combination therapy of low-dose PSL and AZA. During the follow-up period of 30 months after the combination therapy, there was no serious side effects, thus resulting in sufficient tolerability. Hoyles et al. reported that AZA was effective as a maintenance therapy for SSc-IP after combination therapy of steroids and IVCY [6]. Dheda et al. have performed combination therapy of low-dose steroids and AZA for 11 cases of SSc-IP and reported that the effects of "improved" (FVC% improved by 10% or more than the base line) in 5 patients and "stable" (FVC% improved by 10% or less) in 3 patients were obtained [9]. When the 8 cases of Dheda et al. and the present case are compared, the 8 cases of Dheda et al. showed a mean duration for IP of 18.45 ± 4.52 months and a mean FVC% of 54.25 ± 3.53%, whereas the present case showed a duration for IP of 171 months and a FVC% of 45.1%, and is a case in which the respiratory function was damaged for a much longer period of time. As in our case, there is a possibility that even SSc-IP in which the respiratory function was severely damaged for a long period of time may improve with combination therapy of a low-dose steroid and AZA, and it is believed to be worth attempting.

In the present case, no obvious side effects due to steroids and AZA were observed. AZA has fewer serious side effects than CPA and there is a possibility that it can be used for a long period of time. However, AZA may also possibly cause side effects such as digestive symptoms, bone marrow suppression, hepatic damage, and increased susceptibility to infection although less severe than those of CY. Dheda et al. have also reported that among the 11 cases of SSc-IP in which AZA was used, side effects of nausea in 1 case and decreased WBC in 1 case were observed, and, therefore, it is necessary to pay attention to the expression of side effects in using AZA for SSc-IP.

As in the present case, combination therapy of a low-dose steroid and AZA is also effective for cases of SSc-IP in which the respiratory function has been severely damaged for a long period of time, indicating that it was a treatment method that could be used for a long period of time. However, because there are still only a few cases in which AZA is used for SSc-IP, it is necessary to evaluate the efficacy and safety after the future accumulation of more cases.

References

[1] A. Bérezné, D. Valeyre, B. Ranque, L. Guillevin, and L. Mouthon, "Interstitial lung disease associated with systemic sclerosis: what is the evidence for efficacy of cyclophosphamide?" *Annals of the New York Academy of Sciences*, vol. 1110, pp. 271–284, 2007.

[2] Y. Hamaguchi, M. Hasegawa, M. Fujimoto et al., "The clinical relevance of serum antinuclear antibodies in Japanese patients with systemic sclerosis," *British Journal of Dermatology*, vol. 158, no. 3, pp. 487–495, 2008.

[3] K. B. Highland and R. M. Silver, "Clinical aspects of lung involvement: lessons from idiopathic pulmonary fibrosis and the scleroderma lung study," *Current Rheumatology Reports*, vol. 7, no. 2, pp. 135–141, 2005.

[4] D. P. Tashkin, R. Elashoff, P. J. Clements et al., "Cyclophosphamide versus placebo in scleroderma lung disease," *The New England Journal of Medicine*, vol. 354, no. 25, pp. 2655–2666, 2006.

[5] D. Khanna, D. E. Furst, P. J. Clements, D. P. Tashkin, and M. H. Eckman, "Oral cyclophosphamide for active scleroderma lung disease: a decision analysis," *Medical Decision Making*, vol. 28, no. 6, pp. 926–937, 2008.

[6] R. K. Hoyles, R. W. Ellis, J. Wellsbury et al., "A multicenter, prospective, randomized, double-blind, placebo-controlled trial of corticosteroids and intravenous cyclophosphamide followed by oral azathioprine for the treatment of pulmonary fibrosis in scleroderma," *Arthritis and Rheumatism*, vol. 54, no. 12, pp. 3962–3970, 2006.

[7] G. Raghu, W. J. Depaso, K. Cain et al., "Azathioprine combined with prednisone in the treatment of idiopathic pulmonary fibrosis: a prospective double-blind, randomized, placebo-controlled clinical trial," *American Review of Respiratory Disease*, vol. 144, no. 2, pp. 291–296, 1991.

[8] V. V. Yurovsky, F. M. Wigley, R. A. Wise, and B. White, "Skewing of the CD8+ T-cell repertoire in the lungs of patients with systemic sclerosis," *Human Immunology*, vol. 48, no. 1-2, pp. 84–97, 1996.

[9] K. Dheda, U. G. Lalloo, B. Cassim, and G. M. Mody, "Experience with azathioprine in systemic sclerosis associated with interstitial lung disease," *Clinical Rheumatology*, vol. 23, no. 4, pp. 306–309, 2004.

7

A Case of Systemic Lupus Erythematosus Presenting as Guillain-Barré Syndrome

Helen Chioma Okoh, Sandeep Singh Lubana, Spencer Langevin, Susan Sanelli-Russo, and Adriana Abrudescu

Icahn School of Medicine at Mount Sinai, Queens Hospital Center, Jamaica, NY 11432, USA

Correspondence should be addressed to Helen Chioma Okoh; helenokohc@gmail.com

Academic Editor: Suleyman Serdar Koca

Systemic lupus erythematosus (SLE) is an autoimmune systemic disease with multiple organ involvement with high morbidity and mortality rate. Among the severe potential fatal complications are those of the central and peripheral nervous system which usually develop during the course of the disease and very rarely from the outset of the disease. We are reporting a rare case of Miller-Fisher (MFS) variant of Guillain-Barré syndrome (GBS) as the first manifestation of SLE in a 41-year-old female who progressed to flaccid paralysis with no neurological improvement with initial immunosuppressive therapy, plasmapheresis, and first cycle of intravenous immunoglobulin (IVIG) but with remarkable and complete recovery after the second 5-day course of IVIG.

1. Introduction

Neuropsychiatric systemic lupus erythematosus (NPSLE) as described by the American College of Rheumatology (ACR) research committee includes 19 neuropsychiatric syndromes divided into neurologic syndromes of the central, peripheral, and autonomic nervous system and the psychiatric syndromes observed in patients with SLE in which other causes have been excluded. These symptoms may precede the onset of SLE or can occur at any time during the course of SLE [1]. Peripheral nervous system involvement occurs in 3–18% [2]. Guillain-Barré syndrome which is classified under the peripheral involvement has been rarely associated with SLE. We report a case of Miller-Fisher variant of Guillain-Barré syndrome presenting as the initial presentation of SLE and while the nonneurological manifestations, renal function, and SLE serology resolved with immunosuppressive therapy and plasmapheresis, the MFS symptoms did not improve and the patient remained dependent on mechanical ventilation and endogastric tube feeding. Complete recovery was only achieved after the 2nd cycle of IVIG which was given approximately 2 months after the 1st cycle while only on prednisone maintenance daily dose.

2. Case Report

Patient is a 41-year-old female originally from Nigeria, immigrated to the United States 9 years ago with no past medical history, who presented to the emergency department with worsening lower extremity weakness and swelling for 3 months. She also complained of 2 days of right eye swelling with diplopia and blurry vision and 1-day history of an inability to walk. Patient reported a flu-like illness with diarrhea prior to symptoms 5 months ago. She works as a house remodeler and denied any exposure to mold, asbestos, heavy metals, and silica. She gave no history of skin rashes, mouth ulcers, hair loss, photosensitivity, or arthralgia. On initial physical examination vital signs were stable; oxygen saturation was 98% on room air. There was no evidence of skin rash, she denied joint tenderness, and there was no palpable swelling. Heart lungs and abdominal exam revealed no abnormalities. There was bilateral lower extremity pitting edema. The neurological exam revealed that she was alert and oriented x3, followed commands, and had no aphasia with intact comprehension and fluent speech. Cranial nerve examination revealed anisocoria right > left, extra ocular muscles intact, and no nystagmus and the rest of cranial nerves were normal.

Waveforms

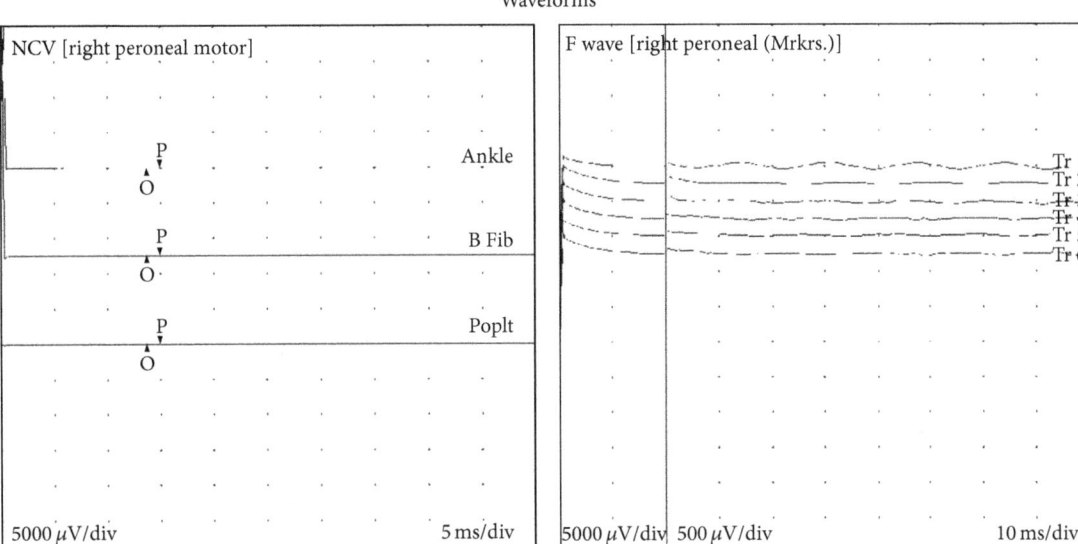

FIGURE 1: Nerve conduction studies (see Table 1). Findings: evaluation of the right peroneal motor nerve showed prolonged distal onset latency (13.8 ms), reduced amplitude (Ankle, 0.0 mV), reduced amplitude (B Fib., 0.0 mV), and reduced amplitude (Poplt., 0.0 mV). F wave studies indicate that the right peroneal F wave has no response.

Motor exam revealed 2/5 strength in the proximal upper extremities (abduction and flexion) and 5/5 in wrist flexion and extension. Hip flexion was 2/5 on the right and 3/5 on the left. Knee extension and flexion, dorsiflexion, and plantar flexion were 5/5 bilaterally. Reflexes were equal and symmetric in upper extremities but diminished in lower extremities.

Laboratory data revealed leukopenia 4.3 K/mcl and anemia with Hg/Hct at 6.6/19.5 g/dL, respectively; platelets were within normal limit. Liver function panel was also within normal limits except albumin at 2.3 g/dL. Prealbumin was low at 8.1 mg/dL and BUN/creatinine was at 29/1.29 mg/dL, respectively. Urinalysis revealed protein of 300 and RBC of 11–25/hpf. Head CT, MRI brain, and C-spine and T-spine CT scans revealed no abnormalities. CT thorax was obtained which revealed moderate bibasilar pleural effusion and moderate pericardial effusion. Echocardiography revealed ejection fraction of 60%.

Four days after admission, the patient's neurological status worsened. She became progressively weaker and lethargic and was only able to state her name. She had difficulty swallowing, speaking, taking deep breaths, and coughing. She was intubated for airway protection and placed on nasogastric tube (NGT) feeding. Neurologist evaluated the patient; exam was notable for absent reflexes in addition to progressive lower extremity weakness; GBS was suspected. She also developed ophthalmoparesis with inability of the eyes to cross the midline bilaterally. Stool studies were negative for *Campylobacter jejuni* and were guaiac negative. Lumbar puncture and plasma exchange were recommended. Cerebral spinal fluid (CSF) analysis revealed protein of 35 mg/dL; WBC was 8/cumm. Oligoclonal bands and myelin basic protein were absent, with Anti-GQ-1 antibody titers less than 1 : 100. West Nile viral titers were negative. Nerve conduction studies revealed absence of F wave response in right peroneal nerve,

prolonged distal onset latency, and severe conduction block (Figure 1); although CSF results were inconsistent with GBS as the protein was not elevated, a diagnosis was made clinically. Treatment with plasma exchange was begun 5 days after admission. She received 5 plasma exchanges with no improvement.

Due to the presence of leukopenia, pericardial and pleural effusions, proteinuria, and hematuria SLE work-up was sent with results showing the following: +ANA titers of 1 : 2560 4+ speckled, Anti-ds-DNA positive titer 1 : 80, and AntiSmith ab positive >8, low C3 and C4 levels at <40 mg/dL and <10 mg/dL, respectively. Serum antiribosomal P antibodies positive >8, serum antineuronal antibodies were negative, and lupus anticoagulant and anticardiolipin antibodies were negative. Patient fulfilled ACR SLE criteria and Pulse SoluMedrol therapy 1 gm daily for 3 consecutive days was started 7 days after admission. Renal function was rapidly deteriorating with anuria at 67 mL in 24 hours and worsening of BUN/creatinine to 50/3.29 mg/dL, respectively; hemodialysis (HD) was started 8 days after admission. Renal biopsy was performed which showed evidence of membranous and focal lupus nephritis [ISN/RPS 2004 classification lupus nephritis, classes III (A) and V], acute tubular necrosis (Figure 3).

SoluMedrol was given on alternate days with plasma exchange and hemodialysis to avoid removal and maintain optimal serum levels of steroids. SoluMedrol was continued as maintenance therapy on 120 mg IV daily.

Cyclophosphamide 500 mg every 2 weeks as per EURO Lupus protocol was started 10 days after admission due to lupus nephritis. Patient failed multiple weaning trials and subsequently needed PEG tube and tracheostomy tube. Plasma exchange was stopped after 5 sessions on day 14 of admission due to the absence of improvement in neurological status. Patient was started on IVIG on day 17 of admission.

TABLE 1: (a) Motor summary table. (b) F wave studies.

(a)

Site	NR	Onset (ms)	Norm. onset (ms)	O-P Amp. (mV)	Norm. O-P Amp.	Site 1	Site 2	Delta-0 (ms)	Dist. (cm)	Vel. (m/s)	Norm. Vel. (m/s)
				Right peroneal motor (Ext. Dig. Brev.)							
Ankle		**13.8**	<6	**0.0**	>3	B Fib.	Ankle	0.0	0.0		>40
B Fib.		13.8		**0.0**	>3	Poplt.	B Fib.	0.0	0.0		>40
Poplt.		13.8		**0.0**	>3						

(b)

NR	F-Lat. (ms)	Lat. Norm. (ms)	L-R F-Lat. (ms)	L-R Lat. Norm.
		Right peroneal (Mrkrs.) (EDB)		
NR		<60		<4

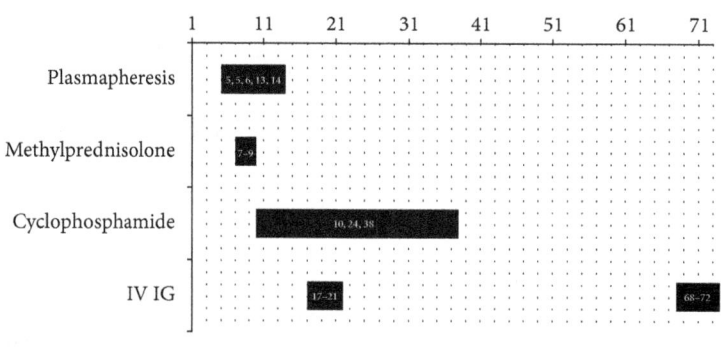

Treatment administered on days

FIGURE 2

Patient received 1st course of IVIG 0.4 g/kg/day for 5 days concomitantly with SoluMedrol maintenance therapy on 120 mg IV daily and cyclophosphamide. Renal function began to improve with resolution of anuria; hemodialysis was discontinued. Due to significant SLE serology improvement with normalized C3 and C4 and negative ds DNA and improved renal function off hemodialysis, SoluMedrol was tapered to 40 mg IV daily.

Cyclophosphamide was terminated after the 3rd dose, 39 days after admission as the patient developed pancytopenia and fever with pneumonia and worsening of the sacral decubitus ulcer. In view of SLE with positive antiribosomal P protein and lack of improvement in the neurological/GBS symptoms (no improvement in muscle strength, ophthalmoparesis, or reflexes) and with patient still being dependent on mechanical ventilation and PEG tube feeding, a 2nd course of IVIG was started 2 g/kg divided over 5 days. Her weight was 60 kg and she was started on a 2nd course of IVIG 24 g/day, 68 days after admission. The choice of therapy and the onset of treatment are summarized in Figure 2.

Significant daily improvement in motor function and reflexes started to occur. Patient was able to start bedside physical therapy. Tracheostomy tube was subsequently removed as well as PEG tube. Patient was transferred to the inpatient acute rehabilitation unit for 2 weeks and was discharged home 131 days after initial presentation on prednisone 20 mg

daily. Patient was seen in the rheumatology and neurology clinics within 1 month after discharge, with no significant residual motor or sensory deficits, walking without support, and asymptomatic for weakness. C3 and C4 levels were normalized at 100 mg/dL and 22.6 mg/dL, respectively. The patient was noted to have hematuria and low complement levels on subsequent clinic visits 2 months after and was started on mycophenolate mofetil in addition to prednisone.

3. Discussion

Guillain-Barré syndrome (GBS) is clinically defined as an acute peripheral neuropathy causing limb weakness that progresses over a time period of days or, at the most, up to 4 weeks. GBS is considered to be an autoimmune disease triggered by a preceding bacterial or viral infection. *Campylobacter jejuni*, cytomegalovirus, Epstein-Barr virus, and *Mycoplasma pneumoniae* are commonly identified antecedent pathogens [11]. The exact cause is unknown. Diagnosis of GBS includes clinical, serological, and electrophysiological criteria. The subtypes include acute inflammatory demyelinating polyneuropathy (AIDP) and acute motor axonal neuropathy (AMAN), acute motor and sensory axonal neuropathy (AMSAN), and Miller-Fisher variant with AIDP as the most common form of GBS in western countries and account for 85–90% of the patients with GBS. Miller-Fisher variant is

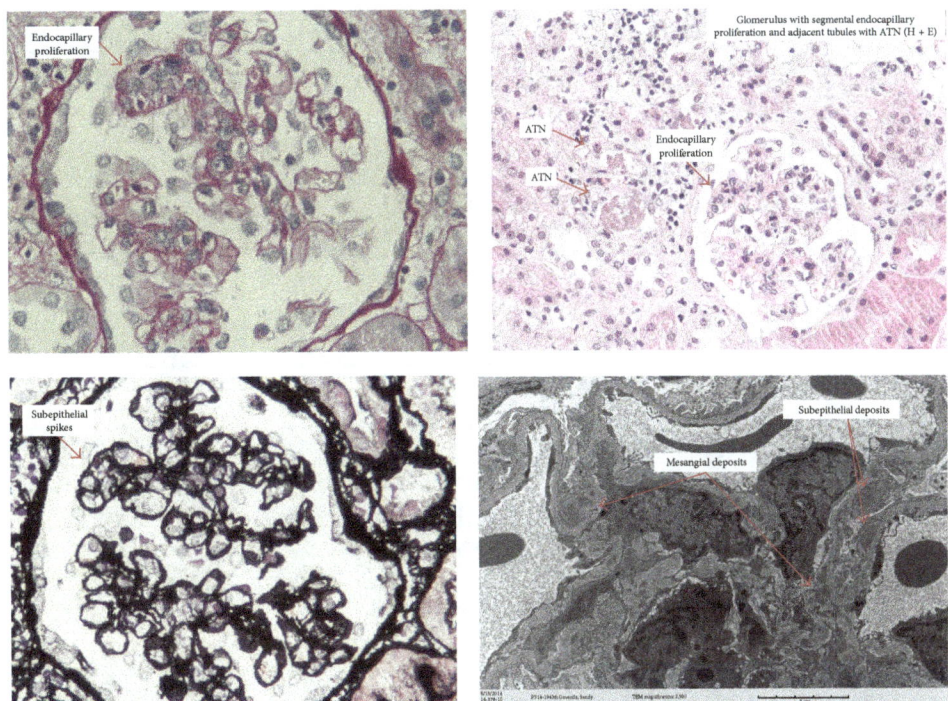

FIGURE 3: Kidney biopsy: membranous and focal lupus nephritis [ISN/PPS 2004 classification lupus nephritis, classes III (A) and V]; acute tubular necrosis.

characterized by a unique clinical triad of ophthalmoplegia, ataxia, and areflexia [12]. MFS variant is closely associated with antibodies against ganglioside GQ1b. The patient was diagnosed with SLE presenting as Miller-Fisher variant of Guillain-Barré despite Anti-GQ1b antibodies, *Campylobacter jejuni*, and CSF protein elevation being negative. The diagnosis of MFS still remains a clinical one [7]. Cranial nerve examination revealed anisocoria R > L, extra ocular muscles intact, and no nystagmus and the rest of cranial nerves were normal (Figure 1); although CSF results were inconsistent with GBS as the protein was not elevated, a diagnosis was made clinically and with the support of electroneuromyography.

Systemic lupus erythematosus (SLE) is an autoimmune disease of unknown etiology characterized by the presence of autoantibodies with involvement of multiple organ systems. Neuropsychiatric systemic lupus erythematosus (NPSLE) as described by the American College of Rheumatology (ACR) research committee includes 19 neuropsychiatric syndromes divided into neurologic syndromes of the central, peripheral, and autonomic nervous system and the psychiatric syndromes observed in patients with SLE in which other causes have been excluded These symptoms may precede the onset of SLE or can occur at any time during the course of SLE [1]. Peripheral nervous system involvement occurs in 3–18% [2].

Guillain-Barré syndrome as the initial presentation of SLE has been reported in only a few cases. [3, 4]. Some were treated with plasmapheresis and steroids with full recovery [3] or steroids, plasmapheresis, and cyclophosphamide with partial recovery [4] or had full recovery to only cyclophosphamide and steroids after failed initial treatment with IVIG

and plasmapheresis [5] or had full recovery with cyclophosphamide and steroids after failed treatment with IVIG [6]. Reports from the literature document that some have had response to IVIG [7] or steroids only [8], 5 courses of plasmapheresis after failed treatment with IVIG, steroids, and cyclophosphamide [9], or 2 courses of plasmapheresis after failed treatment with IVIG and steroids [2]. Varying responses have been noted with each patient encountered and no universal treatment guidelines have yet been established. About 10% of GBS patients deteriorate after initial improvement or stabilization following IVIG or plasmapheresis treatment, a condition termed "treatment-related clinical fluctuation" [13]. However, no suggestions have been made regarding repeated treatment in this subgroup. A second course of IVIG was given as there was a case of severe unresponsive Guillain-Barré syndrome which responded to a repeat treatment of IVIG 2 g/kg given over 5 days, 14–21 days after presentation [10]. Therapeutic and outcome data have been summarized in Table 2.

An ongoing RCT (SID-GBS) to study the effects of a second course of IVIG in patients with poor prognosis is still ongoing in Netherlands [14]. A 2nd course of IVIG was given in this patient 51 days after the initial dose because of the absence of neurological improvement after the first course of IVIG and plasmapheresis despite the fact that, serologically, SLE seemed to be improving with normalization of C3 and C4 titers and Anti-ds-DNA. If a 2nd course of IVIG had been given sooner, perhaps an earlier response might have been elicited and possibly limiting hospital stay. Plasmapheresis and IVIG are both recommended treatments for GBS and both are considered equally effective. Corticosteroids alone

TABLE 2

Case report	Treatment	Outcome
Hsu et al. [3]	Plasma exchange and steroids	Ambulation 2 weeks after therapy
Chaudhuri et al. [4]	Plasma exchange, steroids, and cyclophosphamide	Ambulation with persistent foot drop bilaterally 4 months after admission
Santiago-Casas et al. [5]	Plasmapheresis + IVIG with no response. Cyclophosphamide + steroids with response after four weeks	Full clinical remission after four months of therapy
Van Larrhoven et al. [6]	IVIG with no response. Cyclophosphamide + high doses steroids with response	Resolution of symptoms began on day 45 to inpatient rehab on day 74. Symptoms resolved by day 90
Tan et al. [7]	IVIG	Follow-up at 2 months revealed a completely normal exam
Echaniz-Laguna et al. [8]	Steroids	Complete resolution of symptoms by day 40
Bingisser et al. [9]	IVIG, cyclophosphamide, and steroids with no response. Plasma exchange ×5 with response	After fifth plasma exchange patient's symptoms completely resolved
Hess et al. [2]	IVIG + steroids, with no response. Plasma exchange ×2 with response	Residual mild proximal weakness, otherwise neurologically normal
Farcas et al. [10]	IVIG. Retreatment with a second course of IVIG	Complete recovery

do not alter the outcome of GBS [11]. We recommended from this case report when a diagnosis of SLE is made and is complicated by concurrent GBS with no neurological improvement after IVIG, plasmapheresis, or cyclophosphamide to consider a 2nd course of 5 days of IVIG with concomitant steroid use.

References

[1] "The American College of Rheumatology nomenclature and case definitions for neuropsychiatric lupus syndromes," *Arthritis & Rheumatism*, vol. 42, no. 4, pp. 599–608, 1999.

[2] D. C. Hess, E. Awad, H. Posas, K. D. Sethi, and R. J. Adams, "Miller Fisher syndrome in systemic lupus erythematosus," *Journal of Rheumatology*, vol. 17, no. 11, pp. 1520–1522, 1990.

[3] T.-Y. Hsu, S.-H. Wang, C.-F. Kuo, T.-F. Chiu, and Y.-C. Chang, "Acute inflammatory demyelinating polyneuropathy as the initial presentation of lupus," *American Journal of Emergency Medicine*, vol. 27, no. 7, pp. 900.e3–900.e5, 2009.

[4] K. R. Chaudhuri, I. K. Taylor, R. M. Niven, and R. J. Abbott, "A case of systemic lupus erythematosus presenting as Guillain-Barre syndrome," *British Journal of Rheumatology*, vol. 28, no. 5, pp. 440–442, 1989.

[5] Y. Santiago-Casas, R. A. Peredo, and L. M. Vilá, "Efficacy of low-dose intravenous cyclophosphamide in systemic lupus erythematosus presenting with Guillain-Barré syndrome-like acute axonal neuropathies: report of two cases," *Lupus*, vol. 22, no. 3, pp. 324–327, 2013.

[6] H. W. M. Van Larrhoven, A. Rooyer Fergus, B. G. M. van Engelen et al., "Guillain–Barré syndrome as presenting feature in a patient with lupus nephritis," *Nephrology Dialysis Transplantation*, vol. 16, no. 4, pp. 840–842, 2001.

[7] H. Tan, I. Caner, O. Deniz, and M. Büyükavci, "Miller fisher syndrome with negative anti-GQ1b immunoglobulin G antibodies," *Pediatric Neurology*, vol. 29, no. 4, pp. 349–350, 2003.

[8] A. Echaniz-Laguna, F. Battaglia, R. Heymann, C. Tranchant, and J.-M. Warter, "The Miller Fisher syndrome: neurophysiological and MRI evidence of both peripheral and central origin in one case," *Journal of Neurology*, vol. 247, no. 12, pp. 980–982, 2000.

[9] R. Bingisser, R. Speich, A. Fontana, J. Gmur, B. Vogel, and T. Landis, "Lupus erythematosus and Miller-Fisher syndrome," *Archives of Neurology*, vol. 51, no. 8, pp. 828–830, 1994.

[10] P. Farcas, L. Avnun, S. Frisher, Y. O. Herishanu, and I. Wirguin, "Efficacy of repeated intravenous immunoglobulin in severe unresponsive Guillain-Barré syndrome," *The Lancet*, vol. 350, no. 9093, p. 1747, 1997.

[11] S. Kuwabara, "Guillain-Barré syndrome: epidemiology, pathophysiology and management," *Drugs*, vol. 64, no. 6, pp. 597–610, 2004.

[12] J. Hernández-Torruco, J. Canul-Reich, J. Frausto-Solís, and J. J. Méndez-Castillo, "Feature selection for better identification of subtypes of Guillain-Barré syndrome," *Computational and Mathematical Methods in Medicine*, vol. 2014, Article ID 432109, 9 pages, 2014.

[13] R. P. Kleyweg and F. G. A. van der Meche, "Treatment related fluctuations in Guillain-Barre syndrome after high-dose immunoglobulins or plasma-exchange," *Journal of Neurology Neurosurgery and Psychiatry*, vol. 54, no. 11, pp. 957–960, 1991.

[14] P. A. van Doorn, "Diagnosis, treatment and prognosis of Guillain-Barré syndrome (GBS)," *La Presse Médicale*, vol. 42, part 2, no. 6, pp. e193–e201, 2013.

8

Gout Initially Mimicking Rheumatoid Arthritis and Later Cervical Spine Involvement

Eduardo Araújo Santana Nunes,[1] Adroaldo Guimarães Rosseti Jr.,[2] Daniel Sá Ribeiro,[3,4] and Mittermayer Santiago[1,4]

[1]*Department of Rheumatology, Santa Izabel Hospital, Praça Almeida Couto 500, 40050-410 Salvador, BA, Brazil*
[2]*Department of Neurosurgery, Santa Izabel Hospital, Praça Almeida Couto 500, 40050-410 Salvador, BA, Brazil*
[3]*Department of Radiology and Image Memorial Radiology Service, Santa Izabel Hospital, Praça Almeida Couto 500, 40050-410 Salvador, BA, Brazil*
[4]*Serviços Especializados em Reumatologia da Bahia, Rua Conde Filho 117, Graça, 40150-150 Salvador, BA, Brazil*

Correspondence should be addressed to Mittermayer Santiago; mbsantiago2014@gmail.com

Academic Editor: Remzi Cevik

Gout is clinically characterized by episodes of monoarthritis, but if not treated properly, it can lead to a chronic polyarthritis, which may eventually mimic rheumatoid arthritis (RA). We present the case of a 59-year-old man, with a history of symmetrical polyarthritis of the large and small joints with later development of subcutaneous nodules, which was initially misdiagnosed as RA, being treated with prednisone and methotrexate for a long period of time. He complained of occipital pain and paresthesia in his left upper limb, and computed tomography (CT) and magnetic resonance imaging (MRI) revealed the presence of an expansive formation in the cervical spine with compression of the medulla. He was admitted for spinal decompressive surgery and the biopsy specimen demonstrated a gouty tophus. Chronic gout can mimic RA and rarely involves the axial skeleton, and thus its correct diagnosis and the implementation of adequate therapy can halt the development of such damaging complications.

1. Introduction

Gout is a common disturbance of purine metabolism, in which the deposition of sodium monourate crystals in the synovial tissue produces acute arthritis of the peripheral joints. Localized urate deposits may also be found in extra-articular sites, or tophi, which in general are present in the later stages of the disease that is commonly found in hands, feet, bursa of the olecranon, and helix of the ear.

Involvement of the axial skeleton is a rare complication of gouty arthritis. We describe a patient with a deforming polyarticular and symmetrical arthritis, with subcutaneous nodules resembling rheumatoid arthritis (RA) that later on developed a severe cervicobrachialgia secondary to a tophaceous deposit in the cervical spine.

2. Case Report

The patient, a 59-year-old Brazilian black man, had been previously diagnosed with RA based on the history of polyarthritis of the large and small joints, morning stiffness, subcutaneous nodules, and joint deformities in his hands and feet. He was taking methotrexate (10 mg/week) and prednisone (5 mg/day) which partially controlled his symptoms. He also suffered from systemic arterial hypertension, which got controlled with captopril (100 mg/day), propranolol (80 mg/day), and hydrochlorothiazide (25 mg/day). Over the last few months the patient experienced severe headaches in the occipital region and cervicalgia with irradiation to the left upper limb, resembling the possibility of atlantoaxial subluxation. On physical examination, it was found that his

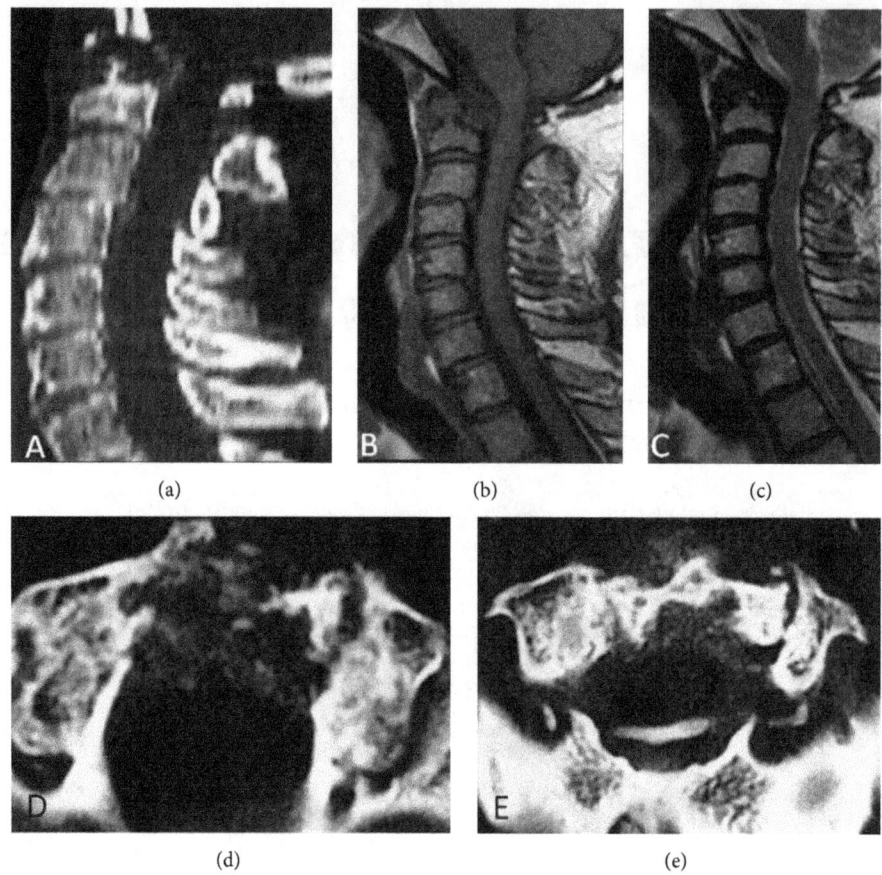

(a)   (b)   (c)

(d)   (e)

FIGURE 1: (a) Sagital computed tomography (CT) image shows a destructive lesion of odontoid process. (b) Sagital T1-weighted spin eco and (c) sagital T2-weighted spin eco demonstrating a hypointense mass with compression of the spinal cord. (d) and (e) Axial CT images of this region with well-defined calcification foci within the mass suggesting microcrystal deposition.

general condition was good, with a blood pressure level of 130/80 mm Hg; he had "swan-neck" deformity of the fingers, "camel back" deformities in his wrists, and fixed deformities in his feet and knees with a significant limitation of movement amplitude both passively and actively. There were several subcutaneous nodules in extension surfaces of his joints, mainly in elbows. There were left brachial paresis graded 4/5, hypertrophy of the left shoulder muscles, and hyperreflexia graded 3/4 in the upper limbs; however, proprioceptive, vibratory, and pain sensitivity were preserved and there were signs of autonomic dysfunction. Cardiovascular and respiratory examinations were unremarkable. The laboratory investigation showed hyperuricemia (8.6 mg/dL), hypertriglyceridemia, and elevation in creatinine values (1.5 mg/dL). The rheumatoid factor (RF) and anti-CCP antibodies were negative. Cervical magnetic resonance imaging (MRI) showed destructive lesion of the odontoid process and computed tomography (CT) revealed part of C1 vertebra with hyperdense foci suggesting microcrystal deposition (Figure 1). Radiographs of the knee, feet, ankle, and hands showed periarticular soft tissue swelling with extensive bone erosions and joint space narrowing with normal bone density (Figure 2). Based on these findings, the diagnosis of tophaceous and mutilans-type gout was established and the use of colchicine and allopurinol was initiated.

The patient was admitted for two neurosurgical procedures: initially occipitocervical arthrodesis and later exeresis of the mass in the odontoid process. The histopathological study demonstrated an accumulation of an acellular amorphous substance with crystals and fibrosis and a granulomatous reaction foreign body type involving the soft parts and bone tissue and the absence of neoplastic cells.

During subsequent evaluations in the outpatient clinic, the patient no longer complained of cervical pain and showed improvement of the left brachial paresis.

3. Discussion

Gout is one of the most ancient clinical entities with evidence of its description dating back to times preceding the descriptions made by Hippocrates [1]. It primarily affects the distal joints of the appendicular skeleton, initially with a monoarticular pattern of involvement and later, particularly when not well treated, becomes polyarticular. It can eventually mimic RA, as in the present case, which was initially treated erroneously as this condition.

There are other descriptions of gout mimicking RA in the literature [2] as well as rare cases of coexisting gout and RA [3]. The latter was not the case with our patient as the bone erosions observed in the radiographs were typical of

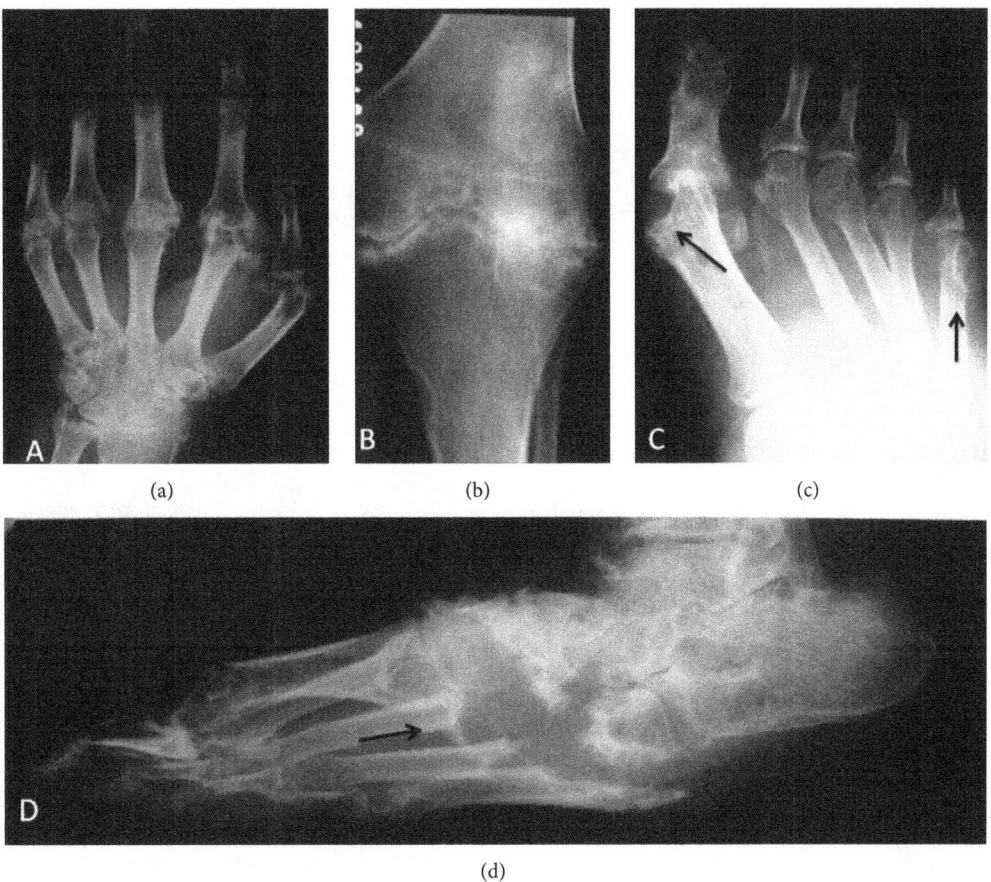

(a)   (b)   (c)

(d)

FIGURE 2: Radiographs of hand (a), knee (b), foot (c), and ankle (d) showing severe destructive changes secondary to tophaceous gout with erosion, soft tissue swelling (tophi), articular space narrowing, and proliferative bone abnormalities. Note the well-defined extra-articular large erosions with overhanging margin and surrounding bone eburnation (arrows). The uniform joint space narrowing with normal bone density in knee and wrist is typical of late gout disease.

gout arthropathy, and the RF and anti-CCP antibodies were negative.

Involvement of the axial skeleton by gouty tophi has been described in the literature in around 100 cases [4] and may be associated with compression of the spinal cord. However, a recently published paper revealed the presence of spinal gout, as identified by CT, in 12 out of 42 (29%) gouty patients, mainly in lumbar and none in cervical spine and there was no association between symptoms and axial gout [5]. Patients may present with a variety of symptoms, such as isolated lumbar or cervical pain or various other neurological syndromes, depending on the level of tophi deposition in the spinal cord. A history of peripheral gout for several months or years preceding the neurological manifestations occurs in the large majority of patients and helps in the clinical diagnosis [6]. Nevertheless, it is worth pointing out that, in the literature, there are reports of gout with axial involvement with nerve compression without a previous history of peripheral arthritis [7]. The concomitant presence of "spinal gout" and the peripheral joint involvement with a rheumatoid-like pattern as seen in our patient is unique. In theory, the spinal complication could probably have been avoided if the diagnosis of gout had not been delayed by

the articular presentation suggestive of RA, and the tophi confounded with rheumatoid nodules and the treatment for gout had been promptly established.

In axial gout, any segment of the spine and its components (vertebral bodies, pedicles, lamina, ligaments, interapophyseal cartilage, and epidural and intradural spaces) may be involved, with lumbar involvement being the most common [8]. The mechanism of compression differs from level to level: (a) at the cervical level, the symptoms of pain and instability are generated by the paravertebral involvement and consequent ligamentous instability; (b) at the thoracic level, it deposits in the extramural space with medullar compression; (c) at the lumbar level, the symptoms result from the radicular compression; (d) at the sacroiliac level, it deposits in the hyaline cartilage of the interarticular space and adjacent bones causing the symptoms [9].

Because of the rarity of axial involvement in gout, before making a diagnosis, it is necessary to exclude other possible etiologies such as spondylodiscitis, infection, and neoplasia [10]. For this purpose, it is necessary to use techniques such as MRI and CT, since plain radiographs are generally negative or may show only degenerative alterations and bone erosions [6, 8–10]. CT can show facet joint erosions that are more consistent with gout than with degenerative alterations [11]. MRI can be very useful in a differential diagnosis since the tophi present a low signal in the pondered sequence in T1 and a low or high heterogeneous signal in the pondered images in T2 (the high signal is owing to the filling of the amorphous center of the tophus with high protein content [7] and the heterogeneity and to the varied levels of calcium deposits in the tophus [12]) and present variable peripheral enhancement after gadolinium administration.

In conclusion, chronic gout can mimic RA and rarely involves the axial skeleton, and thus its correct diagnosis and the implementation of adequate therapy can halt the development of such damaging complications.

Disclosure

Mittermayer Santiago is currently receiving a scholarship from Conselho Nacional de Desenvolvimento Científico e Tecnológico (CNPq).

References

[1] P. Richette and T. Bardin, "Gout," *The Lancet*, vol. 375, no. 9711, pp. 318–328, 2010.

[2] W. A. Read and R. Buxton, "Gout simulating rheumatoid arthritis," *Virginia Medical Monthly*, vol. 75, no. 10, pp. 493–497, 1948.

[3] A. J. Rizzoli, L. Trujeque, and A. D. Bankhurst, "The coexistence of gout and rheumatoid arthritis: case reports and a review of the literature," *Journal of Rheumatology*, vol. 7, no. 3, pp. 316–324, 1980.

[4] L. A. Saketkoo, H. J. Robertson, H. R. Dyer, Z.-U. Virk, H. R. Ferreyro, and L. R. Espinoza, "Axial gouty arthropathy," *American Journal of the Medical Sciences*, vol. 338, no. 2, pp. 140–146, 2009.

[5] F. M. de Mello, P. V. Partezani Helito, M. Bordalo-Rodrigues, R. Fuller, and A. S. Halpern, "Axial gout is frequently associated with the presence of current tophi, although not with spinal symptoms," *Spine*, vol. 39, no. 25, pp. E1531–E1536, 2014.

[6] A. K. Pfister, C. A. Schlarb, and J. F. O'Neal, "Vertebral erosion, paraplegia, and spinal gout," *The American Journal of Roentgenology*, vol. 171, no. 5, pp. 1430–1431, 1998.

[7] R. Dharmadhikari, P. Dildey, and I. G. Hide, "A rare cause of spinal cord compression: imaging appearances of gout of the cervical spine," *Skeletal Radiology*, vol. 35, no. 12, pp. 942–945, 2006.

[8] R. Hausch, M. Wilkerson, E. Singh, C. Reyes, and T. Harrington, "Tophaceous gout of the thoracic spine presenting as back pain and fever," *Journal of Clinical Rheumatology*, vol. 5, no. 6, pp. 335–341, 1999.

[9] M. Draganescu and L. J. Leventhal, "Spinal gout: case report and review of the literature," *Journal of Clinical Rheumatology*, vol. 10, no. 2, pp. 74–79, 2004.

[10] K. Barrett, M. L. Miller, and J. T. Wilson, "Tophaceous gout of the spine mimicking epidural infection: case report and review of the literature," *Neurosurgery*, vol. 48, no. 5, pp. 1170–1173, 2001.

[11] P. Fenton, S. Young, and K. Prutis, "Gout of the spine: two case reports and a review of the literature," *The Journal of Bone and Joint Surgery A*, vol. 77, no. 5, pp. 767–771, 1995.

[12] C.-Y. Hsu, T. T.-F. Shih, K.-M. Huang, P.-Q. Chen, J.-J. Sheu, and Y.-W. Li, "Tophaceous gout of the spine: MR imaging features," *Clinical Radiology*, vol. 57, no. 10, pp. 919–925, 2002.

9

Diffuse Muscular Pain, Skin Tightening, and Nodular Regenerative Hyperplasia Revealing Paraneoplastic Amyopathic Dermatomyositis due to Testicular Cancer

Sarah Norrenberg,[1] Valérie Gangji,[2] Véronique Del Marmol,[1] and Muhammad S. Soyfoo[2]

[1] Department of Dermatology, Hôpital Erasme, Université Libre de Bruxelles, 1070 Bruxelles, Belgium
[2] Department of Rheumatology and Medical Physicine, Hôpital Erasme, Université Libre de Bruxelles, 808 Route de Lennik, 1070 Bruxelles, Belgium

Correspondence should be addressed to Muhammad S. Soyfoo, msoyfoo@ulb.ac.be

Academic Editors: D. R. Alpert, M. Salazar-Paramo, F. Schiavon, and A. Zoli

Paraneoplastic dermatomyositis (DM) associated with testicular cancer is extremely rare. We report the case of a patient with skin tightening, polymyalgia, hypereosinophilia, and nodular regenerative hyperplasia revealing seminoma and associated paraneoplastic DM.

1. Introduction

Dermatomyositis (DM) encompasses a heterogeneous group of multisystemic inflammatory myopathies with variable clinical and laboratory characteristics, affecting mainly the skin and proximal skeletal musculature [1, 2]. The prevalence of DM is between 0.5 and 1 case per 100.000 people [1]. The criteria of Bohan and Peter have been reviewed and newly adapted by A. A. Amato in 2003. This new classification for the idiopathic inflammatory myopathies was approved by the MSG and ENMC workshop [2]. The main subgroups described are the primary idiopathic DM in adults, paraneoplastic DM, amyopathic DM, juvenile DM, overlap syndromes, drug-induced DM, primary idiopathic PM, "inclusion body" myositis, eosinophilic myositis/perimyositis, and orbital myositis with giant cell myocarditis [1, 2]. Principal clinical features include symmetrical proximal muscular weakness, Gottron's papules, Gottron's sign, heliotrope eruption, skin erythema (V-sign erythema, shawl sign), photosensitive poikiloderma, and periungual erythema/telangiectasia [1, 2]. Diagnosis of DM can be made on the basis of biopsy-confirmed classical skin findings, proximal muscle weakness, and elevated muscle enzymes (creatinin Phosphokinase, CPK; Aldolase). Electromyography and/or muscle biopsy can also be performed to confirm active myositis. Amyopathic DM is distinguished from classic DM by the absence of clinically evident myopathy. Furthermore, Stonecipher et al. [3] have defined 3 subgroups of ADM: (1) no subjective or objective evidence of myopathy, (2) no subjective muscle weakness but abnormalities detected by objective tests, (3) subjective muscle weakness but no objective evidence of myopathy.

The relative risk of neoplasia is increased the first year after diagnosis of DM and is about 26/1.000.000 [4]. Variable frequencies of malignancies with DM have been reported in the literature, from 6% to 60% [4–6], around 15% and 34% in Western countries [7]. Dermatomyositis and cancer usually arise within one to five years of one another [8]. The most reported malignancies are nasopharyngeal carcinoma (predominantly in Chinese population), ovarian carcinoma, lung carcinoma, pancreatic carcinoma, lymphomas, breast carcinoma, liver carcinoma, colorectal carcinoma, and gastric carcinoma [3, 5]. The risk of developing a specific type of neoplasia with DM is variable following different populations [4, 6, 8]. Patients with older age at onset of disease (>45 years) and male gender are more likely to develop malignant diseases [5, 7].

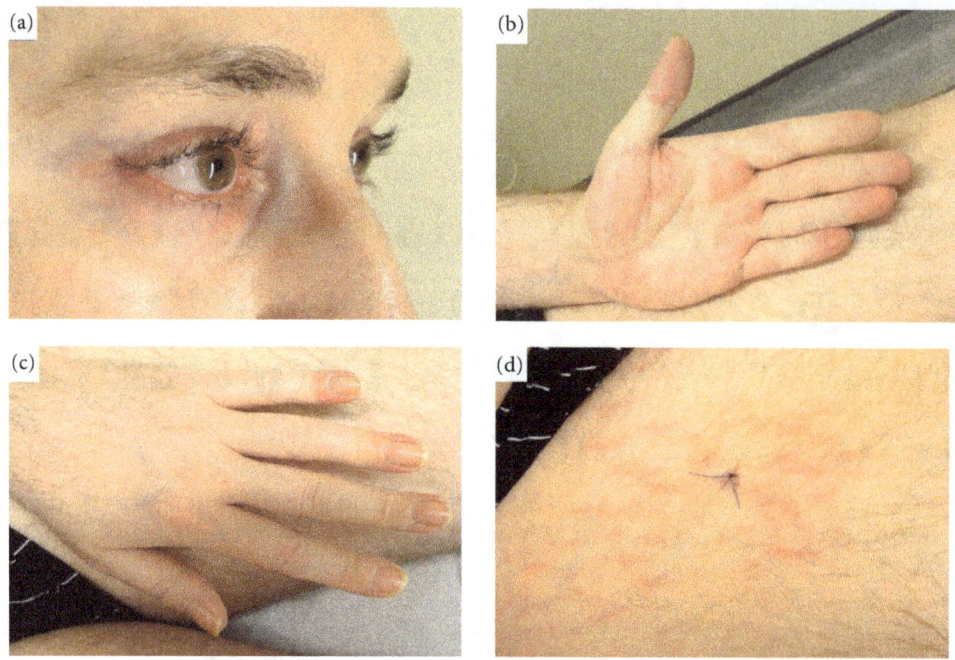

FIGURE 1: Cutaneous features of DM. (a) Heliotrope erythema, (b) palmar erythema, (c) periungual erythema, and (d) flagellate erythema.

We hereby report the case of a patient with fibromyalgia-like syndrome and testicular cancer revealing dermatomyositis.

2. Case Report

A 30-year-old man of Caucasian origin was seen in an outpatient rheumatology clinic for diffuse polyarticular and muscular pain. The patient described important morning stiffness of more than 2 hours, the sensation of skin rigidity, and diffuse myalgia predominating in the proximal muscles. His current medications include tetrazepam 50 mg/d, amitriptyline 75 mg/d (for depression), and oxycodone 80 mg/d. Initial physical examination showed normal vital parameters and absence of synovitis but revealed joint and muscle tenderness. Blood analysis showed normal levels of C-reactive protein and normal erythrocyte sedimentation rate, hypereosinophilia ($700/mm^3$), and increased liver enzymes without increases in CPK levels. Electromyography (EMG) of the left thigh was performed but did not reveal any abnormalities. A liver biopsy was done and showed nodular regenerative hyperplasia (NRH) and no signs of malignancy. Serologies and other investigations were performed to rule out any parasitic infection as well as autoimmune diseases (Sjögren's syndrome and systemic sclerosis). Another EMG and a total body Magnetic Resonance Imaging were performed in 2010, but did not reveal any convincing element in favour of myopathy. Because of worsening physical condition with loss of weight, appetite, and skin tightening, an [18]fluorodeoxyglucose PET-CT was performed and revealed a right testicular hypermetabolic mass, confirmed by ultrasonography. One month later, a large right orchidectomy was performed and histology revealed a pure seminoma of two centimeters, classified pT1NX. The patient condition worsened and he developed palmar erythema, amyotrophy, increased muscular weakness, heliotrope erythema, flagellate erythema on anterior thighs, palmar erythema, and sclerosis-like aspect of the skin (Figure 1). Capillaroscopy showed dermal microvasculitis characterized by tortuosities and diffuse edema. An [18]fluorodeoxyglucose PET-CT scan was performed again and did not show any metastasis but revealed bilateral basal pulmonary infiltrates that were confirmed by a high-resolution computed chest tomography. Pulmonary function tests were performed and showed significantly reduced DLCO compatible with interstitial lung disease. A cutaneous biopsy of the flagellate erythema was done and histological analysis was compatible with a diagnosis of dermatomyositis (Figure 2). Treatment with Methylprednisolone 1 mg/kg daily improved the dermatological features and the liver tests but the muscular pain did not subside. AZA (2 mg/kg/d) was then added but the patient's condition still did not improve.

3. Discussion

We have reported the case of a patient presenting with testicular cancer, hypereosinophilia, and NRH unveiling the diagnosis of amyopathic DM. The diagnosis delay could be attributed to protean clinical and biological manifestations that misled the physicians in charge of the patient. For four years, the patient was believed to have a fibromyalgia-like syndrome because of the appealing symptoms of polymyalgia

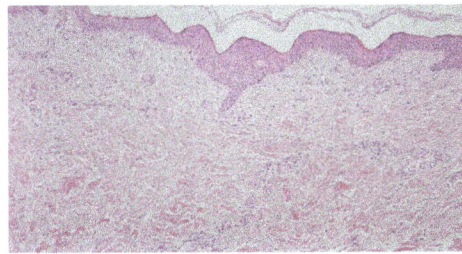

FIGURE 2: The cutaneous biopsy of flagellate erythema (magnification ×10) depicting atrophic epiderma. In the superficial derma, there was a slight inflammatory infiltrate, essentially composed of mononuclear cells and rare telangiectasies.

and myalgia concomitant with the paucity of clinical and biological signs of autoimmune involvement. Early in the disease, the patient presented with high levels of hepatic enzymes and hypereosinophilia, without elevation of CPK. NRH could explain the elevation of hepatic enzymes but the relationship with muscle weakness could not be made at that time. NRH has been described in association with collagen diseases [9], but to our knowledge, this is the first case associated with dermatomyositis. Hypereosinophilia could be linked with neoplasia [10] in the absence of patent evidence of parasitic infection.

Paraneoplastic DM associated with testicular cancer is extremely rare. In their review, Dourmishev et al. [11] reported 11 cases of DM associated with testicular cancer. One new case was also described by Tan et al. [12]. Patients were aged between 24 and 46 years old. There were six cases of nonseminomatous testicular cancer, two malignant teratoma, one intratubular germ-cell tumor, one mix testicular cancer with a pattern of seminoma, and three pure seminoma. Symptoms of DM appeared in seven cases before malignancy, three after orchiectomy and three after orchiectomy and chemotherapy. Half of the patients presented metastasis at diagnosis. All cases showed increased values of CPK, LDH, and liver enzymes that were associated with DM. Disappearance of the DM was totally different from case to case. Some resolved after treatment of cancer while others appeared after treatment as in the present case. Some patients responded to corticosteroids while others did not. Some cases required more effective immunosuppressants such as AZA, HCQ, or methotrexate. The extremely low incidence of paraneoplastic DM associated with seminoma is explained by the rarity of both diseases. The current incidence of testicular tumor is 63/100 000 per year [13]. The death rate is very low [13]. It is found in young male between 15 and 35 years old [12]. This explains the contrast with the age distribution in patients with paraneoplastic DM.

4. Conclusion

Paraneoplastic DM associated with testicular cancer is extremely rare. This is the first case of paraneoplastic amyopathic DM associated with testicular tumor. As in our case, other patients have developed DM after initial treatment of their neoplasia. No pathogenic mechanism

underlying the triggering of DM following treatment of neoplasia has been suggested. This is probably due to the rarity of the phenomenon and the heterogeneous clinical presentation. Furthermore, DM could appear within years before or after diagnosis of malignancy. The disease can spontaneously disappear after treatment of the cancer or could be treated with initial high doses of MPN daily in a decreasing fashion [2]. First line treatment with MPN followed by adjunct of immunosuppressants seems to be the mainstay of treatment even if no randomized controlled trials are available.

References

[1] L. A. Dourmishev, A. L. Dourmishev, and R. A. Schwartz, "Dermatomyositis: cutaneous manifestations of its variants," *International Journal of Dermatology*, vol. 41, no. 10, pp. 625–630, 2002.

[2] J. E. Hoogendijk, A. A. Amato, B. R. Lecky et al., "Workshop report: 119th ENMC international workshop: trial design in adult idiopathic inflammatory myopathies, with the exception of inclusion body myositis, 10–12 October 2003, Naarden, The Netherlands," *Neuromuscular Disorders*, vol. 14, no. 5, pp. 337–345, 2004.

[3] M. R. Stonecipher, J. L. Jorizzo, W. L. White, F. O. Walker, and E. Prichard, "Cutaneous changes of dermatomyositis in patients with normal muscle enzymes: dermatomyositis sine myositis?" *Journal of the American Academy of Dermatology*, vol. 28, no. 6, pp. 951–956, 1993.

[4] A. Airio, E. Pukkala, and H. Isomaki, "Elevated cancer incidence in patients with dermatomyositis: a population based study," *Journal of Rheumatology*, vol. 22, no. 7, pp. 1300–1303, 1995.

[5] Y. J. Chen, C. Y. Wu, and J. L. Shen, "Predicting factors of malignancy in dermatomyositis and polymyositis: a case-control study," *British Journal of Dermatology*, vol. 144, no. 4, pp. 825–831, 2001.

[6] C. L. Hill, Y. Zhang, B. Sigurgeirsson et al., "Frequency of specific cancer types in dermatomyositis and polymyositis: a population-based study," *The Lancet*, vol. 357, no. 9250, pp. 96–100, 2001.

[7] J. P. Callen, "The value of malignancy evaluation in patients with dermatomyositis," *Journal of the American Academy of Dermatology*, vol. 6, no. 2, pp. 253–259, 1982.

[8] B. Sigurgeirsson, B. Lindelof, O. Edhag, and E. Allander, "Risk of cancer in patients with dermatomyositis or polymyositis— a population-based study," *The New England Journal of Medicine*, vol. 326, no. 6, pp. 363–367, 1992.

[9] T. Matsumoto, S. Kobayashi, H. Shimizu et al., "The liver in collagen diseases: pathologic study of 160 cases with particular reference to hepatic arteritis, primary biliary cirrhosis, autoimmune hepatitis and nodular regenerative hyperplasia of the liver," *Liver*, vol. 20, no. 5, pp. 366–373, 2000.

[10] F. Roufosse and P. F. Weller, "Practical approach to the patient with hypereosinophilia," *Journal of Allergy and Clinical Immunology*, vol. 126, no. 1, pp. 39–44, 2010.

[11] L. A. Dourmishev, J. M. Popov, and D. Rusinova, "Paraneoplastic dermatomyositis associated with testicular cancer: a case report and literature review," *Acta Dermatovenerologica Alpina, Pannonica et Adriatica*, vol. 19, no. 1, pp. 39–43, 2010.

10

Takayasu's Arteritis and Crohn's Disease in a Young Hispanic Female

Namrata Singh,[1] Shireesh Saurabh,[2] and Irene J. Tan[3]

[1] Immunology, University of Iowa Hospitals and Clinics, 200 Hawkins Drive, C42 E 10, Iowa City, IA 52241, USA
[2] Mercy Iowa City, 540 E Jefferson Street, Suite 205, Iowa City, IA 52245, USA
[3] Section of Rheumatology, Temple University Hospital, 3200 North Broad Street, Philadelphia, PA 19140, USA

Correspondence should be addressed to Namrata Singh; namrata-singh@uiowa.edu

Academic Editor: Helene Alexanderson

Takayasu's arteritis (TA) and Crohn's disease (CD) are chronic inflammatory granulomatous disorders of undetermined etiology. TA is a large vessel vasculitis with a predilection for the aorta and its branches in young women of Asian descent; whereas CD has characteristic gastrointestinal manifestations more prevalent in young Caucasians. We describe a case of both diseases in a young Hispanic female, review the literature, and impart new insight on possible genetic linkage and the role of interleukin 12 B (IL-12B) as the common autoimmune mechanism and potential therapeutic target in this rare disease combination.

1. Introduction

Takayasu's arteritis (TA) and Crohn's disease (CD) are chronic inflammatory granulomatous disorders of undetermined etiology. TA is a large vessel vasculitis with a predilection for the aorta and its branches; CD, on the other hand, has characteristic gastrointestinal manifestations [1]. TA is most commonly diagnosed in young women of Asian descent whereas CD appears to be more prevalent in young Caucasians.

Here, we report a case of both of these diseases in the same patient.

2. Case Report

A 26-year-old Hispanic female presented for evaluation of nausea, vomiting, abdominal pain, and watery diarrhea of two-week duration. She reported fevers, generalized malaise, and weight loss. She had similar gastrointestinal complaints in the past without any visual loss, weight loss, claudication, or joint pains. Her history was significant for appendicitis in 2003 and a perineal abscess/fistula repair in 2000. She denied smoking, alcohol, or illicit drug use.

Physical examination revealed blood pressure of 126/73 mmHg in the right arm and 114/74 mmHg in the left arm. Her right radial pulse was not palpable and the left one was thready at 70 beats per minute. The femoral and dorsalis pedis pulses were difficult to appreciate bilaterally. An abdominal bruit was noted, as well as tenderness of the right lower quadrant. Musculoskeletal exam was normal except complaint of pain in both arms when raised above her head for more than 6 seconds. The shoulder exam was normal on both sides. Laboratory evaluation (Table 1) was significant for anemia of chronic disease and elevated inflammatory markers. She underwent colonoscopy and the right colon biopsy showed benign colonic mucosa with cryptitis, ulceration, and mild-moderate architectural change, consistent with Crohn's disease. Due to her symptoms of shoulder/arm pain, unequal blood pressure, and pulses in both arms and an abdominal bruit, further imaging studies were pursued. A magnetic resonance angiogram of the chest and abdomen was done and showed severe irregularity and narrowing of the descending thoracic aorta which tapers down from 2 cm transversely at the level of the distal arch to 7.5 mm transversely at the narrowest point just beyond the aortic hiatus. The subclavian arteries were not visualized in their entirety bilaterally during the initial imaging. There was 50% narrowing of the origin of the celiac artery with poststenotic dilatation; renal arteries were normal (Figure 1). At this point, the patient was diagnosed with Takayasu's

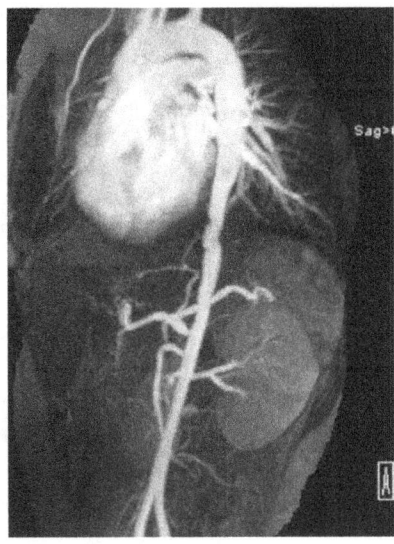

FIGURE 1: Magnetic resonance angiogram of chest and abdomen: severe irregularity and narrowing of the descending thoracic aorta. The subclavian arteries were not visualized in their entirety bilaterally during the initial imaging.

TABLE 1: Labs at the initial evaluation.

Lab	Patient's result	Normal range
Hemoglobin	10.5	11–15.9 g/dL
MCV	75	80–97 fL
WBC	5300	4000–10500/μL
Platelets	359,000	140–415,000/μL
BUN	9	6–20 mg/dL
Creatinine	0.54	0.57–1 mg/dL
AST	28	0–40 IU/L
ALT	40	0–40 IU/L
ESR	48	0–32 mm/hr
CRP	9	0–4.9 mg/L
Hepatitis panel	Negative	
Quantiferon	Negative	

WBC: white blood cells; MCV: mean corpuscular volume; mg/dL: milligrams per deciliter; BUN: blood urea nitrogen; AST: aspartate aminotransferase; ALT: alanine aminotransferase; IU: international units; ESR: erythrocyte sedimentation rate; CRP: C-reactive protein; and mm/hr: millimeters per hour.

arteritis based on the 1990 ACR criteria [2] in addition to Crohn's disease. The absence of recurrent oral and nasal ulcers and episodes of uveitis made Behcet's syndrome less likely. She had no hilar adenopathy; also her levels of serum calcium and angiotensin converting enzyme were normal, so sarcoidosis was low in the differentials. She was treated with pulse methylprednisolone for 3 days and started on adalimumab. A follow-up thoracic and abdominal aortogram 14 months later showed severe tapering of the subclavian arteries bilaterally and stable narrowing and irregularity of the distal aorta (Figure 2). Azathioprine has been added to her regimen; she is currently doing well and her steroids are being tapered.

3. Discussion

The association of TA and CD has been reported worldwide in fewer than 60 patients, mostly from Japan and Europe [3]. We found only 7 prior case reports from the USA [1, 4–9]. Although case reports of the association of Takayasu's arteritis and inflammatory bowel disease began in 1970 [10, 11], the first case of TA associated with CD was described by Yassinger et al. [4]. Kusunoki et al. [3] in 2011 listed 37 cases of individuals with this dual diagnosis found in the literature; of the 32 cases, whose age at diagnosis was noted, 25 cases (78%) had the onset of TA simultaneous with or later than that of CD. In their study of 44 patients with TA, Reny et al. [1] found CD to be present in 9% of the population and they reported that patients with coexistent TA and CD tend to be younger at the time of diagnosis and also tended to have systemic symptoms more frequently than those with TA alone. To our knowledge, no description of an association between anti-Saccharomyces cerevisiae antibodies (a serological marker of inflammatory bowel disease) and TA exists.

This association of TA and CD raises the question of whether it is more than coincidence to encounter these two different granulomatous diseases in the same patient. Interestingly, Maksimowicz-McKinnon and Hoffman [12] have pointed out the common features shared by these diseases despite their different clinical manifestations; both are diseases affecting young females and the pathogenesis of both includes predominantly TH1 lymphocytes and granulomatous inflammation.

Significant CD risk has been associated with genes like NOD2/CARD15, IBD5, and DLG5; IL23 R has also been implicated as a CD susceptibility gene [13]. A pathway analysis using data from the Wellcome Trust Case Control Consortium (WTCCC) uncovered significant associations of CD and IL-12/IL-23 pathway components, harboring 20 genes such as IL12B, JAK2, STAT3, and CCR6 [14]. Glas et al.

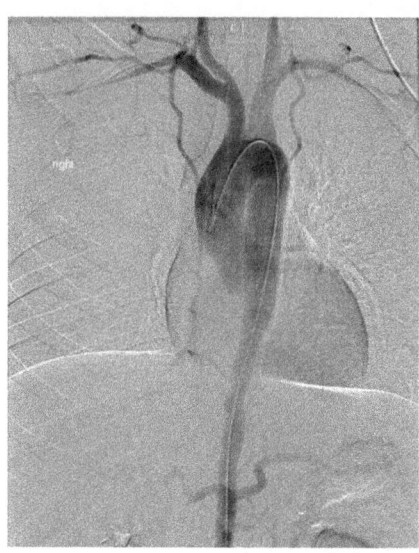

FIGURE 2: Follow-up thoracic and abdominal angiogram 14 months later: severe tapering of the subclavian arteries bilaterally, narrowing, and irregularity of distal aorta. The ascending aorta measured 2.5 cm whereas the distal thoracic aorta measured only 1.2 cm in diameter and tapered to 7.5 mm transversely at the narrowest point just beyond the aortic hiatus.

analyzed IL-12B gene variants regarding association with Crohn's disease and ulcerative colitis in German cohort and found that IL-12 single nucleotide polymorphism rs 6887695 modulates the susceptibility and the phenotype of inflammatory bowel disease [15]. IL-12 promotes the differentiation of naive CD4+ T cells into mature interferon-gamma producing Th1 effector cells and is a potent stimulus of natural killer and CD8+ T cells. In contrast, IL-23, a heterodimeric cytokine composed of a p19 subunit and a p40 subunit of which the latter is shared with IL-12, is required for the generation of memory T cells and drives differentiation of Th17 cells. A common genetic linkage between these diseases was not reported until recently when Terao et al. [16] performed genome scanning of 167 TA cases and 663 healthy controls via Illumina Infinium Human Exome Bead Chip arrays followed by a replication study consisting of 212 TA cases and 1,322 controls. They found that the IL12B (interleukin 12B) region on chromosome 5 and the MLX (Max-like protein X) region on chromosome 17 exhibited significant associations and the detection of these susceptibility loci will provide new insights to the basic mechanisms of TA pathogenesis. Their findings indicate that IL12B plays a fundamental role in the pathophysiology of TA in combination with HLA-B*52:01 and that common autoimmune mechanisms underlie the pathology of TA and other autoimmune disorders such as psoriasis and inflammatory bowel diseases in which IL12B is involved as a genetic predisposing factor. Recently ustekinumab, a monoclonal antibody against IL-12 p40 subunit, was shown to be effective for patients with refractory CD [17]. The findings of Terao et al. raise the possibility of its therapeutic use for TA, and especially for patients with a dual diagnosis of TA and CD, by targeting the IL-12/23 pathway. Currently there are no guidelines on the management of patients with this dual diagnosis. There are case reports of TNF-inhibitor therapy being useful in these patients but few tolerated these biologic agents due to infectious complications. With further insight into the pathogenesis of these granulomatous diseases, we can hope for more effective and targeted therapies.

When providing care for a patient with a known diagnosis of an inflammatory bowel disease like CD, an awareness of the association with TA becomes very important especially because a delay in the diagnosis and then treatment of TA can have serious consequences for the patient including, but not limited to, congestive heart failure and cerebrovascular accidents. It is important for an internist to look for extraintestinal complications or Takayasu's arteritis in patients with IBD when the inflammatory markers are elevated out of proportion to patient's gastrointestinal complaints and their symptomatology/examination does not conform with their known medical problems.

References

[1] S. Ratuapli, M. Mazlumzadeh, S. Gurudu, S. Money, and R. Heigh, "Coexisting crohn's disease and takayasu's arteritis in two patients treated with anti-TNF-α therapies," *Case Reports in Gastroenterology*, vol. 4, no. 1, pp. 35–40, 2010.

[2] W. P. Arend, B. A. Michel, D. A. Bloch et al., "The American College of Rheumatology 1990 criteria for the classification of Takayasu arteritis," *Arthritis and Rheumatism*, vol. 33, no. 8, pp. 1129–1134, 1990.

[3] R. Kusunoki, S. Ishihara, M. Sato et al., "Rare case of Takayasu's arteritis associated with Crohns disease," *Internal Medicine*, vol. 50, no. 15, pp. 1581–1585, 2011.

[4] S. Yassinger, R. Adelman, D. Cantor, C. H. Halsted, and R. J. Bolt, "Association of inflammatory bowel disease and large vascular lesions," *Gastroenterology*, vol. 71, no. 5, pp. 844–846, 1976.

[5] M. Baqir, M. H. U. Usman, H. N. Adenwalla et al., "Takayasu's arteritis with skin manifestations in a patient with inflammatory bowel disease: coincidence or concurrence?" *Clinical Rheumatology*, vol. 26, no. 6, pp. 996–998, 2007.

[6] C. Owyang, L. J. Miller, J. T. Lie, and C. R. Fleming, "Takayasu's arteritis in Crohn's disease," *Gastroenterology*, vol. 76, no. 4, pp. 825–828, 1979.

[7] C. J. Friedman and C. J. Tegtmeyer, "Crohn's disease associated with Takayasu's arteritis," *Digestive Diseases and Sciences*, vol. 24, no. 12, pp. 954–958, 1979.

[8] J. Levitsky, J. R. Harrison, and R. D. Cohen, "Crohns disease and Takayasus arteritis," *Journal of Clinical Gastroenterology*, vol. 34, no. 4, pp. 454–456, 2002.

[9] T. Rustagi and S. Majumder, "Crohn's-Takayasu's arteritis overlap with hypercoagulability: an optimal milieu for ischemic stroke," *Journal of Digestive Diseases*, vol. 12, no. 2, pp. 142–146, 2011.

[10] A. Silverstein and D. H. Present, "Cerebrovascular occlusions in relatively young patients with regional enteritis," *The Journal of the American Medical Association*, vol. 215, no. 6, pp. 976–977, 1971.

[11] M. Soloway, T. W. Moir, and D. S. Linton Jr., "Takayasu's arteritis. Report of a case with unusual findings," *The American Journal of Cardiology*, vol. 25, no. 2, pp. 258–263, 1970.

[12] K. Maksimowicz-McKinnon and G. S. Hoffman, "Crohn's disease plus Takayasu's arteritis: more than coincidence?" *Annales de Médecine Interne*, vol. 154, no. 2, pp. 75–76, 2003.

[13] S. Michail, G. Bultron, and R. W. Depaolo, "Genetic variants associated with Crohn's disease," *Application of Clinical Genetics*, vol. 6, pp. 25–32, 2013.

[14] K. Wang, H. Zhang, S. Kugathasan et al., "Diverse genome-wide association studies associate the IL12/IL23 pathway with Crohn disease," *American Journal of Human Genetics*, vol. 84, no. 3, pp. 399–405, 2009.

[15] J. Glas, J. Seiderer, J. Wagner et al., "Analysis of IL12B gene variants in inflammatory bowel disease," *PLoS ONE*, vol. 7, no. 3, Article ID e34349, 2012.

[16] C. Terao, H. Yoshifuji, A. Kimura et al., "Two susceptibility Loci to Takayasu arteritis reveal a synergistic role of the IL12B and HLA-B regions in a Japanese population," *The American Journal of Human Genetics*, vol. 93, no. 2, pp. 289–297, 2013.

[17] W. J. Sandborn, C. Gasink, L. Gao et al., "Ustekinumab induction and maintenance therapy in refractory Crohn's disease," *The New England Journal of Medicine*, vol. 367, no. 16, pp. 1519–1528, 2012.

11

An Unusual Case of Adult-Onset Still's Disease with Hemophagocytic Syndrome, Necrotic Leukoencephalopathy and Disseminated Intravascular Coagulation

Rajaie Namas,[1] Naveen Nannapaneni,[2] Malini Venkatram,[1] Gulcin Altinok,[3] Miriam Levine,[2] and J. Patricia Dhar[1]

[1] *Department of Internal Medicine, Division of Rheumatology, Wayne State University, Detroit, MI 48201, USA*
[2] *Department of Internal Medicine, Wayne State University, Detroit, MI 48201, USA*
[3] *Department of Radiology, Wayne State University, Detroit, MI 48201, USA*

Correspondence should be addressed to Rajaie Namas; rajainammas@gmail.com

Academic Editors: D. R. Alpert and F. Schiavon

Case. A 34-year-old African-American female with a history of adult-onset Still's disease presented to an outside hospital with oligoarthritis. She experienced a generalized tonic-clonic seizure *en route* via ambulance, was intubated upon arrival, and transferred to the intensive care unit for treatment of suspected pneumonia and sepsis. She subsequently developed generalized cutaneous desquamation that progressed despite the cessation of antibiotics and other potential offending drugs which required transfer to our hospital's burn unit. She was suspected to have reactive hemophagocytic syndrome based on her clinical presentation of fever, rash, polyarthritis, elevated liver enzymes, coagulopathy, splenomegaly, normocytic anemia, thrombocytopenia, hypertriglyceridemia, hyperferritinemia, and hemophagocytosis visualized in bone marrow biopsy specimen. Magnetic resonance imaging demonstrated necrotic demyelination of the deep white matter and corona radiata. The patient developed multiorgan dysfunction and DIC without any other attributable etiology. Despite aggressive broad spectrum therapy and high dose of steroids she progressively deteriorated and eventually expired. *Conclusion*. Previous publications have highlighted the prevalence of necrotic leukoencephalopathy in children with familial hemophagocytic syndrome. Our patient demonstrated some uncommon features complicating her HLH including DIC and necrotic leukoencephalopathy, which are very rare entities in AOSD.

1. Introduction

Still's disease was first described by George Still in 1896. Adult-onset Still's disease (AOSD) describes a similar condition which affects adults and is generally constituted by recurrent high grade fever with concomitant salmon-colored rash of the trunk and extremities, oligo- and later polyarthritis, pharyngitis, splenomegaly, lymphadenopathy, and less commonly pericarditis or pleural effusions [1]. Laboratory evaluation typically demonstrates elevated erythrocyte sedimentation rate, leukocytosis, and elevated liver enzymes [2].

Hemophagocytic syndrome (HS), also termed lymphohistiocytosis (HLH), is a syndrome of immune activation manifested by signs and symptoms of inflammation [3]. HS is diagnosed based on the fulfillment of 5/8 criteria as in Table 1

[4]. Histopathological evaluation demonstrates lymphocytes, macrophages and hemophagocytosis in bone marrow, spleen, cerebral spinal fluid, and liver [4]. Other common clinical manifestations include central nervous system involvement, coagulopathy, liver dysfunction, jaundice, edema, and skin rashes [4]. A variety of CNS manifestations of HS including seizures, ataxia, and meningitis have been reported [5, 6]. HS can be familial as in young children or reactive as in patients with underlying infection, lymphoma, organ transplant, systemic lupus erythematosus, or AOSD [7–9].

2. Case Report

A 34-year-old African-American female was diagnosed with adult-onset Still's disease (AOSD) 3 months prior to this

TABLE 1: Diagnostic criteria of hemophagocytic syndrome.

(1) Fever

(2) Spleenomegaly

(3) Cytopenia in 2 of 3 cell lines

(4) Hypertriglyceridemia

(5) Hemophagocytosis in either bone marrow, lymph nodes or the spleen

(6) Low/absent NK cell activity

(7) Hyperferritinemia ($>500 \, \mu g/L$)

(8) High levels of soluble IL-2

Courtesy from Henter et al. [4].

admission based on episodic fever of unknown origin, gastrointestinal manifestations of episodic diarrhea, vomiting, leukocytosis, oligoarthritis, nonspecific facial rash, weight loss, and elevated ferritin level. Extensive infectious workup was unremarkable. Hematological work up was unremarkable except for leukocytosis, generalized lymphadenopathy and hepatosplenomegaly. A lymph node biopsy demonstrated reactive lymphadenitis and was unremarkable for any hematological malignancy or infection. Upper endoscopy and colonoscopy, including ileal and colon biopsies, and abdominal imaging with CT scan were unremarkable for a primary gastrointestinal disease. Synovial fluid analysis demonstrated an inflammatory fluid pattern. Extensive infectious evaluation with imaging, cultures (sputum, blood, urine, and cervical and all the other potential sources), and serologies for atypical infections including viral and fungal diseases failed to demonstrate an infectious etiology. Synovial cultures were unremarkable for infections including Whipple's disease (*Tropheryma whipplei*). Other autoimmune workups for connective tissue disease and vasculitides were unremarkable. She was eventually diagnosed with Still's disease that was supported by high ferritin levels of 7000 ng/mL which increased to 22000 ng/mL (18–160 ng/mL). Bone marrow biopsy demonstrated mild hemophagocytosis (Figure 1). However, patient did not demonstrate pancytopenia or other features of HS. She responded significantly and rapidly to a trial of prednisone 40 mg daily. Corticosteroid sparing agent such as methotrexate or Kineret (Anakinra) was suggested; however it was unaffordable due to financial constraints and social situation. Attempts to wean her steroid dose under 30 mgs resulted in recurrences many times.

Four days prior to this admission she noted worsening of her oligoarthritis and was evaluated in a local emergency department. She reported compliance with her medication regimen of prednisone 40 mg orally daily. She was discharged on pain medications and antibiotics for a possible urinary tract infection. The next day she was evaluated at another hospital for worsened arthralgia and mental status changes. Her hospital course was further complicated by worsening of her mental status requiring intubation and eventually shock. She was suspected to have pneumonia and was treated with antibiotics and vasopressors for her shock. Cultures were negative for any growth. A computed tomography (CT) of

the head was unremarkable. She was extubated after clinical improvement. However, 5 days later she was noted to develop desquamation of large patches of the skin on her chest, extremities, and abdomen. At this point, potential offending drugs including antibiotics were discontinued due to lack of evidence to support an infectious process and she was transferred to our facility's burn unit with a concern for Stevens-Johnson Syndrome/Toxic Epidermic Necrolysis.

On arrival, she was in moderate distress and found to be stuporous. She was normotensive, tachycardiac, tachypneic, and febrile. Her BMI was $40.7 \, kg/m^2$. She was diffusely edematous, with large patches of denuded skin over the chest, breasts, arms, legs, upper back, and buttocks with nondenuded areas appearing mottled and ecchymotic (Figure 2). There were no mucosal abnormalities. Cardiopulmonary exam revealed tachycardia and diminished breath sounds. Abdominal examination revealed mild splenomegaly with soft consistency. Extremities were cold to palpation without palpable pulses. All fingertips and toes were shriveled and black with dry gangrenous changes (Figure 3). Neurological exam was limited due to mental status changes, but no localizing signs or focal neurological deficit could be identified. The rest of physical exam was unremarkable.

Preliminary labs demonstrated leukocytosis, normocytic anemia, thrombocytopenia, transaminitis, marked elevation of the erythrocyte sedimentation rate, and C-reactive protein and, notably, ferritin levels were profoundly elevated 25,512 ng/mL (normal 18–200). Urine analysis demonstrated moderate hematuria and proteinuria. Urine sediment demonstrated muddy brown casts consistent with acute tubular necrosis. Rheumatoid factor, anti-cyclic citrullinated peptide antibodies (anti-CCP), Extractable Nuclear Antigens (ENA), C and P-ANCA (anti-neutrophil cytoplasmic antibodies), serum protein electrophoresis (SPEP), and urine protein electrophoresis (UPEP) levels were normal. Infectious workup including Epstein-Barr virus (EBV), human immunodeficiency virus (HIV), cytomegalovirus (CMV), rapid plasma reagin (RPR), respiratory syncytial virus (RSV), influenza PCR, hepatitis A, hepatitis B, hepatitis C, Varicella, human T-lymphotropic virus type I and II, herpes simplex virus 1 and 2, human herpesviruses (HHV6, 7, and 8), adenovirus, aspergillus, parvovirus, and Bartonella were all negative. Cultures of the blood, CSF, urine, fungal, mycobacterium, bronchial washings, cervix and rectum, and any other possible source of infection were all negative. Neuron specific enolase level was 13.5 and Interleukin 2 (soluble CD-25) level of 1929 pg/mL (normal 0–1033). Familial HLH and PRF1 gene sequencing was negative.

A chest radiograph demonstrated cardiomegaly with mild pulmonary vascular congestion. Echocardiogram evaluation exhibited mildly decreased left ventricular systolic function with hypokinesis of the inferior and inferolateral walls of the left ventricle. No valvular vegetation was reported. CT of the abdomen revealed splenomegaly with heterogeneous enhancement and areas of hypoattenuation/enhancement along the splenic periphery and mild lymphadenopathy primarily in the upper abdomen and splenic hilum. High-resolution CT of the thorax demonstrated patchy airspace

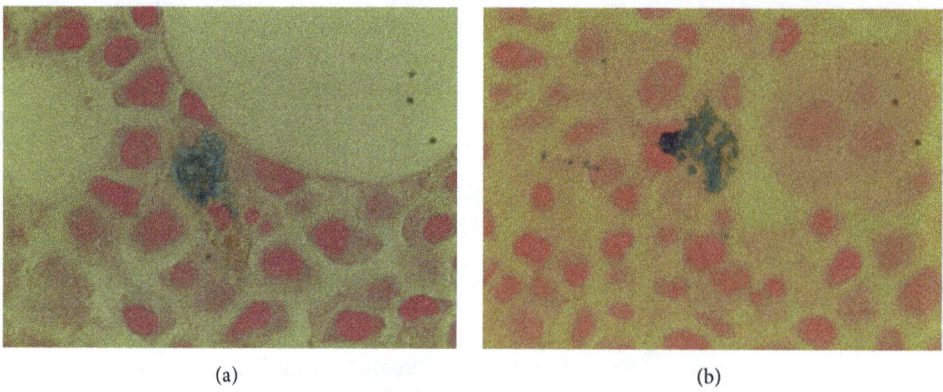

(a)   (b)

FIGURE 1: Bone marrow biopsy demonstrating hemophagocytosis.

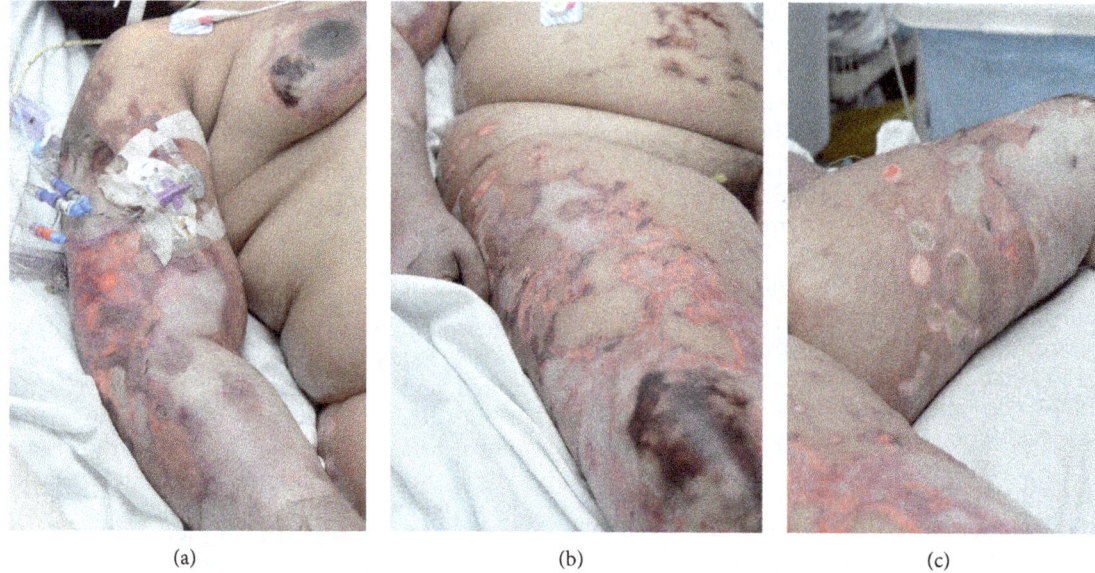

(a)   (b)   (c)

FIGURE 2: Large patches of denuded skin over the chest, breasts, arms, legs, upper back, and buttocks with nondenuded areas appearing mottled and ecchymotic.

opacities in the upper lobes and lower lobes bilaterally, suggestive of acute respiratory distress syndrome.

Magnetic resonance imaging (MRI) of the brain showed an extensive bilateral and symmetric hyperintense T2 signal abnormality and diffusion restriction throughout the deep white matter and corona radiata, sparing the subcortical U fibers without evidence of enhancing lesions, findings which were reported as consistent with necrotic leukoencephalopathy (Figures 4(a)–4(f)). An electroencephalogram was performed revealing diffuse slowing consistent with a moderately severe diffuse encephalopathy.

Bone marrow biopsy demonstrated hemophagocytosis as shown in Figure 1. A skin biopsy performed at the outside hospital demonstrated vascular congestion with mild dermal edema, mild perivascular lymphocytic infiltrate, and rare mast cells.

Patient was started on high dose pulse intravenous steroids. Hematology recommended an aggressive immunosuppressive regimen including intravenous dexamethasone,

etoposide, and intrathecal methotrexate for possible HLH after consultation with additional HLH experts across the country. After initiation of high dose steroids but prior to initiation of etoposide or methotrexate the patient deteriorated, requiring reintubation for acute respiratory distress and vasopressors for shock. She further developed anuric renal failure, lactic acidosis, coagulopathy, and nonsustained ventricular tachycardia requiring an amiodarone drip. At this point, the family decided to avoid further aggressive care and withdraw life support. The patient eventually expired after a progressive downhill course totaling 8 days at our institution.

Postmortem examination was conducted with informed consent from the family and revealed interstitial inflammation in the heart, lungs, gastrointestinal, urinary bladder, and skin. Patchy interstitial and intramuscular fibrosis with multiple vegetation with superimposed organized thrombi in the heart. Cultures of the vegetation were negative. Several microfibrin thrombi were identified in the lumens of small- and medium-sized blood vessels in the lungs. Brain biopsy

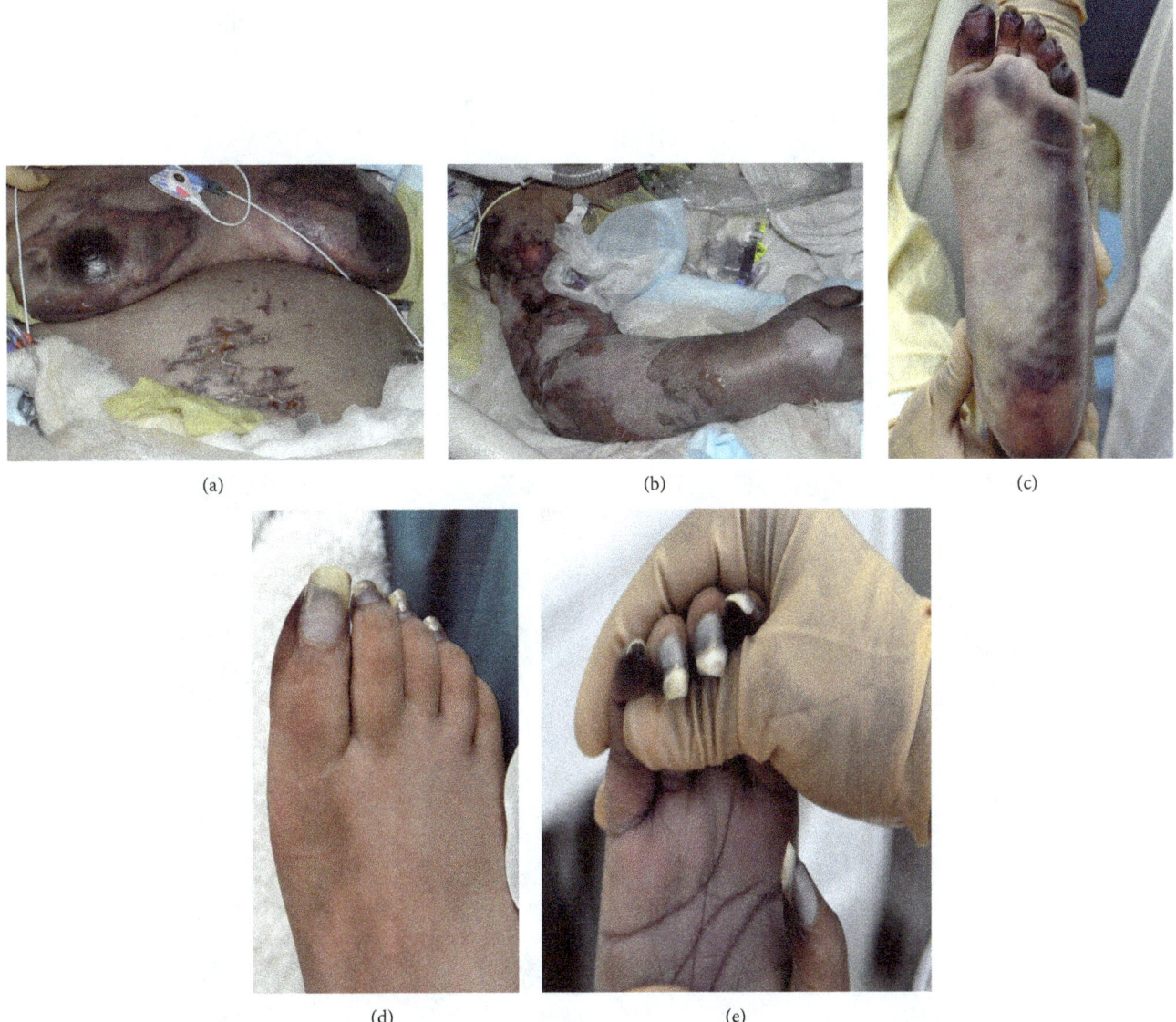

FIGURE 3: Dry gangrenous changes in the fingertips and toes.

revealed extensive Alzheimer type 2 cells with microvascular changes due to reactive inflammatory disease. No infection or tumor was identified in any of the organs.

3. Discussion

Hemophagocytic lymphohistiocytosis (HLH) is a hyperinflammatory syndrome with high mortality [10, 11]. HLH is characterized by acute fever, hepatosplenomegaly, lymphadenopathy, pancytopenia, and raised levels of serum ferritin, triglycerides, and liver enzymes.

Our patient with a recent diagnosis of Still's disease presented with polyarthritis, fever, and encephalopathy with altered mentation, seizures, ischemia resulting in dry gangrene in all extremities, skin desquamation, lymphadenopathy, and splenomegaly. Workup demonstrated anemia, leukocytosis, thrombocytopenia, coagulopathy, elevated inflammatory markers, high ferritin level of 25,000, high triglyceride, and elevated liver enzymes. Imaging demonstrated patchy pulmonary infiltrates suggestive of acute respiratory distress syndrome in the clinical setting of multiorgan failure. Echocardiographic evaluation exhibited mildly decreased left ventricular systolic function with no valvular vegetation reported. Bone marrow smear and biopsy demonstrated hypercellular bone marrow of 80% cellularity with greatly increased myeloid leukemogenesis and decreased erythrocytogenesis without any cellular dysplasia noted and normal appearing of small plasma cells.

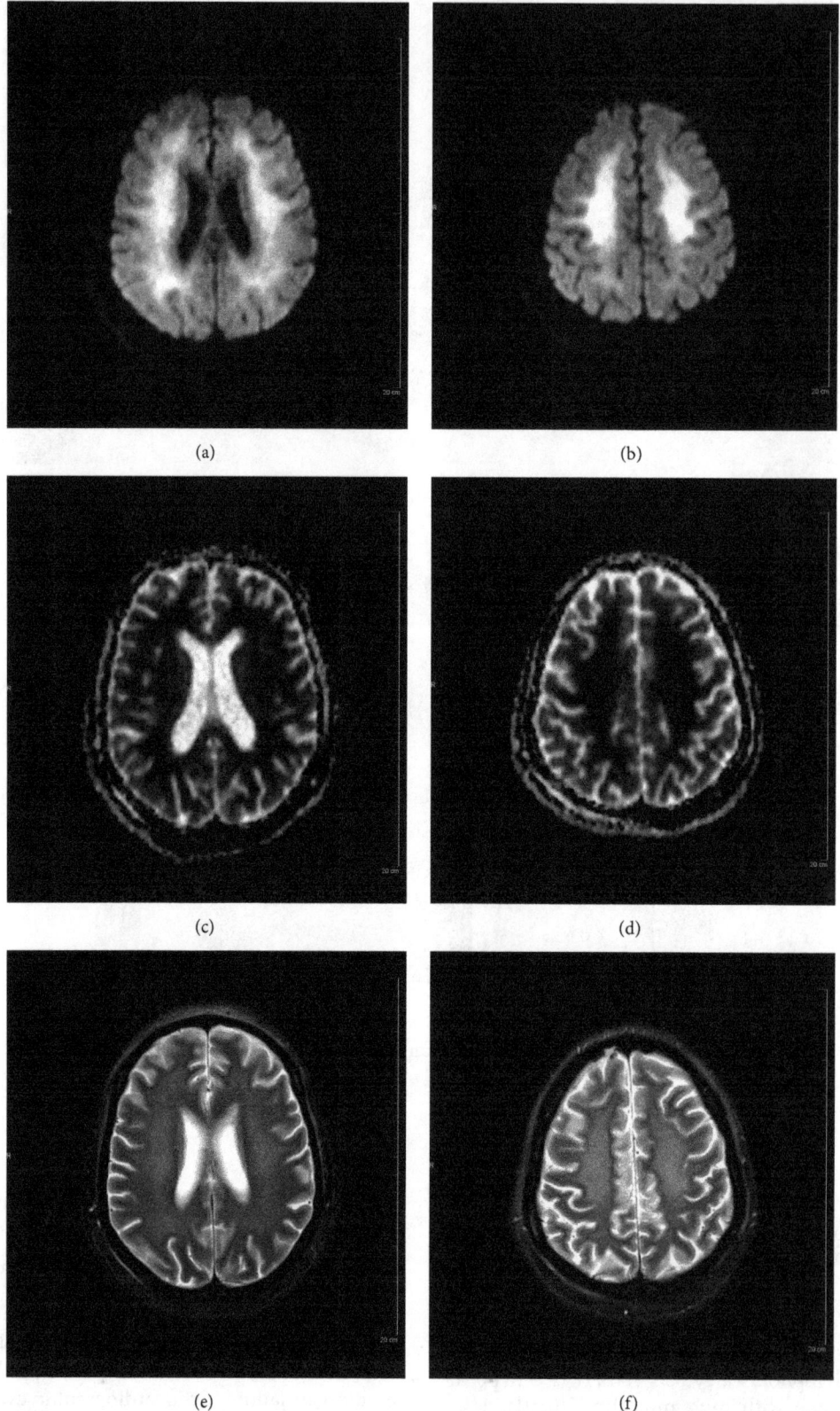

FIGURE 4: (a) DWI, Diffusion weighted images bilateral and symmetric diffusion restriction in the deep white matter. (b) DWI, Diffusion weighted images show bilateral and symmetric diffusion restriction in the corona radiata. (c) ADC map shows loss of the increased signal seen in the DWI images in the bilateral deep white matter. (d) ADC map shows loss of the increased signal seen in the DWI images in the bilateral corona radiata. (e) Axial T2 TSE FS (Blade) acquired in 4 mm thickness, shows hyperintense T2 signal abnormality in the deep white matter. (f) Axial T2 TSE FS (Blade) acquired in 4 mm thickness, shows hyperintense T2 signal abnormality in the corona radiata.

Hemophagocytosis in marrow was noted. An extensive infectious workup was unremarkable for any infectious etiology as a possible explanation of her multiorgan involvement. The diagnosis of HS complicating AOSD in our patient was a result of several clinical findings and laboratory parameters which fulfilled required diagnostic criteria in the absence of an infectious or neoplastic cause for her recent deterioration.

In addition, our patient demonstrated many atypical features aside from HLH complicating AOSD. This includes DIC and necrotizing encephalopathy on imaging which is rarely reported, especially in adults. This was followed by shock and progressive multisystem organ failure. No case has been reported to our knowledge with these two complications occurring concomitantly in an adult patient as a complication of HLH. Further, even prior to this admission our patient manifested with features of GI symptoms of episodic diarrhea every time she had a disease flare reflecting possible GI inflammation which is atypical. She terminally developed multiorgan failure complicating her HLH as supported by autopsy.

Our patient developed HS with months of manifesting with the features of AOSD. Literature review suggested that HS can occur at any time when there is established diagnosis of AOSD. Flare of AOSD and HS are clinically indistinguishable, except for a high frequency of pleuritis and acute respiratory distress syndrome. Laboratory diagnosis may be helpful in making a diagnosis of HS during a flare of AOSD. Leukopenia or thrombocytopenia is uncommon in AOSD. High ferritin level is generally more typical of AOSD. Nevertheless a very high serum ferritin concentration (>10 000 mg/L) is more suggestive of HS complicating AOSD [12]. Raised serum triglyceride level is considered to be a good marker of HS and may be useful in its diagnosis [13] but it has not been specifically analyzed in flare of AOSD. In our patient, serum triglycerides were markedly increased during the diagnosis of HS.

Disseminated intravascular coagulation is a serious complication shared by both HS and AOSD and is associated with high mortality [14–16]. Although it is described more in AOSD case reports, J-B Arlet et al. observed disseminated intravascular coagulation in one third of the patients with AOSD-related HS and was associated with severe liver cytolysis and high mortality.

Our patient developed ischemia and coagulopathy with increased levels of fibrin degradation products, prolongation of prothrombin time and activated partial thromboplastin time, and a low fibrinogen level overall suggesting a diagnosis of DIC in a terminally ill patient with multiorgan dysfunction. Vascular surgery did not suggest the use of vasopressors as the cause of the ischemia. This was further supported by autopsy which demonstrated thrombosis in the lumen of the blood vessels. Although mortality is low in patients with AOSD, most deaths are due to DIC or ARDS, when the diagnosis is associated with HS [2, 17].

Recurrent gastrointestinal symptoms manifesting as a part of clinical flare was another atypical feature of our patient before developing HLH. An extensive workup for primary gastrointestinal diseases contributing to her symptoms such as Whipple's disease and celiac disease was unremarkable.

Multiple endoscopic biopsies with cultures failed to demonstrate anything outside a nonspecific inflammation. Recurrent GI inflammation manifesting as a part of clinical flare is unusual. Predominant GI symptoms are atypical in AOSD but Meeths et al. reported 5 patients who presented with abdominal pain and chronic diarrhea and concluded that severe gastrointestinal symptoms may present before typical clinical manifestations of HLH. This unusual manifestation can add to the diagnostic dilemma and needs to be considered in patients with AOSD. These symptoms likely occurred from the inflammation of the stomach and small intestine. This was previously demonstrated by Zhao et al. by interstitial inflammation in the mucosa of the alimentary canal in postmortem examination in a patient with AOSD [18, 19].

While previous publications have highlighted the prevalence of necrotic leukoencephalopathy in children with familial hemophagocytic syndrome, our adult patient presented with necrotizing leukoencephalopathy in the context of DIC complicating her reactive hemophagocytic syndrome, a far less common presentation [5]. Several case reports indicate that children with necrotic leukoencephalopathy in the setting of hemophagocytic syndrome demonstrated recovery of central nervous system dysfunction [5]; however there is no study evaluating outcomes in adults.

Bone marrow biopsy, often performed to eliminate infection or neoplasm, is less sensitive than bone marrow aspirate. In a study by J-B Arlet et al. bone marrow biopsy was considered to be normal in two thirds of patients, whereas HS was demonstrated in the bone marrow aspirate. This was also noted by others who report positive bone marrow aspirate and negative bone marrow biopsy for HS [13, 20]. Autopsy results revealed interstitial inflammation in the heart, lungs, gastrointestinal, urinary bladder, and skin. Patchy interstitial and intramuscular fibrosis with multiple vegetation with superimposed organized thrombi in the heart. Cultures of the vegetation were negative. Several microfibrin thrombi were identified in the lumens of small- and medium-sized blood vessels in the lungs. Brain biopsy revealed extensive Alzheimer type 2 cells with microvascular changes due to reactive inflammatory disease. No infection or tumor was identified in any of the organs.

To summarize, our patient presented with new onset adult Still's disease manifested with fever, altered mentation, seizures, ischemia resulting in dry gangrene in all extremities, cutaneous denudation, and splenomegaly. Workup demonstrated anemia, thrombocytopenia, leukocytosis, high ferritin, and high triglyceride level with bone marrow changes suggestive of HLH. Course was complicated with DIC considered given the ischemia, coagulopathy, and multiorgan involvement in the absence of any other valid explanation. Brain imaging revealed hyperintense T2 findings and diffusion restriction in the deep white matter bilaterally, consistent with necrotizing leukoencephalopathy. Extensive infectious workup was unremarkable for a possible infectious etiology.

This case underscores the need to be vigilant for these atypical manifestations in HLH including demyelination within the central nervous system, which is a more reported complication in children with familial HLH rather than adults.

Abbreviations

AOSD: Adult-onset Still's disease
HS: Hemophagocytic syndrome
HLH: Hemophagocytic lymphohistiocytosis
GI: Gastrointestinal
CT: Computed tomography
ENA: Extractable nuclear antigens
ANCA: Antineutrophil cytoplasmic antibodies
DIC: Disseminated intravascular coagulation.

Acknowledgment

Thanks to the blessed soul of the patient that gave us all the trust to take care of her medical condition.

References

[1] P. Efthimiou and S. Georgy, "Pathogenesis and management of adult-onset Still's disease," *Seminars in Arthritis and Rheumatism*, vol. 36, no. 3, pp. 144–152, 2006.

[2] J. Pouchot, J. S. Sampalis, F. Beaudet et al., "Adult Still's disease: manifestations, disease course, and outcome in 62 patients," *Medicine*, vol. 70, no. 2, pp. 118–136, 1991.

[3] M. B. Jordan, C. E. Allen, S. Weitzman, A. H. Filipovich, and K. L. McClain, "How I treat hemophagocytic lymphohistiocytosis," *Blood*, vol. 118, no. 15, pp. 4041–4052, 2011.

[4] J.-I. Henter, A. Horne, M. Aricó et al., "HLH-2004: diagnostic and therapeutic guidelines for hemophagocytic lymphohistiocytosis," *Pediatric Blood and Cancer*, vol. 48, no. 2, pp. 124–131, 2007.

[5] E. Haddad, M.-L. Sulis, N. Jabado, S. Blanche, A. Fischer, and M. Tardieu, "Frequency and severity of central nervous system lesions in hemophagocytic lymphohistiocytosis," *Blood*, vol. 89, no. 3, pp. 794–800, 1997.

[6] S. S. Kollias, W. S. Ball Jr., A. A. Tzika, and R. E. Harris, "Familial erythrophagocytic lymphohistiocytosis: neuroradiologic evaluation with pathologic correlation," *Radiology*, vol. 192, no. 3, pp. 743–754, 1994.

[7] A. Hot, M.-L. Toh, B. Coppéré et al., "Reactive hemophagocytic syndrome in adult-onset still disease: clinical features and long-term outcome: a case-control study of 8 patients," *Medicine*, vol. 89, no. 1, pp. 37–46, 2010.

[8] R. Dhote, J. Simon, T. Papo et al., "Reactive hemophagocytic syndrome in adult systemic disease: report of twenty-six cases and literature review," *Arthritis Care and Research*, vol. 49, no. 5, pp. 633–639, 2003.

[9] J. A. Morris, A. R. Adamson, P. J. L. Holt, and J. Davson, "Still's disease and the virus-associated haemophagocytic syndrome," *Annals of the Rheumatic Diseases*, vol. 44, no. 5, pp. 349–353, 1985.

[10] A. H. Filipovich, "Hemophagocytic lymphohistiocytosis and related disorders," *Current Opinion in Allergy and Clinical Immunology*, vol. 6, no. 6, pp. 410–415, 2006.

[11] G. E. Janka, "Hemophagocytic syndromes," *Blood Reviews*, vol. 21, no. 5, pp. 245–253, 2007.

[12] B. Fautrel, G. le Moël, B. Saint-Marcoux et al., "Diagnostic value of ferritin and glycosylated ferritin in adult onset Still's disease," *Journal of Rheumatology*, vol. 28, no. 2, pp. 322–329, 2001.

[13] A. Karras and O. Hermine, "Macrophage activation syndrome," *La Revue de Médecine Interne*, vol. 23, pp. 768–778, 2002.

[14] A. V. Ramanan and R. Schneider, "Macrophage activation syndrome following initiation of etanercept in a child with systemic onset juvenile rheumatoid arthritis," *Journal of Rheumatology*, vol. 30, no. 2, pp. 401–403, 2003.

[15] B. Fautrel, E. Zing, J.-L. Golmard et al., "Proposal for a new set of classification criteria for adult-onset still disease," *Medicine*, vol. 81, no. 3, pp. 194–200, 2002.

[16] O. Lambotte, P. Cacoub, N. Costedoat-Chalumeau, G. le Moel, Z. Amoura, and J.-C. Piette, "High ferritin and low glycosylated ferritin may also be a marker of excessive macrophage activation," *Journal of Rheumatology*, vol. 30, no. 5, pp. 1027–1028, 2003.

[17] U. Emmenegger, U. Frey, A. Reimers et al., "Hyperferritinemia as indicator for intravenous immunoglobulin treatment in reactive macrophage activation syndromes," *The American Journal of Hematology*, vol. 68, no. 1, pp. 4–10, 2001.

[18] D.-B. Zhao, S.-M. Dai, X.-P. Liu, and H. Xu, "Interstitial inflammation in visceral organs is a pathologic feature of adult-onset Still's disease," *Rheumatology International*, vol. 31, no. 7, pp. 923–927, 2011.

[19] M. Meeths, M. Entesarian, W. Al-Herz et al., "Spectrum of clinical presentations in familial hemophagocytic lymphohistiocytosis type 5 patients with mutations in STXBP2," *Blood*, vol. 116, no. 15, pp. 2635–2643, 2010.

[20] M. A. Hamidou, M. Denis, S. Barbarot, D. Boutoille, C. Belizna, and G. le Moël, "Usefulness of glycosylated ferritin in atypical presentations of adult onset Still's disease," *Annals of the Rheumatic Diseases*, vol. 63, no. 5, p. 605, 2004.

12

Pulmonary Arterial Hypertension in Adult-Onset Still's Disease: Rapid Response to Anakinra

Marc Campos and Elena Schiopu

Division of Rheumatology, University of Michigan, P.O. Box 481, Ann Arbor, MI 48109, USA

Correspondence should be addressed to Elena Schiopu, eschiopu@med.umich.edu

Academic Editors: R. Aminov and S. Hamoud

Adult-onset Still's disease (AOSD) is a rare inflammatory condition characterized by spiking quotidian fever, rash, chronic arthralgia, leukocytosis, and occasional pulmonary involvement such as pleural effusion and transient pulmonary infiltrates. Pulmonary arterial hypertension (PAH) is a rare pulmonary complication of AOSD, and we are aware of only 5 cases reported in the literature. We report the case of a 27-year-old woman of Middle Eastern descent, with a 7-year history of AOSD, who developed severe pulmonary arterial hypertension (PAH). After unsuccessful exposure to various immunosuppressive regimens, shortly following the initiation of anakinra, an interleukin-1 (IL-1) receptor antagonist, her disease became quiescent and the PAH resolved. With this case report, we hope to show that anakinra, either by virtue of controlling the overall inflammation in AOSD, or by direct effect on the pulmonary microangiopathy, can improve severe PAH.

1. Introduction

Adult-onset Still's disease (AOSD) is a systemic inflammatory disorder characterized by a variety of clinical features, including intermittent fever, arthritis, evanescent rash, neutrophilic leukocytosis, polyserositis, lymphadenopathy, splenomegaly, and other systemic symptoms [1]. The etiology of AOSD is unknown although a paradigm of genetic predisposition combined with viral triggers has been proposed. The annual incidence has been estimated by a French study to be 0.16 cases per 100,000 persons, with equal representation of the genders [2]. According to the same study, there is a bimodal age distribution, with a first peak at 15–25 years of age, and 36–45 years. Due to the heterogeneity of the presenting symptoms, multiple classification criteria were proposed, but the highest sensitivity for a definite diagnosis of AOSD is claimed by the Yamaguchi criteria [3]. The Yamaguchi criteria require the presence of five features, with at least two being major criteria: there are four major criteria (fever, arthralgias/arthritis, specific rash, and leukocytosis) and a few minor criteria (sore throat, lymphadenopathy, hepato- and splenomegaly, abnormal liver

function tests, negative tests for antinuclear antibody, and rheumatoid factor). Although nonspecific, markedly elevated ferritin levels have been described to help in diagnosis and monitoring in patients with AOSD [4]. Cardiopulmonary disease has been described in 30–40% of the patients with AOSD. Serositis, mild cough, pleuritic chest pain, and dyspnea are the symptoms of lung involvement, while the pathology encompasses acute pneumonitis manifested as transient infiltrates or severe interstitial lung disease [5]. The treatment of AOSD is greatly directed at the inflammatory component. The traditional approach, depending on the severity of the disease, recommended glucocorticoids initiated at 0.5–1 mg/kg/day, followed quickly by a disease-modifying antirheumatic drug (DMARD), such as azathioprine, methotrexate, or leflunomide. The biologic agents have since become the main avenue in patients with steroid-resistant disease, although approximately 70% of the patients respond to steroids alone [6]. Anakinra, a recombinant human IL-1 receptor antagonist, has been shown to rapidly reduce the systemic inflammatory reactions in small series of patients with refractory AOSD [7]. Further, a case series of 25 patients showed rapid resolution of AOSD clinical activity within

6 days and the response was maintained at one year [8]. Newer approaches, including tocilizumab, an anti-IL-6 receptor monoclonal antibody [9] are being proposed.

We report a case of AOSD refractory to glucocorticoids and DMARD combination of azathioprine and hydroxychloroquine, complicated by severe pulmonary arterial hypertension, with rapid response to anakinra, and normalization of the pulmonary pressures. We will review the existing literature and discuss the response to treatment.

2. Case Report

A 27-year-old female of Middle Eastern descent with a history of AOSD for 7 years based on persistent quotidian fevers, evanescent rash, polyarthritis, lymphadenopathy, splenomegaly, leukocytosis, and polyclonal hypergammaglobulinemia was evaluated in our institution for acute onset of severe dyspnea, requiring oxygen supplementation, shortly after a successful pregnancy and uncomplicated delivery. Her rheumatological care for AOSD was conducted in the United Arab Emirates and it included prednisone (unspecified doses), azathioprine, and chloroquine. The patient was initially found to be tachycardic and hypoxic, with a significant cardiac murmur, which prompted an echocardiographic evaluation that revealed the following findings: estimated right ventricular systolic pressure (RVSP) of 100 mmHg, severe tricuspid regurgitation, dilated right atrium, and ventricle and moderate amount of pulmonic valvular regurgitation. Based on these findings, she was referred to the pulmonary hypertension clinic at our institution and hospitalized for further work up.

Her physical examination revealed a cushingoid female in moderate respiratory distress, afebrile, with a pulse of 97 beats/min, a respiratory rate of 20/min, and a blood pressure of 106/78 mmHg, saturating 97% on room air. The lung fields were clear to auscultation, and cardiac examination revealed: right ventricular heave, a loud pulmonic component, and a palpable pulmonary artery, along with a varying murmur of tricuspid regurgitation. The jugular venous distension was up to her earlobes at 45 degrees. There was trace peripheral edema, no evidence of synovitis or rash, and absent hepato- or splenomegaly.

At this time, her medication included prednisone 15 mg/day and azathioprine 50 mg twice daily. The laboratory investigation showed normal C-reactive protein and sedimentation rate, negative hepatitis B and C serology, negative rheumatoid factor and ANA, normal ferritin, complements (C3 and C4) levels, slightly elevated AST and ALT, and normal complete blood count. The chest radiograph showed right atrial and ventricular dilatation and small right pleural effusion. The electrocardiogram showed signs of right axis deviation, right ventricular hypertrophy, and right atrial enlargement, but normal sinus rhythm. She underwent a CT angiography that showed no evidence of pulmonary embolism or interstitial lung disease. The examining cardiologist classified her, based on current symptoms, as New York Heart Association Class IIIB. Based on these preliminary studies, the patient underwent a right and left heart catheterization. Her left heart catheterization revealed completely normal coronary arteries. Presence of pulmonary hypertension was confirmed, based on main pulmonary artery pressure (PAP) of 73/35 mmHg (mean 48 mmHg), pulmonary capillary wedge pressure (PCWP) of 10 mmHg, right atrium pressure of 9 mmHg, cardiac output (CO) by thermodilution was 4.1 L/min, and the calculated pulmonary vascular resistance was 9.3 Wood Units.

The patient was started on amlodipine at 10 mg daily and the rest of immunomodulatory drugs were continued, along with careful monthly clinical follow up. The patient continued to remain dyspneic and she continued to have flares characterized by fevers, rash, and uncontrolled arthralgias (Figure 1). She had moderate improvement of her RVSP by echocardiogram, but her functional class and dyspnea continue to worsen with the flares (Figure 2). Her pulmonary artery pressure continued to stay in the moderate range, prompting increase of the dose of amlodipine to 20 mg daily. A right heart catheterization (RHC) one year following the first one showed PAP of 48/19 mmHg (mean not reported), PCWP of 10 mmHg, and CO of 5.2 L/min. Within another year, her RHC measurements were: PAP of 50/22 (mean of 34 mmHg), PCWP of 9 mmHg, and CO of 6.7 L/min. Despite an overall sense of improvement, the patient continued to have clinical flares and dyspnea. Approximately 5 years from the diagnosis of PAH, following a rocky clinical course, the patient was initiated on anakinra, 100 mg daily, by subcutaneous injections. The patient experienced rapid resolution of her systemic symptoms, and due to the lack of recurrence of her flares, the prednisone was weaned down and stopped within 18 months (Figure 1). She also noticed improvement in her effort tolerance which is evidenced in her performance on six-minute walk tests (Figure 2(a)). She continues to be followed up in the rheumatology clinic on quarterly basis but she is seen only yearly in the pulmonary hypertension clinic.

3. Discussion

We have described a patient with AOSD, refractory to glucocorticoids, who developed severe PAH seven years after the onset of her disease. The PAH seemed to respond to the calcium channel blocker amlodipine, but it was completely resolved upon initiation of IL-1 blockade with anakinra, 5 years later. The patient met the American College of Chest Physicians (ACCP) criteria for prepulmonary hypertension [10]. Based on history, there was no history of sleep disorder, chronic liver disease, HIV infection, anorexigen ingestion, or congenital heart disease. More so, other causes of PAH (such as left heart disease, interstitial lung disease, and chronic thromboembolic lung disease) were excluded by the echocardiogram and the CT angiogram. We feel confident that she had WHO group I PAH.

We performed a literature search to identify described cases of group I PAH in the setting of AOSD. We identified a total of 5 cases described between 1990 and 2011. The first reported case was in 1990, of a 29-year-old woman who developed severe, progressive, precapillary PAH 2.5 years

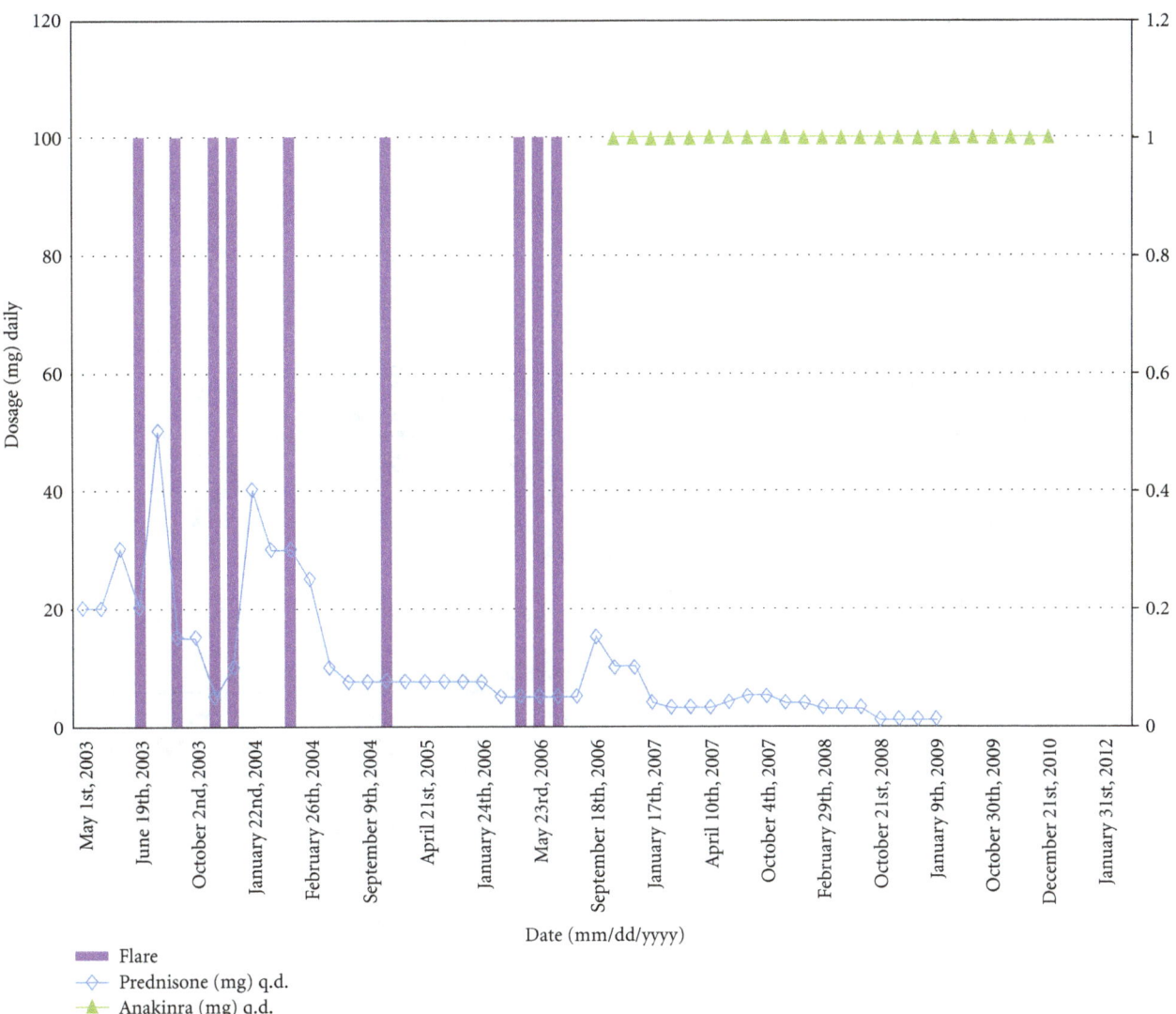

FIGURE 1: Improvement in flares and the decline of the prednisone dose after initiation of anakinra.

after her diagnosis [11]. A retrospective analysis of 19 patients with PAH and various autoimmune diseases was done in northern Taiwan, where PAH has been reported seldom, and revealed that 2 patients had AOSD; in this study, 5 patients died and the RVSP correlated with the levels of serum uric acid ($r = 0.686$, $P = 0.001$) [12]. Another case report described a 29-year-old woman, who 9 years after a diagnosis of AOSD, developed PAH (mean PAP 33 mmHg) responsive to vasodilator infusion, but died 2.5 months later of right heart failure, despite initiation of anakinra [13]. Lastly, a case report from Hyderabad, India, described an 18-year-old female with new onset AOSD who developed severe PAH (mean PAP of 65 mmHg); in the absence of other causes, the authors concluded that the PAH was secondary to the AOSD-related pulmonary microangiopathy [14].

We now report a case of PAH in AOSD which responded rapidly and dramatically to anakinra. Although anakinra was reported to offer rapid control of the systemic manifestations of AOSD [7], there has been no report of improvement of the pulmonary pressures and functional status in a patient with AOSD-PAH. As it is often the case with rare conditions characterized by high symptomatic variability, it is difficult to organize our thoughts when it comes to clinical patterns of causality. It is interesting that our patient, who was diagnosed in 2001, was not exposed to PAH therapy, including the "modern" era (described as starting with the first oral PAH medication in 2002) [15]. Despite availability of PAH-specific therapy, the mortality associated with PAH remains significant [15]. Early diagnosis, classification, and initiation of a disease specific treatment algorithm might improve survival.

Our patient had refractory AOSD, characterized by persistence of flares and elevated inflammatory markers, and in that setting developed PAH. The PAH responded, but not completely, to amlodipine, although her AOSD remained particularly inflammatory. The initiation of IL-1 receptor blockade curtailed both the AOSD and the PAH. It is possible that this was part of the natural history of the disease, as it is described in patients with an intermittent pattern (flares with complete remission between flares and decreasing severity

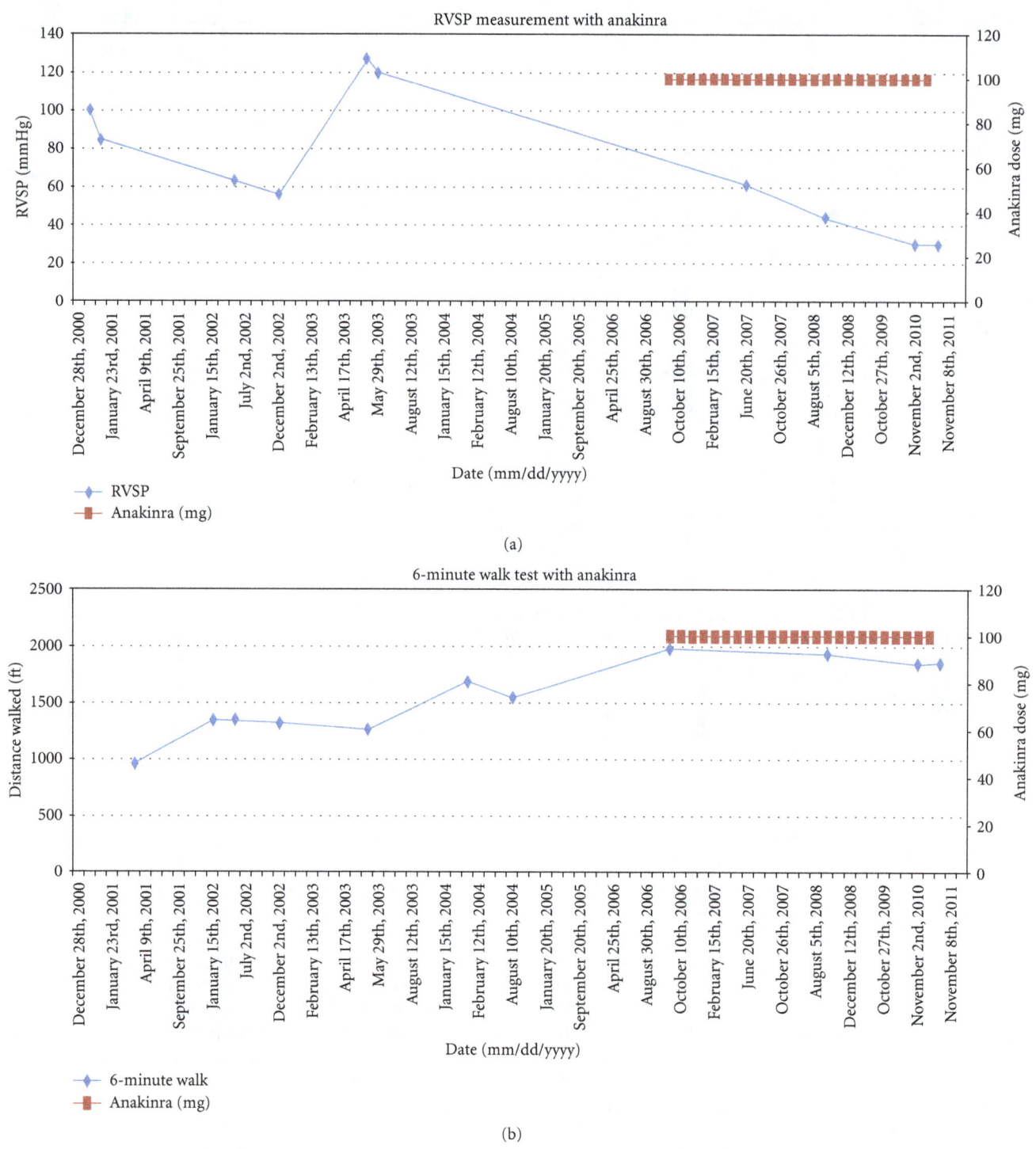

FIGURE 2: (a) Improvement in 6MWT after anakinra initiation; (b) improvement in RVSP after anakinra initiation. 6MWT: six minute walk test; RVSP : right ventricular systolic pressure.

of the flares with time) [16]. However, we believe that the inflammatory burden present in AOSD is most likely the driver for the pulmonary microangiopathy, much like the renal involvement and thrombotic thrombocytopenic purpura in AOSD. It is likely that screening for presence of PAH in patients with AOSD will yield a higher prevalence of AOSD-PAH and will help prevent progressive disease and associated mortality. There is evidence that anakinra lowers pulmonary artery pressure in neonatal surfactant depleted piglet model and further reduces the early proinflammatory pulmonary reaction [17].

The pathophysiology of WHO Group I PAH, specifically PAH associated with autoimmune disorders is unknown. In general, PAH is characterized by proliferation of endothelial cells and expansion of the vascular smooth muscle and adventitial cells, leading to obliteration of the lumen, particularly in the precapillary arterioles [18]. With the increased knowledge about PAH and the ability to recognize its association with autoimmune condition, it is now clearer than ever that autoimmunity plays a significant role in development of PAH. The discussion is starting around regulatory T-cells playing a role in preventing B-cell activity, and potentially leading to the severe angioproliferative pulmonary hypertension that seems to characterize various connective tissue disorders (CTDs). There is a lack of systematic evaluation of how immunosuppressive regimens will affect pulmonary artery pressures in CTD-PAH. It is possible that in CTD-PAH the endothelial cells are apoptosis-resistant, similar to the malignant cells, therefore, much more resistant to traditional PAH therapies [18]. Based on our case, it is likely that immunosuppressives, such as biological agents, alone or in addition to PAH-specific medications, might improve outcomes in AOSD-PAH.

To conclude, we report the first case of anakinra-responsive PAH in the setting of AOSD. We think that PAH should be added as part of the pulmonary manifestations of AOSD, and that clinicians should consider screening for this complication. AOSD should also be added to the WHO Group I PAH secondary to CTDs, and the treatment of AOSD-PAH should be customized to target the inflammatory component of the disease.

References

[1] E. G. Bywaters, "Still's disease in the adult," *Annals of the Rheumatic Diseases*, vol. 30, no. 2, pp. 121–133, 1971.

[2] G. Magadur-Joly, E. Billaud, J. H. Barrier et al., "Epidemiology of adult Still's disease: estimate of the incidence by a retrospective study in West France," *Annals of the Rheumatic Diseases*, vol. 54, no. 7, pp. 587–590, 1995.

[3] M. Yamaguchi, A. Ohta, T. Tsunematsu et al., "Preliminary criteria for classification of adult Still's disease," *The Journal of Rheumatology*, vol. 19, no. 3, pp. 424–430, 1992.

[4] M. Schwarz-Eywill, B. Heilig, H. Bauer, A. Breitbart, and A. Pezzutto, "Evaluation of serum ferritin as a marker for adult Still's disease activity," *Annals of the Rheumatic Diseases*, vol. 51, no. 5, pp. 683–685, 1992.

[5] G. Cheema and F. J Quismorio, "Pulmonary involvement in adult-onset Still's disease," *Current Opinion in Pulmonary Medicine*, vol. 5, no. 5, pp. 305–309, 1999.

[6] J. M. G. W. Wouters and L. B. A. van de Putte, "Adult-onset Still's disease; clinical and laboratory features, treatment and progress of 45 cases," *The Quarterly Journal of Medicine*, vol. 61, no. 235, pp. 1055–1065, 1986.

[7] A. Fitzgerald, S. LeClercq, A. Yan, J. Homik, and C. Dinarello, "Rapid responses to anakinra in patients with refractory adult-onset Still's disease," *Arthritis and Rheumatism*, vol. 52, no. 6, pp. 1794–1803, 2005.

[8] K. Laskari, A. Tzioufas, and H. Moutsopoulos, "Efficacy and long-term follow-up of IL-1R inhibitor anakinra in adults with Still's disease: a case-series study," *Arthritis Research & Therapy*, vol. 13, no. 3, article R91, 2011.

[9] R. Sakai, H. Nagasawa, E. Nishi, A. Okuyama, H. Takei, T. Kurasawa et al., "Successful treatment of adult-onset Still's disease with tocilizumab monotherapy: two case reports and literature review," *Clinical Rheumatology*, vol. 31, no. 3, pp. 569–574, 2012.

[10] L. J. Rubin, "Diagnosis and management of pulmonary arterial hypertension: ACCP evidence-based clinical practice guidelines," *Chest*, vol. 126, no. 1, pp. 7S–10S, 2004.

[11] A. Zen, N. Yamashita, M. Ueda et al., "A case of adult Still's disease with pulmonary hypertension," *Ryumachi*, vol. 30, no. 1, pp. 45–52, 1990.

[12] C. Chen, H. Chen, H. Wang, H. Liao, C. Chou, and D. Huang, "Pulmonary arterial hypertension in autoimmune diseases: an analysis of 19 cases from a medical center in northern Taiwan," *Journal of Microbiology, Immunology and Infection*, vol. 39, no. 2, pp. 162–168, 2006.

[13] E. Mubashir, M. Ahmed, S. Hayat, M. Heldmann, and S. Berney, "Pulmonary hypertension in a patient with adult-onset stills disease," *Clinical Rheumatology*, vol. 26, no. 8, pp. 1359–1361, 2007.

[14] M. Thakare, S. Habibi, S. Agrawal, and G. Narsimulu, "Pulmonary arterial hypertension complicating adult-onset Still's disease" *Clinical Rheumatology*. In press.

[15] M. Humbert, O. Sitbon, A. Chaouat et al., "Survival in patients with idiopathic, familial, and anorexigen-associated pulmonary arterial hypertension in the modern management era," *Circulation*, vol. 122, no. 2, pp. 156–163, 2010.

[16] J. Pouchot, J. S. Sampalis, F. Beaudet et al., "Adult Still's disease: manifestations, disease course, and outcome in 62 patients," *Medicine*, vol. 70, no. 2, pp. 118–136, 1991.

[17] M. Chada, S. Nögel, A. M. Schmidt et al., "Anakinra (IL-1R antagonist) lowers pulmonary artery pressure in a neonatal surfactant depleted piglet model," *Pediatric Pulmonology*, vol. 43, no. 9, pp. 851–857, 2008.

[18] M. Nicolls, L. Taraseviciene-Stewart, P. Rai, D. Badesch, and N. Voelkel, "Autoimmunity and pulmonary hypertension: a perspective," *The European Respiratory Journal*, vol. 26, no. 6, pp. 1110–1118, 2005.

13

Tophaceous Gout of the Patella: A Report of Two Cases

Graeme Hopper,[1] Sanjay Gupta,[1] Sarath Bethapudi,[2] David Ritchie,[2] Elaine MacDuff,[3] and Ashish Mahendra[1]

[1] Trauma and Orthopaedics, Glasgow Royal Infirmary, 84 Castle Street, Glasgow G4 0SF, UK
[2] Radiology, Glasgow Western Infirmary, Dumbarton Road, Glasgow G11 6NT, UK
[3] Pathology, Glasgow Western Infirmary, Dumbarton Road, Glasgow G11 6NT, UK

Correspondence should be addressed to Graeme Hopper, hopperg@doctors.org.uk

Academic Editors: R. Cevik, U. Gresser, and M. A. Hunt

Introduction. Tophaceous gout of the patella is rare and may masquerade as a tumour or tumour-like condition. *Cases.* We report two patients with gout involving the patella, one complicated by a pathological fracture and the other occurring in a bipartite patella in a young adult. *Discussion.* Typical imaging appearances and measurement of serum urate will usually confirm the diagnosis but, occasionally, the serum urate level may be normal in active gout and in such cases, a biopsy will be required. *Conclusion.* Gout of the patella may masquerade as a tumour or tumour-like condition and it is important to consider gout in the differential diagnosis.

1. Introduction

Gout is a relatively common crystal arthropathy caused by chronic hyperuricaemia resulting in the deposition of monosodium urate crystals around joints and tendons. In chronic tophaceous gout, crystals may be deposited in tendons and may cause osseous erosions at their bony attachments. Involvement of the extensor tendon of the knee is not an uncommon site for gout but involvement of the patella is rare and underreported in the literature [1–13]. For patients who present with a patellar lesion, the diagnosis of gout might not be suspected and patients given a provisional diagnosis of infection, tumour, metabolic disease, and degenerative or inflammatory arthropathy. We report two patients with gout involving the patella and discuss the clinical, imaging, and pathological features, differential diagnosis, and management. Patients gave informed consent prior to inclusion in this paper and each author certifies that there is no actual or potential conflict of interests in relation to this paper.

2. Case Reports

2.1. Case 1. A 70-year-old gentleman presented to his general practitioner with a two-month history of pain and swelling involving the anterior aspect of his right knee. He had no past medical history of note and no history of arthropathy or predisposing factors of gout. Radiographs of his right knee showed a faintly and partially mineralised soft tissue mass mainly overlying the superior aspect of the patella as well as a well-defined lytic lesion with marginal sclerosis in the mid patella (Figures 1(a) and 1(b)). Unfortunately, the patient was lost to follow up until he represented to the accident and emergency a year later, having injured his right knee. Radiographs of the knee showed a slightly displaced, comminuted pathological fracture of the patella as well as the previously noted partially mineralised soft tissue mass overlying the patella. The fracture was treated conservatively with a splint (Figures 1(c) and 1(d)). MR imaging confirmed the pathological fracture as well as the prominent prepatellar mass infiltrating the distal quadriceps and proximal patellar tendons (Figures 1(e)–1(h)). The elevated serum urate levels (1.04 mmol/L, normal range <0.40 mmol/L) confirmed active gout but a biopsy was felt justified in view of the unusual site and the need to exclude a coexisting tumour. Subsequent histological examination revealed aggregates of amorphous eosinophilic material surrounded by a palisade of histiocytes and giant cells in keeping with tophaceous gout (Figures 1(i) and 1(j)). This gentleman was referred

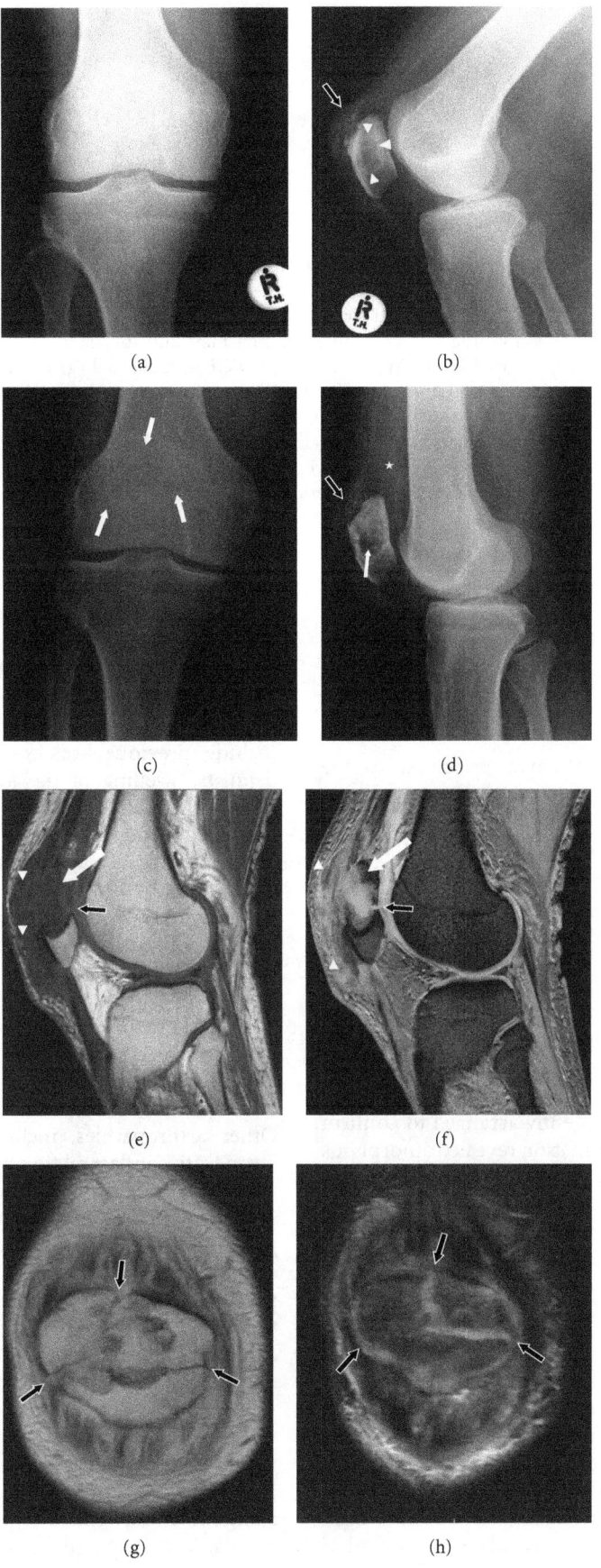

Figure 1: Continued.

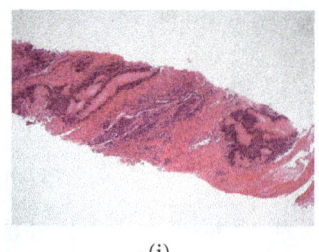
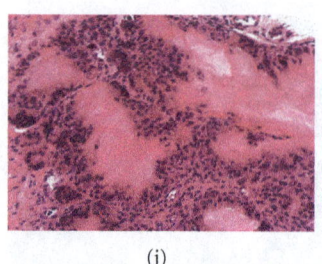

(i)   (j)

FIGURE 1: (a) AP and (b) lateral radiographs of right knee demonstrate diffuse faint calcification involving the insertion of the quadriceps tendon at the upper pole of the patella (black arrow). Note the well-defined lytic lesion with marginal sclerosis (arrowheads) in the patella and prepatellar soft tissue swelling. (c) AP and (d) lateral radiographs of the right knee a year later show a comminuted pathological fracture of the mid patella involving the lytic lesion (white arrows) with associated joint effusion (star). The faint calcification within the distal quadriceps is again noted (black arrow). Sagittal (e) T1-WSE and (f) T2-WGE and coronal (g) PDSE and (h) STIR MR images confirm a comminuted pathological fracture of the mid and upper patella (black arrows) involving the patellar lesion (white arrows) that displays nonspecific features. However, there is a prominent inhomogeneous soft tissue mass in the prepatellar region, some of which displays low signal intensity (SI) on all sequences that corresponds to the mineralisation noted on the radiographs (arrowheads). (i) Core biopsy at low power and (j) core biopsy at high power, stained with H&E. There are aggregates of amorphous eosinophilic material surrounded by a palisade of histiocytes and giant cells in keeping with tophaceous gout.

back to his GP for appropriate medical management of gout with colchicine and allopurinol. He was reviewed one year later in the oncology clinic, his symptoms had improved significantly, and radiographs demonstrated satisfactory healing of his fracture.

2.2. *Case 2.* A 34-year-old gentleman presented to the orthopaedic department with a two-month history of anterior knee pain and swelling involving his left knee. He had no past medical history of note, no history of arthritis or predisposing factors of gout such as obesity, high blood pressure, high cholesterol levels, and heavy alcohol use. Radiographs of his left knee showed a well-defined slightly expansile, lytic lesion involving the patella (Figures 2(a) and 2(b)). MR imaging showed a slightly inhomogeneous lesion involving the superolateral aspect of the patella with soft tissue infiltration around the patellar attachment of the lateral retinaculum (Figures 2(c)–2(g)). Serum urate levels were slightly raised at 0.54 mmol/L. An ultrasound-guided biopsy of this lesion was subsequently arranged to confirm the diagnosis. Histological examination revealed amorphous material consistent with gout (Figures 2(h) and 2(i)). This gentleman was referred back to his GP for appropriate medical management of gout with colchicine and allopurinol and has had no reported adverse outcomes.

3. Discussion

Tophaceous gout of the patella was first reported in 1955 by Peloquin [10]. They presented a patient who was found to have erosion of the patellar cortex at surgery. Greenberg described the first reported pathological fracture of the patella due to underlying gout in 1986 [5]. Further pathological fractures of the patella due to gout have been published in [1, 2, 11]. Other reports include a nonunion of a patellar fracture as a result of gout [4] and a painful bipartite patella secondary to a gouty tophus [3]. Recht et al.

reported seven patients with gouty tophi of the patella and concluded that osteolytic lesions of the superolateral portion of the patella with an associated soft tissue mass should raise the possibility of gout [13]. Reber et al. reported three cases of patellar gout, one in a bipartite patella [12].

The classical history and examination findings of gout include previous attacks of gouty arthritis, tophaceous deposits, swelling of the joint, and occasional pain. Our reported patients did not have any history of gout but presented with a two-month history of pain and swelling involving the knee. Routine blood tests should include evaluation of serum urate and raised levels will confirm the diagnosis. However, occasionally, the serum urate may be normal during acute gout and in such cases evaluation of synovial fluid or biopsy may be required [14]. Radiographs of the extensor complex of the knee may show soft tissue swelling and mineralisation as in Case 1 but involvement of the patella is rare and raises the possibility of other pathology including tumours, infection, other arthropathies, and metabolic disorders [7–9, 15]. Other arthropathies, including rheumatoid arthritis and seronegative inflammatory arthropathies, osteoarthritis, and calcium pyrophosphate disease are often associated with subarticular changes including geodes and cysts but neither patient gave a history of a known arthropathy and there was no other evidence of arthropathy on the imaging studies of the affected knee joints. The differential also includes bone tumours but tumour-like lesions of the patella are more common than tumours and benign tumours more common than malignant tumours. In patients less than 40 years of age, chondroblastoma and giant cell tumour of bone are the most common diagnoses whereas over the age of 40 years, the most common diagnoses are gout and metastatic disease [15]. Radiologically, there is often difficulty in differentiating benign from malignant lesions. The relative small size of the patella, lack of physeal zones, and absence of periosteum make radiological assessment more difficult. Mineralisation in a patellar lesion may be found with gout and various

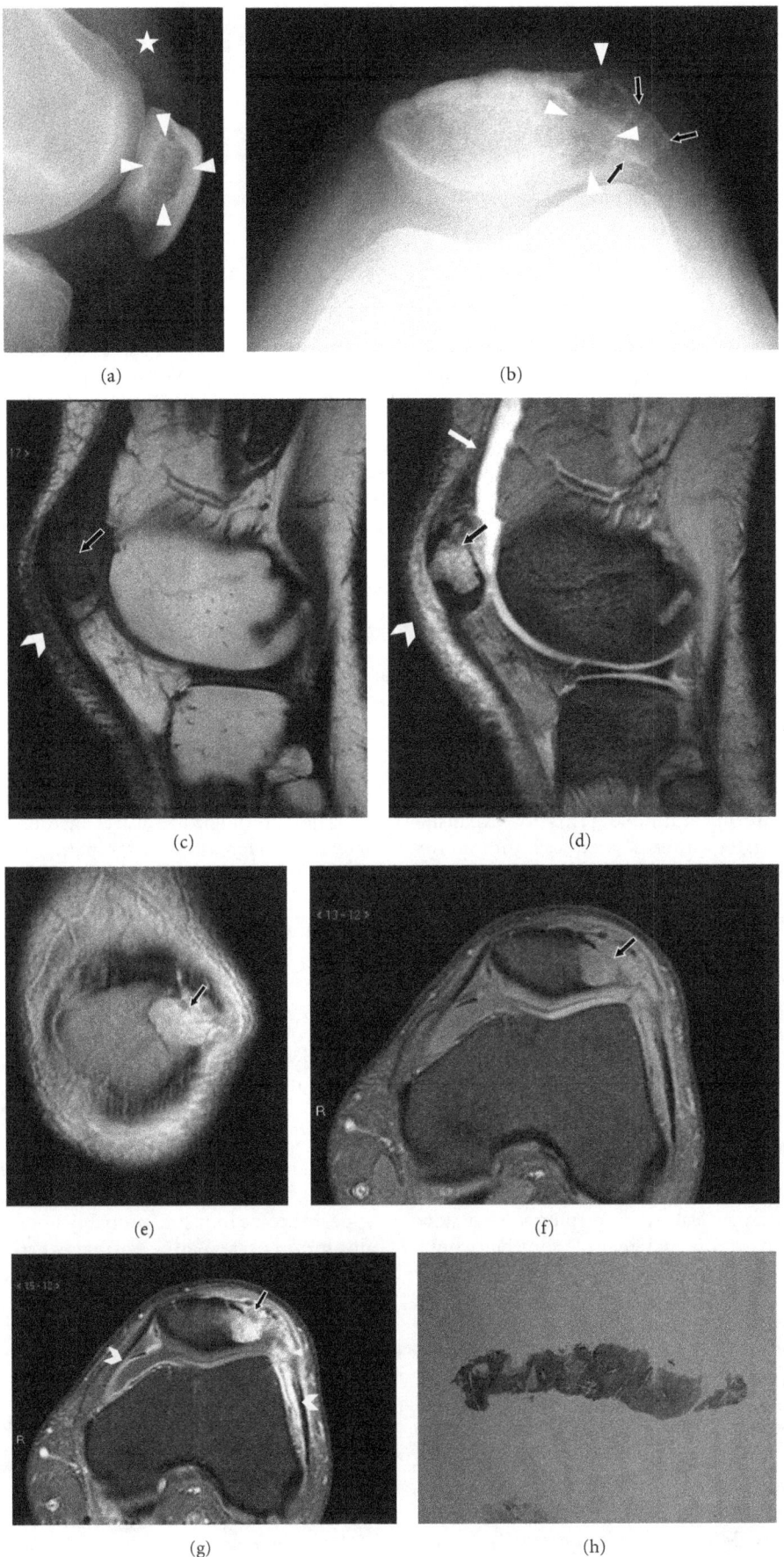

(a)

(b)

(c)

(d)

(e)

(f)

(g)

(h)

Figure 2: Continued.

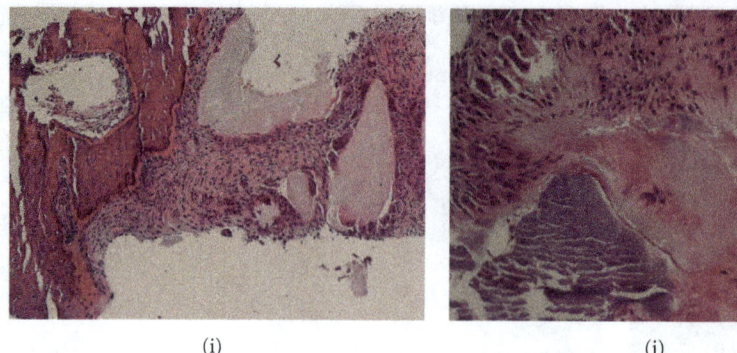

(i)   (j)

FIGURE 2: (a) Lateral and (b) sky line view radiographs of the patella demonstrate a well-defined slightly expansile lytic lesion with sclerotic margin in the mid lateral aspect of the patella (arrowheads) and knee joint effusion (star). On the skyline view, there is also evidence of a bipartite patella (black arrows). Sagittal (c) T1-WSE and (d) T2-WGE and (e) coronal T2-WSE MR images demonstrate a well-defined mass in the patella (black arrows) that displays intermediate SI on T1-W and moderately increased SI on T2-W MR images. Note the prepatellar bursitis (chevrons) and reactive joint effusion (white arrow). Axial T1-WSE fat saturated (f) before and (g) after gadolinium MRI images, show avid enhancement of the patellar lesion (black arrows), involvement of the adjacent lateral parapatellar soft tissues and lateral retinaculum (arrowhead), and enhancing reactive synovitis (chevrons). (h) Core biopsy at low power, (i) core biopsy at medium power, and (j) core biopsy at high power stained with H&E. There are aggregates of amorphous eosinophilic material with a surrounding foreign body giant cell and histiocyte reaction consistent with gout.

neoplasms including chondroblastoma, osteoid osteoma, and osteoblastoma, osteosarcoma but these tumours tend to occur in the second decades and gout would be most unusual in this age group unless there was a history of renal disease or genetic disorders associated with hyperuricaemia. A focal lesion in the patella may also be due to acute haematogenous osteomyelitis but this again is usually found in the immature patella and is very rare in adulthood [15]. An expansile lytic lesion should suggest either a giant cell tumour or brown tumour due to hyperparathyroidism and both of these diagnoses were considered in Case 2. Gout in a patient of 34 years is unusual and may be associated with obesity, high blood pressure, high cholesterol levels, and heavy alcohol abuse but none of these predisposing factors were present. Although the serum urate level was slightly elevated in Case 2, a biopsy was felt justified in view of the patient's relatively young age. Soft tissue involvement may occur with malignant lesions, including metastases, lymphomas, and sarcomas as well as gout but the presence of mineralisation within the soft tissue mass adjacent to the patella and in particular, the extensor tendon is more suggestive of gout. Furthermore, the marginal sclerosis around the intrapatellar lesions on the radiographs is a benign feature in keeping with a slow growing lesion as opposed to a malignant lesion that would usually have a more ill-defined zone of transition between lesion and normal bone. Pigmented villo-nodular synovitis (PVNS) and synovial osteochondromatosis (SOC) could also be considered in the differential diagnosis as these conditions may involve tendon sheaths and can cause intraosseous erosions with marginal sclerosis. However, mineralisation is not a feature of PVNS and involvement of the extensor tendon of the knee in SOC is very rare. Cross-sectional imaging may be helpful in lesion characterisation and staging. CT is very sensitive at detecting mineralisation and cortical destruction and MR imaging is the most accurate imaging technique for assessing soft tissue extent. The MR

signal characteristics of gouty tophi are nonspecific with low/intermediate signal intensity (SI) on T1-weighting and variable SI on T2-weighting. Low SI foci on T2-weighting may be due to haemosiderin deposition or mineralisation, as in Case 1. Although the serum urate level was also elevated in Case 1, a biopsy was felt justified in view of the unusual site and the need to exclude a coexisting tumour.

The pathological features of tophaceous gout are characteristic. Macroscopic examination reveals a nodular chalky appearance. Polarised microscopy of a fresh imprint demonstrates positively birefringent needle shaped crystals. These crystals are lost during processing for H&E examination. Instead, histologically, there are nodular aggregates of amorphous material surrounded by a palisade of histiocytes and multinucleated giant cells.

In conclusion, gout of the patella is a rare but recognised condition. We have presented two cases, one complicated by a pathological fracture and other occurring in bipartite patella in a male of 34 years. Gout of the patella may masquerade as a tumour or tumour-like condition and it is important to consider gout in the differential diagnosis. In patients with raised serum urate levels and typical imaging appearances, a biopsy is probably not required but, occasionally, serum urate may be normal in active gout and a cytological or histological proof will be required in such cases.

References

[1] A. J. Aboulafia, B. Prickett, and L. Giltman, "Displaced pathological patella fracture due to gout," *Orthopedics*, vol. 22, no. 5, pp. 543–545, 1999.

[2] P. Engelhardt and F. Buschor, "Pathological fracture of the patella secondary to gout, a case report," *Zeitschrift fur Rheumatologie*, vol. 52, no. 4, pp. 241–243, 1993.

[3] H. Enomoto, N. Nagosi, E. Okada, N. Ota, S. Iwabu, and S. Kamiishi, "Hemilaterally symptomatic bipartite patella

associated with bone erosions arising from a gouty tophus: a case report," *Knee*, vol. 13, no. 6, pp. 474–477, 2006.

[4] R. Espinosa-Morales and A. Escalante, "Gout presenting as non-union of a patellar fracture," *Journal of Rheumatology*, vol. 24, no. 7, pp. 1421–1422, 1997.

[5] D. C. Greenberg, "Pathological fracture of the patella secondary to gout. A case report," *Journal of Bone and Joint Surgery A*, vol. 68, no. 8, pp. 1286–1288, 1986.

[6] M. J. Kransdorf, R. P. Moser, T. N. Vinh, J. Aoki, and J. J. Callaghan, "Primary tumors of the patella: a review of 42 cases," *Skeletal Radiology*, vol. 18, no. 5, pp. 365–371, 1989.

[7] R. L. Linscheid and D. C. Dahlin, "Unusual lesions of the patella," *Journal of Bone and Joint Surgery A*, vol. 48, no. 7, pp. 1359–1366, 1966.

[8] M. Mercuri and R. Casadei, "Patellar tumors," *Clinical Orthopaedics and Related Research*, no. 389, pp. 35–46, 2001.

[9] P. Melloni, R. Valls, M. Yuguero, and M. Larrosa, "Unusual imaging manifestations of intraosseous tophaceous gout of the patella," *Journal of Rheumatology*, vol. 32, no. 5, pp. 959–961, 2005.

[10] L. U. Peloquin, "Graham JH. Gout of the patella, report of a case," *The New England Journal of Medicine*, vol. 253, no. 22, pp. 979–980, 1955.

[11] M. D. Price, R. F. Padera, M. B. Harris, and M. S. Vrahas, "Pathologic fracture of the patella from a gouty tophus," *Clinical Orthopaedics and Related Research*, no. 445, pp. 250–253, 2006.

[12] P. Reber, X. Crevoisier, and B. Noesberger, "Unusual localisation of tophaceous gout: a report of four cases and review of the literature," *Archives of Orthopaedic and Trauma Surgery*, vol. 115, no. 5, pp. 297–299, 1996.

[13] M. P. Recht, F. Seragini, J. Kramer, M. K. Dalinka, K. Hurtgen, and D. Resnick, "Isolated or dominant lesions of the patella in gout: a report of seven patients," *Skeletal Radiology*, vol. 23, no. 2, pp. 113–116, 1994.

[14] N. Schlesinger, J. M. Norquist, and D. J. Watson, "Serum urate during acute gout," *Journal of Rheumatology*, vol. 36, no. 6, pp. 1287–1289, 2009.

[15] J. Singh, S. L. James, H. M. Kroon, K. Woertler, S. E. Anderson, and A. M. Davies, "Tumour and tumour-like lesions of the patella—a multicentre experience," *European Radiology*, vol. 19, no. 3, pp. 701–712, 2009.

14

Rapidly Destructive Inflammatory Arthritis of the Hip

Jenny Shu,[1] Ian Ross,[2] Bret Wehrli,[3] Richard W. McCalden,[4] and Lillian Barra[1,5]

[1] *Department of Medicine, Division of Rheumatology, Western University, London, ON, Canada N6A 5W9*
[2] *Department of Diagnostic Radiology, Western University, London, ON, Canada N6A 5W9*
[3] *Department of Pathology, Western University, London, ON, Canada N6A 5A5*
[4] *Department of Orthopaedic Surgery, Western University, London, ON, Canada N6A 5A5*
[5] *Division of Rheumatology, Arthritis Centre, Monsignor Roney Building, St. Joseph's Health Care London, 268 Grosvenor Street, London, ON, Canada N6A 4V2*

Correspondence should be addressed to Lillian Barra; lillian.barra@sjhc.london.on.ca

Academic Editor: Gregory J. Tsay

Rapidly destructive coxarthrosis (RDC) is a rare syndrome that involves aggressive hip joint destruction within 6–12 months of symptom onset with no single diagnostic laboratory, pathological, or radiographic finding. We report an original case of RDC as an initial presentation of seronegative rheumatoid arthritis (RA) in a 57-year-old Caucasian woman presenting with 6 months of progressive right groin pain and no preceding trauma or chronic steroid use. Over 5 months, she was unable to ambulate and plain films showed complete resorption of the right femoral head and erosion of the acetabulum. There were inflammatory features seen on computed tomography (CT) and magnetic resonance imaging (MRI). She required a right total hip arthroplasty, but arthritis in other joints showed improvement with triple disease modifying antirheumatic drugs (DMARD) therapy and almost complete remission with the addition of adalimumab. We contrast our case of RDC as an initial presentation of RA to 8 RDC case reports of patients with established RA. Furthermore, this case highlights the importance of obtaining serial imaging to evaluate a patient with persistent hip symptoms and rapid functional deterioration.

1. Introduction

Rapidly destructive coxarthrosis (RDC) of the hip joint was initially coined in 1970 [1] to describe a rare syndrome that involved rapid and total deterioration of both the acetabular and femoral aspects of the hip joint [2]. The joint destruction is usually unilateral, occurs within 6–12 months of symptom onset, and has similar radiographic features of, but not consistent clinically with septic arthritis [3]. However, RDC is an idiopathic condition with no single diagnostic laboratory, pathological, or radiographic finding [4]. Several underlying pathogeneses proposed in the past include crystal deposition [5], neuropathic Charcot arthropathy [6], primary osteonecrosis [1], a subset of osteoarthritis [7], subchondral insufficiency fracture [8], and inflammatory arthritis [3, 9–11]. There have only been 8 case reports of patients with RDC ad preexisting rheumatoid arthritis (RA) (disease duration 2–20 years), some of whom were also treated with DMARDs and/or biologic therapy and required total hip arthroplasty [3, 9–11]. We report the first case of RDC as an initial presentation of seronegative RA.

2. Case Presentation

A 57-year-old Caucasian woman was referred to our rheumatology outpatient center from the orthopedics service for assessment of a possible inflammatory etiology for her rapidly destructive arthritis. Table 1 summarizes the major clinical, lab, and imaging findings. She initially presented with 6 months of progressive right hip and groin pain with no preceding trauma or chronic steroid use. There was a leg length discrepancy with the right leg 3 cm shorter and severe limitation of the right hip and some decreased range of motion on internal and external rotation of her left hip. She did not have any neurovascular compromise. Over 5 months, she became severely disabled and was unable to ambulate. With respect to her other joints, she had chronic

TABLE 1: Major clinical, lab, and imaging findings.

---

(1) Rapid progressive right hip destructive arthritis

(2) Morning stiffness greater than 1 hour

(3) Maximum active joint count of 11

(4) Chronic metatarsal phalangeal joints arthritis with erosions, periarticular osteopenia on imaging of hands

(5) Right knee arthritis with no imaging evidence of crystal arthropathy

(6) Erythrocyte sedimentation rate (ESR) of 56 mm/h and C-reactive protein (CRP) 106.4 mg/L, antinuclear antibody (ANA) was weakly positive at 1:80, with a negative rheumatoid factor (RF), anticitrullinated peptide (anti-CCP), antidouble stranded DNA (anti-dsDNA), and extractable nuclear antigen (ENA) screen

(7) Two incidental pulmonary nodules

(8) A soft tissue calcified mass in the right sacroiliac (SI) fossa and right gluteal muscles

(9) Presence of extracellular calcium pyrophosphate dehydrate (CPPD) crystals in right hip joint, negative synovial biopsy for crystals

(10) Biopsy showed chronic inflammation, fibrosis, multinucleated giant cell reaction with dystrophic calcification, and reactive synovial proliferation

---

pain in her metatarsal phalangeal joints (MTPs) and toes for approximately 3 years with progressive deformities, with recent episodes of swelling. Subsequent to her right hip pain, she also developed right knee pain with multiple episodes of warmth and swelling. Morning stiffness in affected joints was approximately 2 hours. Her initial swollen joint count (SJC) was 8 out of 66 joints examined, involving her right knee and multiple metatarsal phalangeal joints (MTPs). Over the next few visits, her swollen joint count of her small joints reached 11. There was also an unintentional 50-pound (lb) weight loss since the onset of her illness, partially due to decreased appetite secondary to pain.

Initial diagnostic work-up was significant for elevated inflammatory markers, weakly positive antinuclear antibody (ANA) and otherwise negative autoimmune markers including both rheumatoid factor (RF) and anticitrullinated peptide (anti-CCP) (Table 1). All cultures, including three sets of anaerobic and aerobic cultures and one set of systemic fungal and mycobacterial culture, were negative. Metabolic panel showed normal renal, thyroid, and liver function. Angiotensin-converting enzyme (ACE) serum level was within normal limits. Malignancy work-up was negative: serum and urine electrophoresis, CEA, CA-125, total body position-emission tomography (PET) scan, and bone scan were all within normal range. Two incidental pulmonary nodules were found on computed tomography (CT) thorax with focal ground glass appearance, but negative for malignancy on bronchoscopy and on repeat imaging. CT abdomen and pelvis was negative for any abdominal masses and showed a soft tissue calcified mass in the right sacroiliac (SI) fossa and right gluteal muscles.

Initial plain films of her right hip and pelvis showed femoral head lucencies compatible with subchondral cysts (but no definite fracture) and moderate diffuse articular joint space loss with flattening of the femoral head (Figure 1(a)). Over a 5-month span, there was complete destruction of the right femoral head, erosion of the right acetabulum, and lateral subluxation of the proximal femur (Figure 1(b)). CT pelvis with contrast (Figure 1(c)) showed fragmented bone within the acetabular fossa, which was remnants of the femoral head resorption process. Magnetic resonance imaging (MRI) of the right hip showed extensive synovial hypertrophy consistent with inflammatory arthritis (Figure 2). There were also minimal bone marrow edema and a fluid collection in the iliopsoas bursa extending posteriorly to the sciatic notch and enlargement of the hip joint capsule (Figure 2). X-rays of her feet revealed erosive changes in the MTPs and X-rays of her hands showed periarticular osteopenia in her metacarpal phalangeal (MCP) joints and ulnar deviation. There were degenerative changes on imaging of her knees, shoulders, and spine.

Three right hip aspirations were attempted with sufficient sample in only one attempt, which showed bloody fluid, 0.6 nucleated cells (17% neutrophils), and presence of only extracellular but not intracellular calcium pyrophosphate dehydrate (CPPD) crystals. Synovial biopsy did not reveal any crystals. Historically, CPPD crystal deposition disease can cause such acutely destructive disease on imaging and pathology [5], but the most common sites of CPPD joint involvement are the knees, wrists, and symphysis pubis with hip involvement being rarer with a prevalence of 5% [12]. This patient's plain-film images of her hands, knees, and pelvis were helpful in that there were no typical features of crystal arthropathy such as cartilage or joint capsule calcification and her blood work was also negative for an underlying metabolic precipitant of CPPD. Furthermore, single joint aspiration of her right knee showed no crystals, with bloody fluid and 35 nucleated cells (96% neutrophils).

The major differential diagnosis of this atypical case of destructive arthritis is outlined in Table 2. The patient's initial plain films showed evidence of degenerative changes but very unlikely to be primary osteoarthritis given the atypical symmetric joint space narrowing on plain imaging, complex joint effusion, and synovial thickening with chronic inflammatory changes on biopsy. She also did not have any evidence of a subchondral insufficiency fracture, which has been linked to the pathogenesis of the rapid destruction of osteoarthritic joints [8]. Other potential etiologies that could rarely cause such severe arthritis were considered on the differential including systemic diseases such as multicentric histiocytosis and sarcoidosis, but the patient lacked any other features of these diseases. Her neurovascular status was intact throughout and no evidence of a neurological problem or predisposing factors such as diabetes to cause Charcot's or neuropathic arthropathy. An avascular type necrosis (AVN) with subsequent inflammation was possible, but unusual without a history of steroidal use prior to her initial presentation or other risk factors for AVN. The imaging was also not classic for AVN and the patient did not have monoarthritis. Although seronegative, she did not have any inflammatory back pain, dactylitis, enthesitis, DIP involvement, inflammatory bowel disease, psoriasis, or other

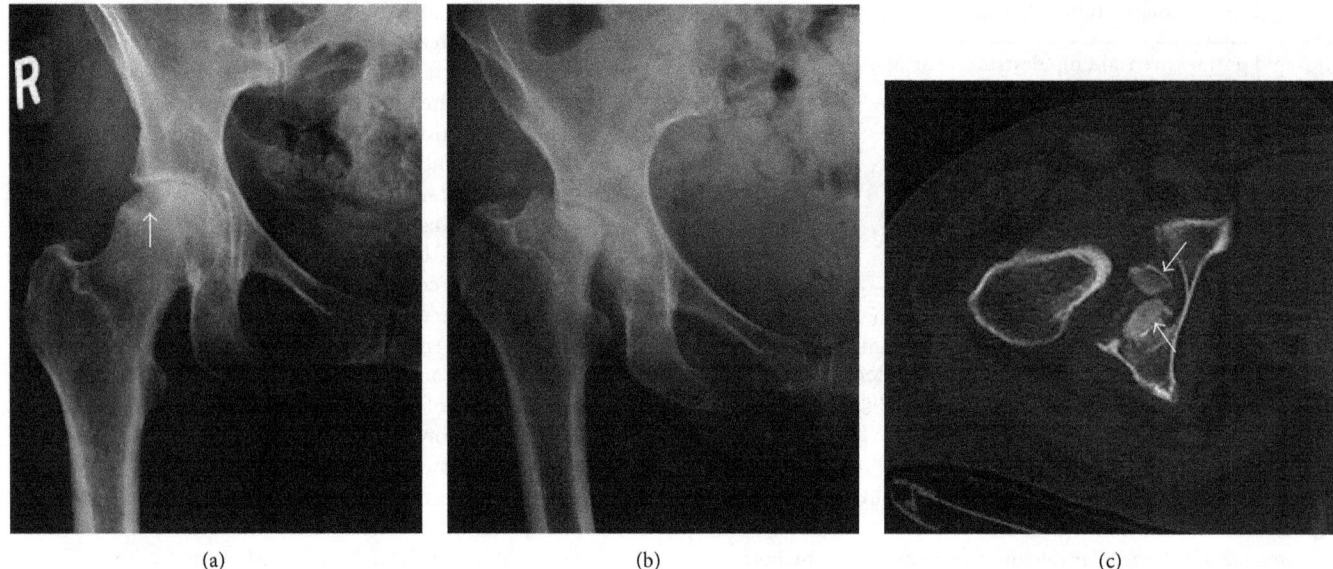

FIGURE 1: (a) AP radiograph of the right hip. A focal area of subchondral lucency is present involving the superolateral aspect of the right femoral head (arrow). (b) The follow-up radiograph taken 5 months later reveals near complete destruction of the femoral head. (c) CT scan of the right hip in the axial plane shows loss of the femoral head with two bone fragments within the hip joint (arrows).

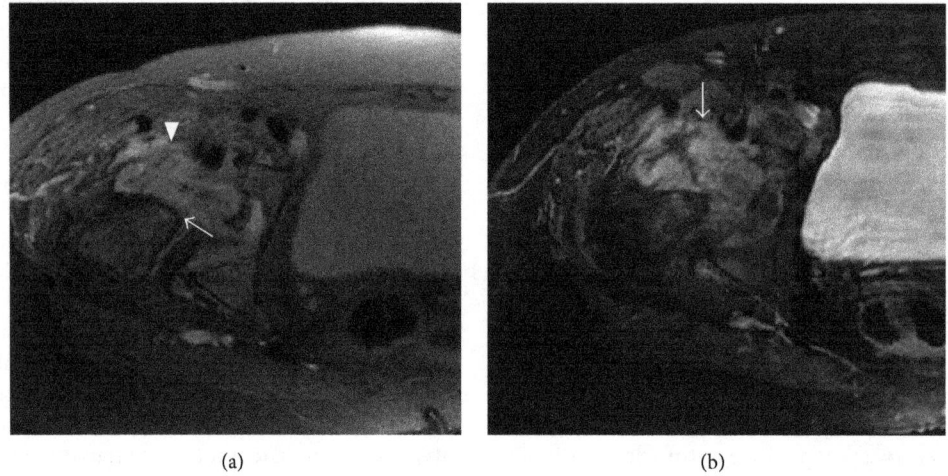

FIGURE 2: (a) Axial proton density with fat saturation sequence through the right hip joint (a) shows destruction of the femoral head (arrow) and a complex joint effusion (arrowhead). (b) Axial T1 fat saturated sequence after gadolinium reveals synovial thickening and enhancement (arrow).

features of seronegative spondyloarthropathy. X-rays of her spine and CT pelvis did not show evidence of sacroiliitis.

In order to definitively differentiate between chronic sepsis, malignancy, and a chronic inflammatory process, an open biopsy of the hip was performed by the orthopaedic service, which showed overall morphology with features of chronic inflammation, fibrosis, multinucleated giant cell reaction with dystrophic calcification, and reactive synovial proliferation (Figure 3). Cultures of synovial tissue were negative for fungus and mycobacteria, ruling out tuberculosis. Although the biopsy results were not specific for an exact etiology of rapid joint destruction, we were able to exclude neoplastic, infectious, osteoarthritis, and osteonecrotic etiologies.

An inflammatory etiology was most likely given multiple swollen joints, elevated inflammatory markers, constitutional symptoms, evidence of inflammatory features on imaging, and other causes excluded. Hence, a diagnosis of seronegative rheumatoid arthritis (RA) was ultimately made, fulfilling 4/7 of the 1987 RA American College of Rheumatology (ACR) classification criteria [13] and scoring 6 points for the 2010 ACR//European League Against Rheumatism (EULAR) classification criteria [14] (Table 3). Given the extent of right hip destruction, the patient received a total hip arthroplasty with good results. To prevent destruction of her other joints, triple disease modifying antirheumatic drugs (DMARD) therapy with hydroxychloroquine 400 mg daily, leflunomide

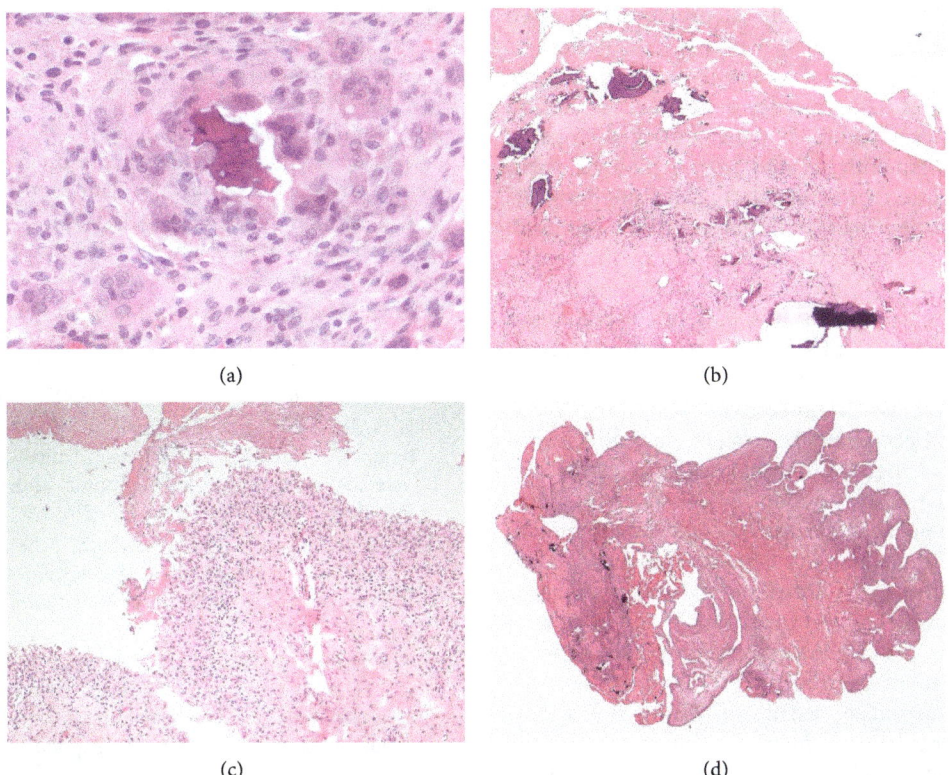

FIGURE 3: (a) Papillary, hyperplastic, chronically inflamed synovium is shown with abundant fibrin covering the surface and multiple fragments of bone being degraded by histiocytes and multinucleated giant cells. (b) At higher magnification, fibrin is seen on the surface of the synovium with a hyperplastic synovium consistent with chronic inflammation. (c) Fibrin and bone are detailed at 40x magnification showing multiple bone fragments which is typical of a rapidly destructive joint process. (d) Bone is seen being further broken down by multinucleated giant cells.

TABLE 2: Major differential diagnosis of rapidly destructive coxarthrosis.

(1) Infectious particularly mycobacterial and fungal
(2) Crystal arthropathy
(3) Avascular necrosis
(4) Inflammatory such as rheumatoid arthritis
(5) Degenerative
(6) Neuropathic
(7) Seronegative spondyloarthropathy
(8) Multicentric histiocytosis
(9) Sarcoidosis
(10) Neoplastic

TABLE 3: Rheumatoid arthritis classification criteria.

(a) 1987 American College of Rheumatology (ACR)

Morning stiffness > 1 hour (1)
Arthritis of 3 or more joint areas (1)
Symmetric arthritis (1)
Radiographic changes (1)
Total: 4/7

(b) 2010 ACR/European League of Rheumatism (EULAR)

Greater than 10 small joints (4)
Abnormal CRP and ESR (1)
Symptoms > 6 weeks (1)
Total: 6 points

Table 3 details the clinical classification criteria of rheumatoid arthritis (RA) that the patient fulfills as part of the 1987 American College of Rheumatology criteria (A) and 2010 American College of Rheumatology/European League of Rheumatism criteria (B). Only the features the patient had that met criteria are shown with the number of points in brackets.

20 mg daily, and methotrexate 25 subcutaneously weekly was initiated. For symptom relief, she was given an 80 mg intramuscular Depo-Medrol injection and joint injection to her right knee. At her 2-month follow-up visit, she had significantly reduced swelling of her knees and MTP's with much symptomatic relief. Adalimumab was added because of incomplete response and patient had further improvement. Over a 6-month period, SJC decreased from 8 to 1/66.

3. Discussion

Inflammatory arthritis is a rare cause of RDC with only 8 case reports of patients with preexisting RA [3, 9–11]. Likewise, our case is the first with RDC as an initial presentation of RA. In contrast to this patient, seven of the cases were in patients with well-established rheumatoid arthritis (disease duration between 7 and 20 years) who all required total hip arthroplasties [3, 9, 10]. Another case [11] had a similar presentation with early RA of 2-year disease duration, but details on treatment were unavailable. All previously reported cases were of Japanese patients; whereas our patient is Caucasian. There was one case of a 45-year-old Japanese man with a 7-year history of RA refractory to betamethasone and methotrexate who developed RDC and an enlarged iliopsoas bursa and was subsequently treated with a biologic agent (etanercept) in addition to arthroplasty with good results [9]. Similarly, our patient had resolution of joint swelling in her knee and MTPs on subcutaneous weekly methotrexate, leflunomide, and hydroxychloroquine and adalimumab.

Another atypical feature of this patient's presentation was an associated benign soft tissue mass with enhancement involving the articular region, acetabulum, sacroiliac region, and anterior pelvis (Figure 2). A previous case report [11] has found evidence of iliopsoas bursitis in a patient with RA who developed rapidly destructive inflammatory hip arthritis with MRI findings similar to this patient who had a soft tissue mass that enhanced post gadolinium and was consistent with bursitis (Figure 2). Three other previous case reports also had nonmalignant inflammatory soft tissue masses on imaging [3, 9]. Iliopsoas bursitis has also been seen in other cases of RDC [8] and suggests evidence of an inflammatory process. A possible mechanism may be the overproduction of synovial fluid exerting intra-articular pressure weakening the capsule and allowing the protrusion of the synovial membrane of the hip joint into the iliopsoas bursa, which was seen with other cases of RDC of inflammatory etiology in patients with RA [11].

Total hip arthroplasties have been used as a treatment modality for severe RDC with good response in a retrospective review of total hip arthroplasties performed on patients with RDC [4]. However, thorough preoperative work-up should be completed to exclude contraindications to total hip arthroplasties particularly neoplasia, infection, and neuroarthropathy [4].

To conclude, rheumatoid arthritis is a rare cause of rapidly destructive coxarthrosis (RDC). We present the first case report of RDC as the initial presentation of seronegative rheumatoid arthritis in a 57-year-old woman who required right total hip arthroplasty, but whose other active joints had a good response to DMARD and biologic therapy. This case also highlights the importance of obtaining serial imaging to evaluate a patient with persistent hip symptoms and rapid functional deterioration.

References

[1] M. Postel and M. Kerboull, "Total prosthetic replacement in rapidly destructive arthrosis of the hip joint," *Clinical Orthopaedics and Related Research*, vol. 72, pp. 138–144, 1970.

[2] K. Flik and J. H. Vargas, "Rapidly destructive hip disease: a case report and review of the literature.," *The American journal of orthopedics*, vol. 29, no. 7, pp. 549–552, 2000.

[3] K. Yoshino, S. Momohara, K. Ikari et al., "Acute destruction of the hip joints and rapid resorption of femoral head in patients with rheumatoid arthritis," *Modern Rheumatology*, vol. 16, no. 6, pp. 395–400, 2006.

[4] A. Kuo, K. A. Ezzet, S. Patil, and C. W. Colwell Jr., "Total hip arthroplasty in rapidly destructive osteoarthritis of the hip: a case series," *HSS Journal*, vol. 5, no. 2, pp. 117–119, 2009.

[5] C. J. Menkes, F. Simon, F. Delrieu, M. Forest, and F. Delbarre, "Destructive arthropathy in chondrocalcinosis articularis.," *Arthritis and Rheumatism*, vol. 19, pp. 329–348, 1976.

[6] S. D. Slowman-Kovacs, E. M. Braunstein, and K. D. Brandt, "Rapidly progressive Charcot arthropathy following minor joint trauma in patients with diabetic neuropathy," *Arthritis and Rheumatism*, vol. 33, no. 3, pp. 412–417, 1990.

[7] Z. S. Rosenberg, S. Shankman, G. C. Steiner, D. K. Kastenbaum, A. Norman, and M. G. Lazansky, "Rapid destructive osteoarthritis: clinical, radiographic, and pathologic features," *Radiology*, vol. 182, no. 1, pp. 213–216, 1992.

[8] T. Yamamoto and P. G. Bullough, "The role of subchondral insufficiency fracture in rapid destruction of the hip joint: a preliminary study," *Arthritis & Rheumatology*, vol. 43, no. 11, pp. 2423–2427, 2000.

[9] T. Yoshioka, A. Tachihara, T. Koyama, K. Iwakawa, M. Sakane, and H. Nakamura, "Rapidly destruction of the hip joint associated with enlarged iliopsoas bursa in a patient with refractory rheumatoid arthritis," *Journal of Nippon Medical School*, vol. 75, no. 4, pp. 233–238, 2008.

[10] H. H. Yun, S. Y. Song, S. B. Park, and J. W. Lee, "Rapidly destructive arthropathy of the hip joint in patients with rheumatoid arthritis," *Orthopedics*, vol. 35, no. 6, pp. e958–e962, 2012.

[11] T. Matsumoto, T. Juji, and T. Mori, "Enlarged psoas muscle and iliopsoas bursitis associated with a rapidly destructive hip in a patient with rheumatoid arthritis," *Modern Rheumatology*, vol. 16, no. 1, pp. 52–54, 2006.

[12] A. Abhishek, S. Doherty, R. Maciewicz, K. Muir, W. Zhang, and M. Doherty, "Chondrocalcinosis is common in the absence of knee involvement," *Arthritis Research and Therapy*, vol. 14, article R205, no. 5, 2012.

[13] F. C. Arnett, S. M. Edworthy, D. A. Bloch et al., "The American Rheumatism Association 1987 revised criteria for the classification of rheumatoid arthritis," *Arthritis and Rheumatism*, vol. 31, no. 3, pp. 315–324, 1988.

[14] D. Aletaha, T. Neogi, and A. J. Silman, "2010 Rheumatoid arthritis classification criteria: an American College of Rheumatology/European League Against Rheumatism collaborative initiative (Annals of the Rheumatic Diseases (2010) 69, (1580–1588))," *Annals of the Rheumatic Diseases*, vol. 69, no. 9, pp. 1580–1588, 2010.

15

Marked Multiple Tendinitis at the Onset of Rheumatoid Arthritis in a Patient with Heterozygous Familial Hypercholesterolemia: Ultrasonographic Observation

Takeshi Suzuki and Akiko Okamoto

Division of Rheumatology, Mitsui Memorial Hospital, 1 Kandaizumi-cho, Chiyoda-ku, Tokyo 101-8643, Japan

Correspondence should be addressed to Takeshi Suzuki; suzuki-rheum@mitsuihosp.or.jp

Academic Editor: Tsai-Ching Hsu

A 59-year-old woman who had been diagnosed with heterozygous familial hypercholesterolemia developed rheumatoid arthritis (RA). She presented with marked tendinitis of the Achilles tendons, patellar tendons, and finger extensor tendons at the onset of RA. Ultrasonographic examination revealed that tendon lesions were predominantly tendinitis rather than paratenonitis, and that the tendinitis was of the noninsertional variety, rather than the insertional variety. Preexisting tendon xanthomas might have contributed to the unusually dominant noninsertional tendinitis of multiple tendons.

1. Introduction

The prevalence of rheumatoid arthritis (RA) is relatively constant at 0.5 to 1.0% in many populations [1]. The estimated prevalence of RA is 1.0% of the entire Japanese population aged ≥16 to <75 years [2]. Familial hypercholesterolemia (FH) is a genetic disorder associated with severe hypercholesterolemia, atherosclerosis, and xanthomas at various sites in which the primary defect is a mutation in the low-density lipoprotein receptor [3, 4]. Although homozygous FH is a very rare disease with a poor prognosis, heterozygous FH (HeFH) is a relatively common disorder with a prevalence of approximately 0.2% in most countries, including Japan [5]. The frequency of the incidental association of HeFH and RA is estimated to be around one per 50,000 adults. Despite this, only one case has been reported in the English literature [6]. Herein, we report a case of HeFH presenting with marked multiple tendinitis at the onset of RA.

2. Case Presentation

A 59-year-old Japanese woman was referred to our hospital in May 2012 due to posterior ankle pain and anterior knee pain in both legs. She had been diagnosed with hypertension and HeFH at the age of 57. At that time, her total cholesterol was 458 mg/dL (11.8 mmol/L), triglycerides 237 mg/dL (2.67 mmol/L), low-density lipoprotein cholesterol (LDL-C) 359 mg/dL (9.4 mmol/L), and high-density lipoprotein cholesterol 45 mg/dL (1.18 mmol/L). She had a family history of hypercholesterolemia and premature coronary heart disease (CHD) but had no family history of RA. She had no past history of CHD but had a severe stenosis of the left internal carotid artery. She had been treated with 2 mg of pitavastatin for two years and 10 mg of ezetimibe for six months at the time of her initial visit to our hospital. Her serum LDL-C level was reduced to around 260 mg/dL (6.7 mmol/L) by the administration of pitavastatin and was further reduced to around 170 mg/dL (4.4 mmol/L) by adding ezetimibe. Her cholesterol levels had been stable for the last six months.

She had experienced pain in the bilateral Achilles tendons for six weeks and in the bilateral knees and the metacarpophalangeal (MCP) joint of the left third finger for four weeks at the time of her initial visit to our hospital. Physical examination revealed bilateral arcus cornea. Swelling and thickening of the bilateral Achilles tendons were observed along the midportion of the tendon. There was tenderness on palpation along the Achilles tendons from the midportion to the distal insertion into the calcaneal bone. There was also

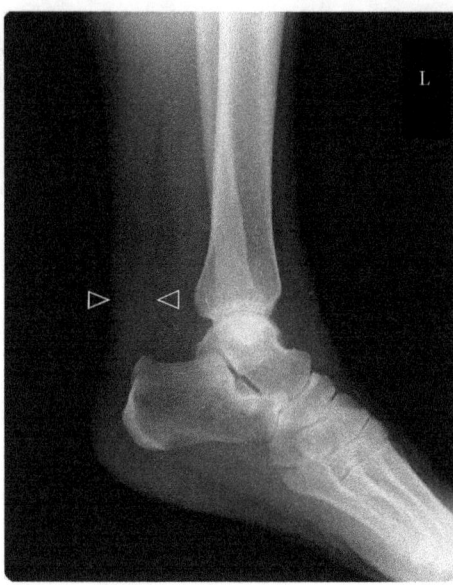

FIGURE 1: X-ray of the ankle. X-ray of the ankles showed thickening of the bilateral Achilles tendons [left side (arrows heads): 20 mm, right side (not shown): 19 mm].

tenderness on palpation of the bilateral tibial tuberosities and the right medial epicondyle of the humerus. As for small joints, there was tenderness on palpation of the first and fifth metatarsophalangeal (MTP) joints of the right foot and the second MTP joint of the left foot. The dorsal aspect of the third MCP joint of the right hand and the second MCP joint of the right hand had no tenderness but was swollen. Nodular thickening of the extensor tendon of the third digit of the right hand was also noted.

Laboratory examination revealed an erythrocyte sedimentation rate of 118 mm/h, a C-reactive protein level of 2.06 mg/dL, a rheumatoid factor of 49.3 U/mL (normal <15), an anti-CCP2 antibody level >300 U/mL (normal <4.5), and a matrix metalloproteinase 3 level of 62.3 ng/mL (normal <59.7). X-ray imaging of the hands, feet, ankles, and knees revealed neither bone erosion nor enthesophytes. X-rays of the ankles showed widening of soft tissue shadow suggestive of thickening of the bilateral Achilles tendons (Figure 1).

Musculoskeletal ultrasonography (US) disclosed marked multiple tendinitis in the legs and fingers. Gray-scale US (GSUS) images of the Achilles tendon revealed a markedly swollen tendon with a rounded cross section (Figure 2(a)). The tendon appearance was inhomogenous and predominantly hypoechoic with loss of the fibrillar pattern (Figures 2(b)–2(d)). Power Doppler US (PDUS) revealed markedly increased vascularity of the Achilles tendons. Increased blood flow was observed both inside and at the periphery of the tendons (Figures 2(e)-2(h)). The vessels appeared to enter from the ventral aspect of the tendon through the Kager's fat. These abnormal appearances in both GSUS and PDUS were recognized bilaterally and found predominantly along the midportion of the Achilles tendon rather than at the level of the tendon insertion on the calcaneus. No remarkable thickening of the paratenon was observed. Neither bony

irregularity of the calcaneus nor retrocalcaneal bursitis was detected. No other ankle lesions, including talocrural joint synovitis, subtalar joint synovitis, tibialis posterior tenosynovitis, or peroneal tenosynovitis, were detected.

US findings of the knees were similar to those of the ankles. GSUS revealed focal thickening of the patellar tendon with inhomogenous and hypoechoic appearance and loss of the fibrillar pattern along the distal portion of the tendon (Figure 3(a)). PDUS revealed markedly increased blood flow in the hypoechoic areas inside of the tendon observed by GSUS (Figure 3(b)). These abnormal appearances were recognized bilaterally and found predominantly along the distal portion of the patellar tendon rather than at the level of the tendon insertion on the tibial tuberosity. Neither bony irregularity of the tibia nor infrapatellar bursitis was detected. Except for the patellar tendon lesions, mild synovitis was observed in the bilateral suprapatellar pouch. In the hands, GSUS revealed focal thickening of the finger extensor tendons with hypoechoic appearance and loss of the fibrillar pattern in the dorsal aspect of the right third MCP joint and the left second and fourth MCP joint. PDUS revealed increased blood flow around the hypoechoic areas of the extensor tendons (Figure 3(c)). Except for the extensor lesions, mild synovitis was observed in the right second MCP joint.

The hypoechoic areas detected inside of the Achilles tendons, patellar tendons, and finger extensor tendons presumably correspond to tendon xanthomas with or without tendinosis. The markedly increased blood flow inside and/or around the hypoechoic areas cannot be explained solely by slowly developed neovascularization into the tendon xanthomas. It is evident that there occurred a highly active tendinitis, which is considered a subacute inflammatory process.

In the feet, synovial thickening with hyperemia, which was consistent with RA, was detected in the first, second, third, and fifth MTP joints of the right foot and the first and second MTP joints of the left foot (Figure 3(d)). According to the 2010 RA classification criteria, she was classified as having RA and methotrexate was started [7]. Three months later, swelling and tenderness on palpation of the bilateral Achilles tendons and patellar tendons were resolved, although thickening of the bilateral Achilles tendons persisted.

3. Discussion

RA is a chronic inflammatory disease that predominantly affects the synovial membranes lining the joints and tendon sheaths. The affected synovium is proliferative and erosive in character. In addition to synovial tendon sheaths, tendons are also occasionally involved in RA. Our previous study regarding the US findings of Achilles tendon-related involvement in RA found that retrocalcaneal bursitis was the most common pathology and was frequently observed in early RA patients [8]. Achilles paratenonitis was relatively rare and tended to be observed in early RA. As for tendinitis, insertional tendinitis, enthesitis of the Achilles tendon tended to be observed in established RA patients. Noninsertional tendinitis of the Achilles tendon was less common and was almost equally observed between early RA and established RA.

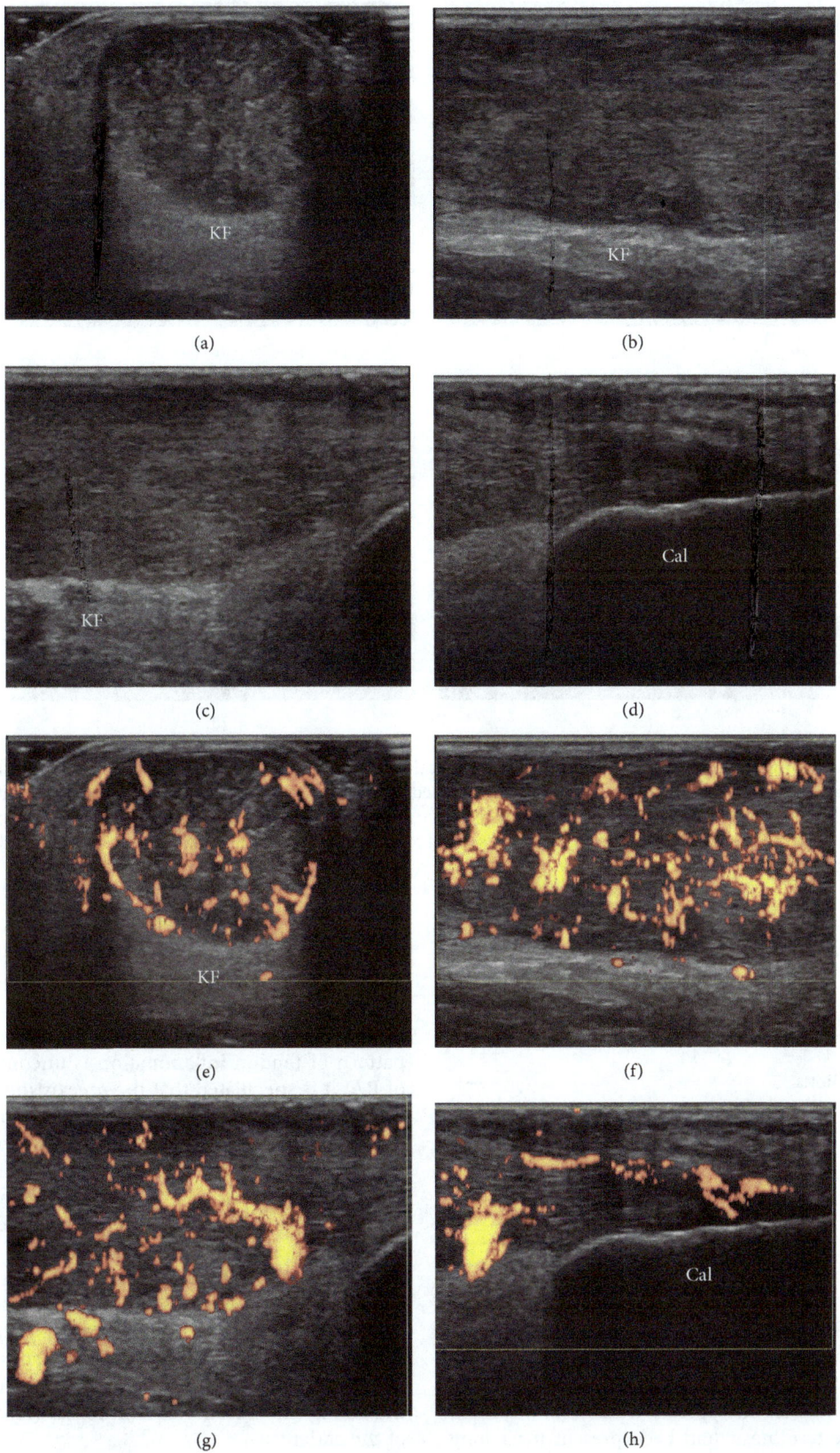

FIGURE 2: Ultrasound findings of the Achilles tendon. Gray-scale ((a)–(d)) and power Doppler ((e)–(h)) ultrasonograms of the right Achilles tendon (AT). Transverse scans at the midportion ((a), (e)) and longitudinal scans at the midportion ((b), (f)), at the level of retrocalcaneal bursa ((c), (g)), and at the insertion into the calcaneal bone ((d), (h)) of the right AT. Similar findings were also observed in the left AT (not shown). KF Kager's fat pad, Cal calcaneus.

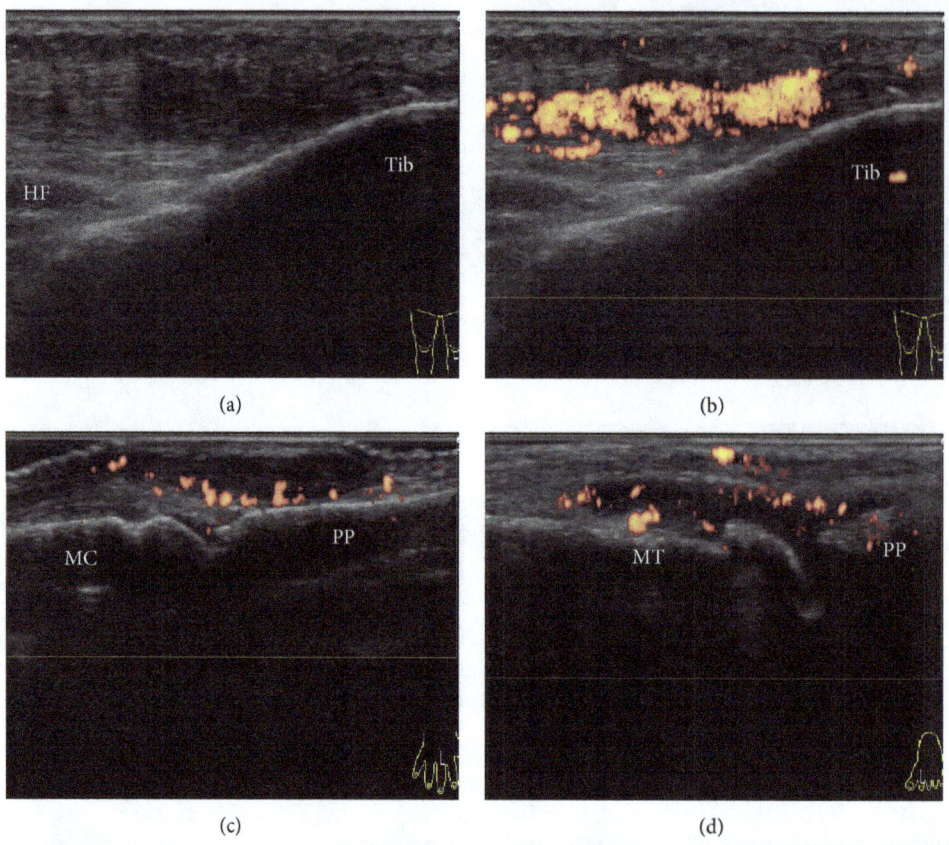

FIGURE 3: Ultrasound findings of knees, fingers, and toes. (a) Gray-scale and (b) power Doppler ultrasonograms of the longitudinal scan of the distal right patellar tendon (PT). Similar findings were also observed in the left PT (not shown). (c) Power Doppler ultrasonograms of the longitudinal scan of the extensor tendon and metacarpophalangeal joint of the third finger of the left hand. (d) Power Doppler ultrasonograms of the longitudinal scan of the metatarsophalangeal joint of the second toe of the left foot. HF Hoffa's fat pad, Tib Tibia, MC metacarpal bone, PP proximal phalange, MT metatarsal bone.

TABLE 1: The degree of ultrasound pathologies at the onset of rheumatoid arthritis in the present case.

Pathology	Degree
Tendinosis	+++
Noninsertional tendinitis	+++
Paratenonitis	++
Insertional tendinitis (enthesitis)	+
Joint synovitis	+
Tenosynovitis	−
Bursitis	−

The overall US findings of this case and the degree of each pathology are summarized in Table 1. Although the US examination was performed in the very early phase of RA, the degree of Achilles and patellar tendinosis was high, suggesting that the tendinosis had been present for a long time. The main cause of the tendinosis is thought to be the xanthomas due to genetically determined HeFH rather than the tendinitis due to the newly occurring RA. The patient presented with marked tendinitis in multiple tendons, including the Achilles tendons, patellar tendons, and finger extensor tendons, at the onset of RA. Our examination revealed that tendon lesions were predominantly tendinitis rather than paratenonitis, and that the tendinitis was of the noninsertional variety, rather than the insertional variety. Because this pattern of tendon inflammation is uncommon at the onset of RA, it is speculated that the preexisting tendinosis due to HeFH modified the manifestation of tendon pathology.

In HeFH patients, xanthoma formation inside tendons such as the Achilles tendons and thickening of the tendons are frequently observed. US examination is known to be very useful for evaluating tendon involvement in patients with HeFH, although the descriptions of US findings have varied over the decades. Recently, Tsouli et al. reported the GSUS findings of Achilles tendons among 80 untreated adult patients with HeFH [9]. According to the report, an abnormal echostructure with a diffuse heterogeneous echo pattern was observed in 52.5% of the patients and focal hypoechoic lesions indicating the presence of xanthomas were observed in 10% of the patients.

It has been reported that neovessels inside the tendon xanthomas can be detected by PDUS [10, 11]. As for Achilles tendon xanthomas, PDUS reveals increased vascularity in the "avascular zone" where the blood supply is normally very poor. The flow signals are typically observed along the ventral aspect of the Achilles tendon. It has been confirmed that the PD signals represent neovascularization into the tendon xanthomas by histological observations in the excised specimen of a HeFH patient and in heritable hyperlipidemic rabbit models [11, 12].

Grassi et al. recently proposed that PD signals in patients with early arthritis may be related to increased perfusion of nutritional vessels at the level of either bone-perforating canals and/or the fat pad [13]. Such a phenomenon may imply that preexisting vascularity to joint components functions as a gateway to articular inflammation at the beginning of RA. It would be interesting to speculate that the unusually prominent tendinitis in this patient at the onset of RA was induced by the unusual preexisting hypervascularity in the tendons due to tendon xanthomas.

Is there a causal association between genetically determined HeFH and the development of RA in this patient? An incidental association seems highly plausible because of the absence of literature on their coexistence (there has only been one case report) [6]. It is known, however, that patients with HeFH are prone to rheumatic complaints. Klemp et al. interviewed and examined 48 patients with HeFH and reported that 21% had a history of oligoarthritis and 10% had a history of polyarthritis but none had clinical evidence of RA or other arthropathies [14]. The pretreatment cholesterol levels were significantly higher in HeFH patients with musculoskeletal manifestations than in those without. It was also shown that the musculoskeletal manifestations in HeFH patients improved after receiving lipid-lowering treatment. Artieda et al. have shown that macrophages from HeFH patients exhibit a differential gene expression profile characterized by increased plasma tryptase, TNF-α, IL-8, and IL-6 expression [15]. This proinflammatory predisposition of macrophages may contribute to the tendency of HeFH patients to present with musculoskeletal manifestations.

Although we cannot completely deny the possibility, it is unlikely that lipid-lowering agents induced her tendinitis for the following reasons. (1) While it has been reported that most statin-induced tendinopathy occurred within the first year of administration [16], pitavastatin had been maintained on constant dose for two years in the present case. (2) While there is a hypothesis that the rapid lowering of cholesterol can provoke exacerbations of tendinopathy [10], her serum LDL-C had been stable at slightly high levels for six months prior to the onset of tendinitis.

In conclusion, here we report a case of HeFH presenting with marked tendinitis in multiple tendons at the onset of RA. Preexisting tendon xanthomas might contribute to the unusually dominant noninsertional tendinitis of the Achilles tendons, patellar tendons, and finger extensor tendons. Although it was a very rare case, the observation by PDUS throws some light on the role of existing vessels in the initial phase of rheumatoid inflammation.

References

[1] A. J. Silman and J. E. Pearson, "Epidemiology and genetics of rheumatoid arthritis," *Arthritis Research and Therapy*, vol. 4, supplement 3, pp. S265–S272, 2002.

[2] H. Yamanaka, N. Sugiyama, E. Inoue, A. Taniguchi, and S. Momohara, "Estimates of the prevalence of and current treatment practices for rheumatoid arthritis in Japan using reimbursement data from health insurance societies and the IORRA cohort (I)," *Modern Rheumatology*, vol. 24, no. 1, pp. 33–40, 2014.

[3] M. S. Brown and J. L. Goldstein, "A receptor-mediated pathway for cholesterol homeostasis," *Science*, vol. 232, no. 4746, pp. 34–47, 1986.

[4] J. L. Goldstein, H. H. Hobbs, and M. S. Brown, "Familial Hypercholesterolemia," in *The Metabolic Basis of Inherited Disease*, C. R. Scriven, A. L. Beaudit, W. S. Sly, and D. Valle, Eds., pp. 1981–2030, McGraw-Hill, New York, NY, USA, 1995.

[5] T. Teramoto, J. Sasaki, S. Ishibashi et al., "Familial hypercholesterolemia," *Journal of Atherosclerosis and Thrombosis*, vol. 21, no. 1, pp. 6–10, 2014.

[6] B. Josipovic, D. Jablanovic, A. Josipovic, R. Nedeljkovic, and S. Ilic, "Unrecognized seropositive RA and SS in a patient with associated familial hypercholesterolemia type IIa and osseous xanthoma of the proximal femur," *Clinical and Experimental Rheumatology*, vol. 21, no. 5, pp. 678–679, 2003.

[7] D. Aletaha, T. Neogi, A. J. Silman et al., "2010 Rheumatoid arthritis classification criteria: an American college of rheumatology/European league against rheumatism collaborative initiative," *Annals of the Rheumatic Diseases*, vol. 69, no. 9, pp. 1580–1588, 2010.

[8] T. Suzuki and A. Okamoto, "Ultrasound examination of symptomatic ankles in shorter-duration rheumatoid arthritis patients often reveals tenosynovitis," *Clinical and Experimental Rheumatology*, vol. 31, no. 2, pp. 281–284, 2013.

[9] S. G. Tsouli, V. Xydis, M. I. Argyropoulou, A. D. Tselepis, M. Elisaf, and D. N. Kiortsis, "Regression of Achilles tendon thickness after statin treatment in patients with familial hypercholesterolemia: an ultrasonographic study," *Atherosclerosis*, vol. 205, no. 1, pp. 151–155, 2009.

[10] M. Abate, C. Schiavone, V. Salini, and I. Andia, "Occurrence of tendon pathologies in metabolic disorders," *Rheumatology*, vol. 52, no. 4, pp. 599–608, 2013.

[11] J. H. Ahn, T. J. Chun, and S. Lee, "Nodular excision for painful localized achilles tendon xanthomas in type II hyperlipoproteinemia: a case report," *Journal of Foot and Ankle Surgery*, vol. 50, no. 5, pp. 603–606, 2011.

[12] A. Nakano, M. Kinoshita, R. Okuda, T. Yasuda, M. Abe, and M. Shiomi, "Pathogenesis of tendinous xanthoma: histopathological study of the extremities of Watanabe heritable hyperlipidemic rabbits," *Journal of Orthopaedic Science*, vol. 11, no. 1, pp. 75–80, 2006.

[13] W. Grassi and E. Filippucci, "Rheumatoid arthritis: diagnosis of RA—we have a dream," *Nature Reviews Rheumatology*, vol. 9, no. 4, pp. 202–204, 2013.

[14] P. Klemp, A. M. Halland, F. L. Majoos, and K. Steyn, "Musculoskeletal manifestations in hyperlipidaemia: a controlled study," *Annals of the Rheumatic Diseases*, vol. 52, no. 1, pp. 44–48, 1993.

[15] M. Artieda, A. Cenarro, C. Junquera et al., "Tendon xanthomas in familial hypercholesterolemia are associated with a differential inflammatory response of macrophages to oxidized LDL," *FEBS Letters*, vol. 579, no. 20, pp. 4503–4512, 2005.

16

Serum Cytokine Concentrations in a Patient with Rheumatoid Arthritis on Etanercept Therapy Who Subsequently Developed Pneumocystis Pneumonia

Masao Sato,[1] Masao Takemura,[2] Ryuki Shinohe,[3] and Katsuji Shimizu[1]

[1] Department of Orthopaedic Surgery, Gifu University School of Medicine, 1-1 Yanagido Gifu, Gifu 501-1194, Japan
[2] Department of Informative Clinical Medicine, Gifu University School of Medicine, 1-1 Yanagido Gifu, Gifu 501-1194, Japan
[3] Department of Orthopadeic Surgery, Nishimino Welfare Hospital, 986 Oshikoshi Yoro, Gifu 503-1394, Japan

Correspondence should be addressed to Masao Sato, sat@air.linkclub.or.jp

Academic Editors: S. S. Koca, J. Mikdashi, and L. Schachna

We report a rheumatoid arthritis patient who was treated with etanercept. Serum levels of tumor-necrosis-factor- (TNF-) *alpha*, soluble-tumor-necrosis-factor receptor- (sTNFR-) I and -II, interleukin- (IL-) 6, and IL-1 beta were measured by ELISA before and during the course of therapy. While the serum levels of IL-6 and IL-1 beta dropped rapidly following the initiation of therapy, the concentrations of TNF-alpha and sTNFR-II steadily increased to a plateau. Although significant clinical efficacy was observed, etanercept had to be discontinued when after 12 weeks of therapy the patient was found to have pneumocystis pneumonia.

1. Introduction

Rheumatoid arthritis (RA) is an autoimmune inflammatory disease in which cytokines, such as tumor-necrosis-factor- (TNF-) *alpha* and interleukin- (IL-) 1, are thought to play a major role in the pathogenesis. Consequently, several publications have focused on the serum and/or synovial fluid levels of various inflammatory cytokines in patients with RA, psoriatic arthritis, and ankylosing spondylitis, with the clinical utility of such measurements being advocated [1, 2]. Recently, TNF-*alpha* inhibitors have been found to induce a rapid and sustained attenuation of disease activity in patients with RA. We describe here a patient with RA treated with a TNF-*alpha* inhibitor, etanercept for 12 weeks before discontinuation of therapy for pneumocystis pneumonia (PCP). The serum concentrations of TNF-*alpha*, sTNFR-I and -II, IL-6, and IL-1 beta were measured before, during, and after etanercept therapy.

2. Case Presentation

A 54-year-old Japanese man who had been diagnosed with RA for 8 years according to the 1987 American Rheuma-tism Association classification criteria for RA was admitted with polyarthritis. He complained of pain and swelling in the wrists, fingers, and knees and had difficulty walking without assistance. He claimed to have morning stiffness lasting about 3 hours. Past medical history included a left total knee arthroplasty complicated by a traumatic fracture of the left distal femur postoperatively and a cerebral infarction with residual right hemiparesis. His medication regimen included sulfasalazine (1000 mg/day), bucillamine (300 mg/day), mizoribine (150 mg/day), and prednisolone (10 mg/day). The Steinbrocker stage was IV and functional class was 4. He was unable to stand unassisted due to bilateral knee pain. Swelling and tenderness were present in the proximal interphalangeal and metacarpophalangeal joints of both hands and fingers, as well as in the wrists and knees. Right-sided muscle weakness was observed. Laboratory findings were as follows: white blood cell count 8800/mm^3 (75.6% neutrophils, 19.5% lymphocytes, 2.9% monocytes, 0.3% eosinophils, 0.2% basophils), hemoglobin 10.7 mg/dL, platelets $48.7 \times 10^4/\mu$L, erythrocyte sedimentation rate (ESR) 75 mm/h, C-reactive protein (CRP) 3.58 mg/dL, rheumatoid factor (RF) 219.6 IU/mL, and anticyclic citrullinated peptide antibody (ACPA) 189 IU/mL. Serum β-D-glucan was negative. The purified protein derivative skin test for tuberculosis was negative.

Treatment was initiated with subcutaneous injections of etanercept 25 mg twice a week. Blood samples were collected before the first dose (at baseline), 24 hours after the first injection (day 1), daily until day 8, and weekly thereafter. Specimens were centrifuged at 3000 rpm and the sera stored at $-80°$C until the assay was performed. TNF-*alpha*, TNFR-I and -II, IL-6, and IL-1 beta concentrations were measured using commercial ELISA kits.

After initiating etanercept, the patient's clinical condition improved markedly, with swelling and tenderness of the wrists and finger joints significantly better. He was able to stand with the aid of crutches despite residual hemiparesis. The duration of morning stiffness dropped to below 30 minutes. The 28-joint count Disease Activity Score (DAS28) dropped significantly within the first 4 weeks and continued to decrease (DAS28 = 8.09, 5.37, 4.73, and 4.60, at baseline, 4 weeks, 8 weeks, and 12 weeks, resp.), achieving the European League Against Rheumatism (EULAR) moderate response criteria. The CRP dropped to below 0.30 mg/mL within the first 2 weeks of therapy. Subsequently, the oral immunosuppressive regimen of sulfasalazine, bucillamine, and mizoribine was discontinued after initiation of treatment. Prednisolone was reduced to 5 mg/day.

After 12 weeks of treatment with etanercept, the patient developed a nonproductive cough along with a fever of $38°$C. Serum β-D-glucan was found to be positive, and sputum polymerase chain reaction (PCR) was positive for pneumocystis (Figure 1). Etanercept was discontinued, and an antifungal regimen initiated.

Preceding etanercept therapy, the serum IL-6 levels were found to be elevated, correlating with the high CRP value and high clinical disease activity. Conversely, the serum level of TNF-*alpha* was nondetectable (<0.2 pg/mL); the sTNFR-I, -II, and IL-1 beta values were not found to be significantly elevated (Figure 2). After initiation of etanercept, there was a rapid decline in the IL-6 and CRP levels, whereas the levels of TNF-*alpha* and sTNFR-II increased significantly within 24 hours after administration of the first dose to a plateau after 2 weeks (range: 100 pg/mL to 170 pg/mL) and 6-7 weeks (range: 300 ng/mL to 700 ng/mL), respectively. The sTNFR-I and IL-1-beta levels remained relatively unchanged (sTNFR-I levels at baseline, 3.56 ng/mL; 4 weeks, 3.36 ng/mL; 8 weeks, 2.93 ng/mL; 12 weeks, 3.58 ng/mL). At week 12, concurrent to the patient developing clinical symptoms of PCP, the levels of IL-6, CRP, and TNF-*alpha* showed an acute peak, which tapered downward over the following 3 weeks with the institution of an appropriate antifungal regimen (Figures 3 and 4).

3. Discussion

Several cytokines, chemokines, and matrix metalloproteinases with serum levels that correlate with the disease activity of RA have been reported. Furthermore, a favorable clinical response following the administration of TNF-*alpha*

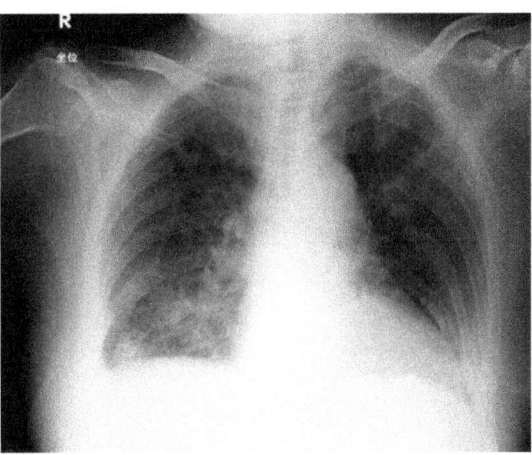

FIGURE 1: Chest radiograph revealed bilateral ground-glass infiltrates and reticular shadows.

inhibitors was shown to be accompanied by the reduced serum levels of these inflammatory mediators [3].

Etanercept is a recombinant fusion protein consisting of two p75 receptors and the Fc domain of the human IgG1 that binds to both soluble and cell-bound TNF-*alpha* [4]. Although etanercept is known to reduce disease activity and inhibit bone and joint destruction in patients with RA [4], it is not clear if and how etanercept modulates the serum levels of TNF-*alpha*, TNFR-I, and TNFR-II. We previously demonstrated that serum TNFR-II concentrations in RA patients ($n = 45$) not on biologics were significantly higher than in healthy controls ($n = 80$) (7.28 ± 4.16 ng/mL versus 4.40 ± 0.88 ng/mL) [5]. In the patient reported here, the serum TNFR-II concentration was elevated to more than 500 ng/mL during treatment with etanercept, with return to baseline levels after discontinuation of treatment. Since etanercept is composed in part by the p75 TNF receptor, the ELISA assay might be detecting (a component of) etanercept as TNFR-II.

TNF-*alpha* concentrations were elevated within 24 hours of etanercept therapy in the present patient and remained high until the cessation of etanercept treatment, which supports previous reports that TNF-*alpha* concentrations are elevated during etanercept therapy [6]. We could explain this rise in serum TNF-*alpha* by the possibility that the assay might be measuring TNF-*alpha* that is bound to etanercept. Etanercept has an approximately 50-fold greater affinity for human recombinant TNF-*alpha* in a binding inhibition assay and is approximately 1000 times more efficient than monomeric soluble TNFR. In addition, etanercept has a 5- to 8-fold longer plasma half-life compared with naturally occurring soluble TNFR. [7, 8]. Etanercept-bound TNF-*alpha* is known to be immunoreactive although without biological activity [6]. In this case, even though TNF-*alpha* as measured by the ELISA was elevated during the course of treatment, disease activity was well inhibited. The levels of CRP were clearly lower during the course of treatment.

Mori et al. reported that etanercept lowered the TNFR-I, IL-6, and IL-1 beta serum concentrations in juvenile idiopathic arthritis patients. The concentrations of IL-6 at

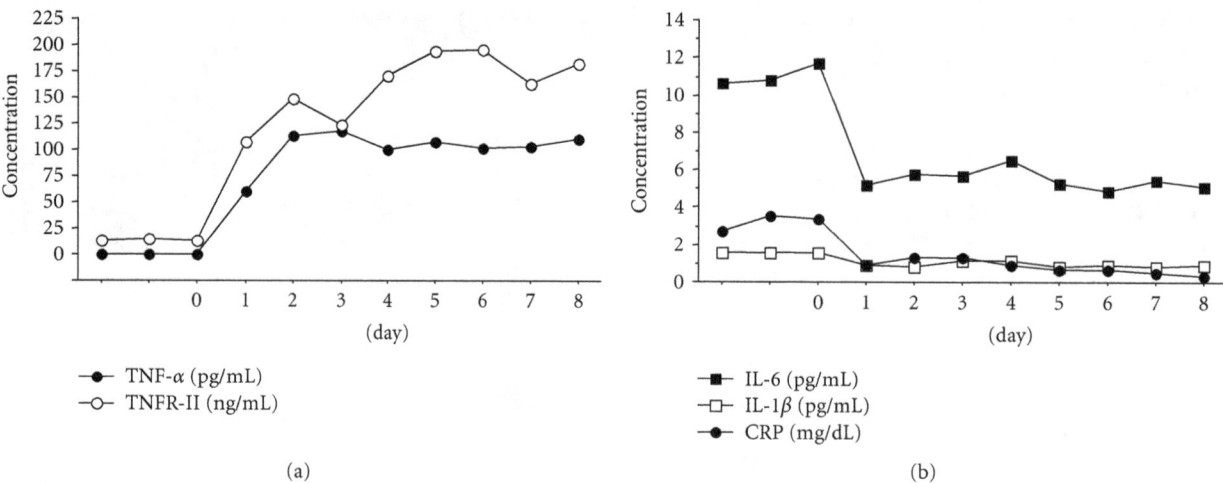

FIGURE 2: Time course of serum cytokines concentrations from baseline to 8 days. (a) TNF-*alpha* was not detectable in baseline samples. One day after the start of etanercept therapy TNF-*alpha* was measurable by ELISA. TNF-*alpha* levels became steady within 2 days of etanercept therapy. TNFR-II concentrations became elevated after the start of etanercept therapy. Within the first week of etanercept therapy, TNFR-II reached levels ranging from 160 ng/mL to 190 ng/mL. (b) Serum IL-6, IL-1 beta, and CRP concentrations were decreased just after the initiation of treatment.

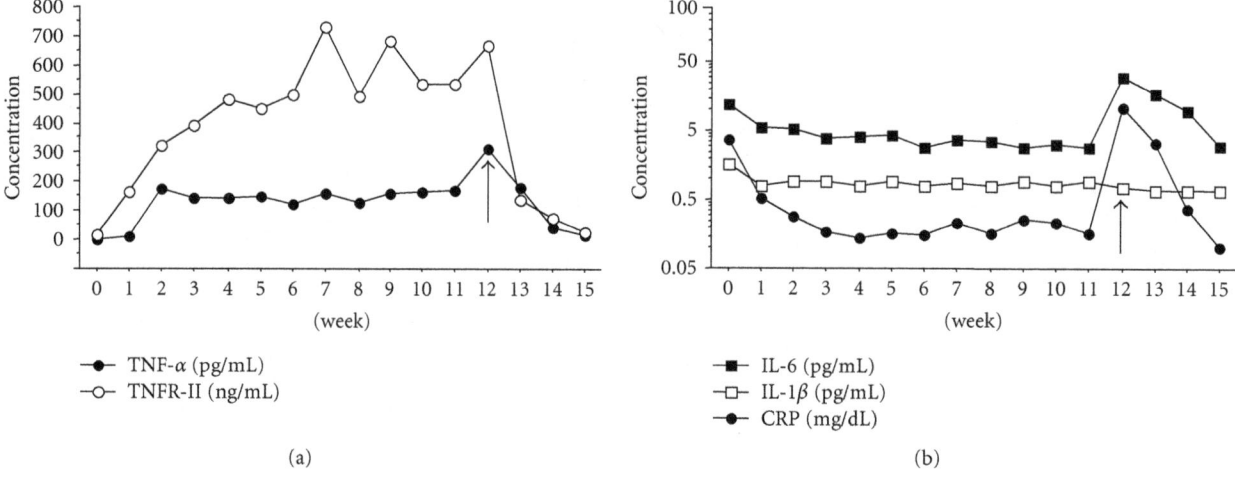

FIGURE 3: Time course of serum cytokines concentrations. (a) TNF-*alpha* concentration increased between weeks 1 and 2 after the initiation of etanercept therapy then remained steady ranging from 100 pg/mL to 170 pg/mL. At 12 weeks, the patient developed PCP and the TNF-*alpha* value increased steeply (arrow). With cessation of etanercept, the TNF-*alpha* concentration immediately returned to pretreatment levels. Four weeks after the initiation of therapy, the TNFR-II concentration became steady, ranging from 300 ng/mL to 700 ng/mL. With cessation of etanercept due to the PCP, TNFR-II concentration returned to pretreatment levels. (b) On the other hand, at week 12, the levels of IL-6, CRP, and TNF-*alpha* showed an acute peak (arrow), which tapered downward over the following 3 weeks with the institution of an appropriate antifungal regimen.

weeks 2, 4, 8, and 12 of IL-1 beta at week 4 and of TNFR-I at week 12 were significantly lower than before treatment [9]. Our data did not show remarkable changes in TNFR-I concentrations, but serum IL-6 and IL-1 beta concentrations were markedly decreased during the course of treatment. Trials have shown that etanercept therapy had significant clinical efficacy in patients with RA [10, 11]. It was suggested that clinical efficacy of etanercept was due to the reduction in CRP, IL-6, and IL-1 beta concentrations.

In general, therapies using biological agents have been highly effective in the treatment of RA. However, cases with serious adverse events have also been reported. Biologics may mask the clinical symptoms of infection because they diminish the production of acute inflammatory proteins [12]. In the case discussed here, CRP and IL-6 levels were found to be elevated when the patient developed PCP. Furthermore, the serum concentration of TNF-*alpha* increased by more than 300 pg/mL. Previously reported was a patient with high concentrations of TNF-*alpha* on etanercept therapy with development of gastric outlet obstruction, suggesting that serum TNF-*alpha* may rise in the early phase of the pneumonia, gastrointestinal obstruction, and other

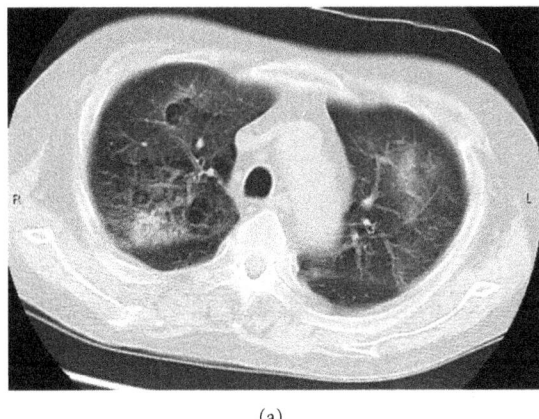

(a)

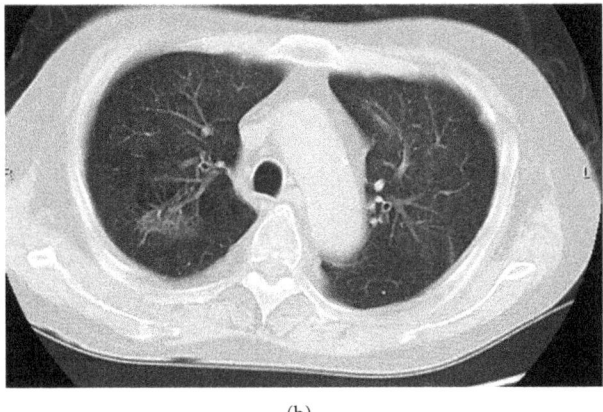

(b)

FIGURE 4: (a) Computed tomography scans on the day patient diagnosed as PCP showed infiltrates and reticular shadows. (b) The shadows disappeared after treatment with antifungal agents.

infectious/inflammatory complications [6]. Furthermore, we considered that endogenous TNF-*alpha* itself accounted for the majority of the elevated concentration of TNF-*alpha* at the time of pneumonia in this case. On the other hand, TNF-*alpha* concentrations were steady after the start of etanercept therapy until the cessation of the drug. This phenomenon might demonstrate that the TNF-*alpha* levels reflected the proper drug dosage in the course of etanercept treatment.

In conclusion, although TNF-*alpha* and TNFR-II concentrations measured by ELISA might consist of the TNF-etanercept complex and even etanercept itself, these concentrations could reflect the microenvironments in the course of etanercept therapy. Monitoring TNF-*alpha* levels might provide much information in terms of avoiding serious adverse events and evaluating clinical efficacy.

References

[1] H. Amital, V. Barak, R. E. Winkler, and A. Rubinow, "Impact of treatment with infliximab on serum cytokine profile of patients with rheumatoid and psoriatic arthritis," *Annals of the New York Academy of Sciences*, vol. 1110, pp. 649–660, 2007.

[2] C. Romero-Sánchez, W. H. Robinson, B. H. Tomooka et al., "Identification of acute phase reactants and cytokines useful for monitoring infliximab therapy in ankylosing spondylitis," *Clinical Rheumatology*, vol. 27, no. 11, pp. 1429–1435, 2008.

[3] K. L. Hyrich, K. D. Watson, A. J. Silman, D. P. M. Symmons, and The BSR Biologics Register, "Predictors of response to anti-TNF-α therapy among patients with rheumatoid arthritis: results from the British Society for Rheumatology Biologics Register," *Rheumatology*, vol. 45, no. 12, pp. 1558–1565, 2006.

[4] M. Feldmann, "Development of anti-TNF therapy for rheumatoid arthritis," *Nature Reviews Immunology*, vol. 2, no. 5, pp. 364–371, 2002.

[5] M. Sato, M. Takemura, R. Shinohe et al., "Soluble tumor necrosis factor receptor levels in sera and joint fluids of rheumatoid arthritis patients," *Rinsho Riumachi*, vol. 15, pp. 313–318, 2003 (Japanese).

[6] S. Madhusedan, M. Foster, S. R. Muthuramalingam et al., "A phase II study of etanercept (Enbrel), a tumor necrosis factor a inhibitor in patients with metastatic brest cancer," *Clinical Cancer Research*, vol. 10, pp. 6528–6534, 2004.

[7] L. W. Moreland, M. H. Schiff, S. W. Baumgartner et al., "Etanercept therapy in rheumatoid arthritis: a randomized, controlled trial," *Annals of Internal Medicine*, vol. 130, no. 6, pp. 478–486, 1999.

[8] A. Alldred, "Etanercept in rheumatoid arthritis," *Expert Opinion on Pharmacotherapy*, vol. 2, no. 7, pp. 1137–1148, 2001.

[9] M. Mori, S. Takei, T. Imagawa et al., "Pharmacokinetics, efficacy, and safety of short-term (12 weeks) etanercept for methotrexate-refractory polyarticular juvenile idiopathic arthritis in Japan," *Modern Rheumatology*, vol. 15, no. 6, pp. 397–404, 2005.

[10] L. Klareskog, D. van der Heijde, J. P. de Jager et al., "Therapeutic effect of the combination of etanercept and methotrexate compared with each treatment alone in patients with rheumatoid arthritis: double-blind randomised controlled trial," *The Lancet*, vol. 363, no. 9410, pp. 675–681, 2004.

[11] D. van der Heijde, L. Klareskog, V. Rodriguez-Valverde et al., "Comparison of etanercept and methotrexate, alone and combined, in the treatment of rheumatoid arthritis: two-year clinical and radiographic results from the TEMPO study, a double-blind, randomized trial," *Arthritis & Rheumatism*, vol. 54, no. 4, pp. 1063–1074, 2006.

[12] N. Miyasaka, T. Takeuchi, and K. Eguchi, "Guidelines for the proper use of etanercept in Japan," *Modern Rheumatology*, vol. 16, no. 2, pp. 63–67, 2006.

17

Report of a Rare Case of Gorham-Stout Disease of Both Shoulders: Bisphosphonate Treatment and Shoulder Replacement

Eike Garbers,[1] Falk Reuther,[1] and Gunther Delling[2]

[1] Klinik für Unfallchirurgie und Orthopaedie, DRK Kliniken Berlin Koepenick, Salvador-Allende-Straße 2-8, 12559 Berlin, Germany
[2] Institut für Pathologie Hannover, Berliner Allee 48, 30175 Hannover, Germany

Correspondence should be addressed to Eike Garbers, eike.garbers@gmail.com

Academic Editors: R. Cevik, C. Pineda, C. Saadeh, and F. Schiavon

Massive osteolysis known as Gorham-Stout disease is a rare idiopathic disorder typically affecting long bones in a unifocal pattern. Angiomatosis is strongly connected to the osteolysis. Weather angiomatosis is the cause or the result of osteolysis is subject of intense discussion (Kawasaki et al. (2003), Möller et al. (1999), Radhakrishnan and Rockson (2008)). There are about 200 cases described since 1955. Our patient is a 77-year-old female patient with osteolyses of both shoulders involving the proximal humerus, lateral clavicle, and the glenoid. Under bisphosphonate therapy, the progressive osteolysis stopped on the right side and showed progression on the left. With the patient complaining about severe rest pain and impaired function, we performed surgical reconstruction by implantation of total shoulder prosthesis three months after onset of symptoms. Our case shows a possibility of primary and early surgical reconstruction with good clinical outcome.

1. Introduction

Osteolyses are common findings on plain X-rays of the skeletal system. Most commonly, they are seen as secondary osteolyses due to an underlying hereditary, metabolic, or neoplastic condition [1, 2]. From these secondary osteolyses, we differentiate the rare group of idiopathic primary osteolyses. Hardegger et al. classified these in five groups as shown in Table 1 [1].

The Gorham-Stout disease (GSD; synonyms: massive osteolysis, vanishing bone disease) is a rare condition of unknown etiology characterized by semispecific histological findings and a typical radiological and clinical pattern resulting in progressive destruction and resorption of bony structures [3]. Typical histological findings include local osteoclastic hyperactivity and proliferation of small thin-walled arterial or lymphatic vessels (angiomatosis) [3–7]; radiological features include massive progressive osteolysis that does not respect anatomical borders and spread from the primary focus to adjoining bones [2, 8]. The idiopathic osteolysis is self-limiting after a variable amount of time. There is no specific treatment described yet; symptomatic therapy includes bisphosphonate medication, alpha-2b-interferon, radiation therapy, and surgical procedures as resection and endoprosthetic operation [9–12].

GSD was defined first by Gorham and Stout in 1955, where the authors suspected the local angiomatosis to result in a local hyperemia resulting in an alteration of the balance of osteoblastic and osteoclastic activity thus leading to massive osteolysis. In many cases, a minor trauma was described as an initiating event for the osteolysis and the authors hypothesized that the proliferation of a local angiomatosis might be triggered by a trauma mechanism [3].

The age of onset is variable; in about 200 reported cases, the majority were younger patients; there were no familiar disposition and no gender specific distribution. Typical unifocal localizations are the skull (18.3%), the pelvis (17.7%), the shoulder girdle (16.0%), the lower (14.9%), and the upper limb (11.4%); less often the spine, ribs, and the sternum were reported to be affected. The overall lethality is about 13.3%; involvement of the thorax typically including a chylothorax result in a poor prognosis with a lethality of

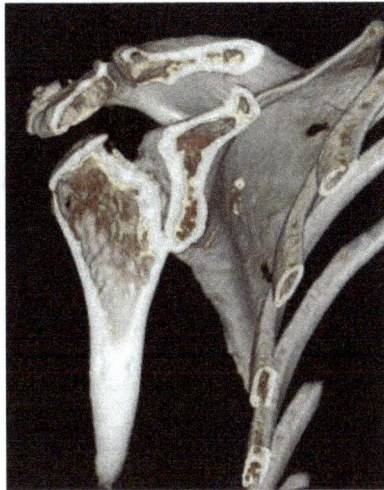

FIGURE 1: 3D reconstructed CT scan showing osteonecrosis of the humeral head, the acromion, lateral clavicle, and the glenoid in Gorham-Stout disease.

TABLE 1: Classification of idiopathic osteolyses [1].

Type 1: Hereditary multifocal osteolyses with dominant inheritance

Type 2: Hereditary multifocal osteolyses with recessive inheritance

Type 3: Nonhereditary multifocal osteolyses with nephropathia

Type 4: Gorham-Stout syndrome

Type 5: Winchester syndrome

TABLE 2: Criteria for the diagnosis of Gorham-Stout-disease [13].

(i) Positive histology (angiomatosis)

(ii) Absence of cellular atypicalities

(iii) Minimal or no osteoplastic reaction

(iv) Local progressing resorption of bone

(v) Absence of ulcerations

(vi) Absence of visceral involvement

(vii) Radiological finding of osteolysis

(viii) Ruling out of hereditary, metabolic, neoplastic, infectious, or immunological etiology

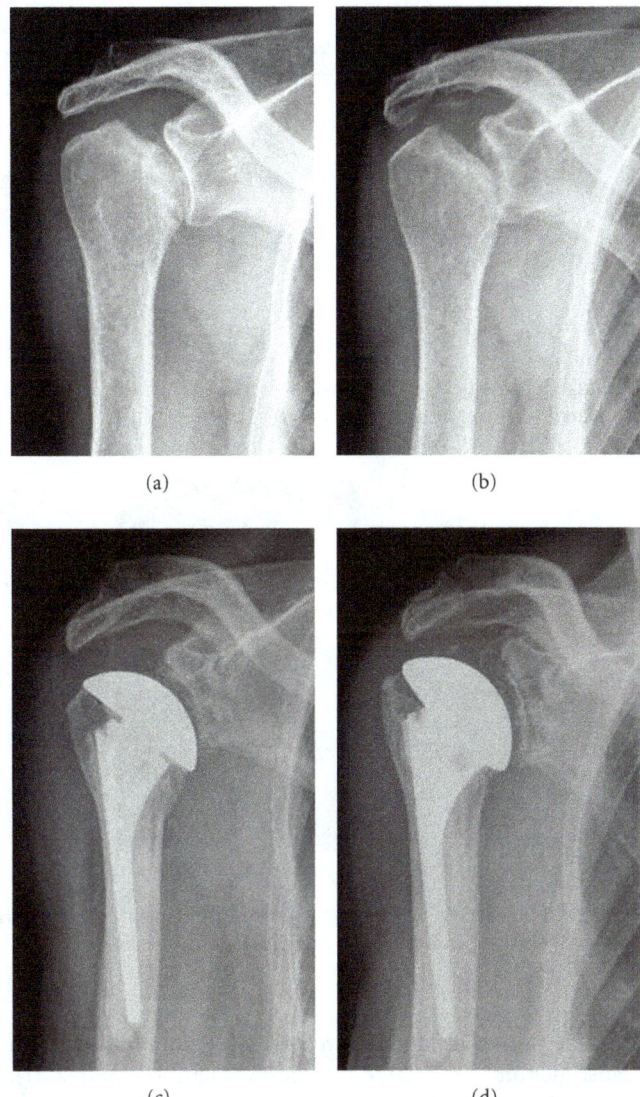

(a)

(b)

(c)

(d)

FIGURE 2: Plain true a.p. X-rays of the right shoulder on first admission in 12/2007 (a), after disease limitation under bisphosphonate therapy in 03/2008 (b), postoperative after implantation of total shoulder prosthesis (c), 1-year followup showing no progression of the osteolyses and no signs of loosening of the prosthesis (d).

52% [13–15]. Diagnostic criteria for the GSD are given in Table 2 and include radiological, histological, and clinical features after ruling out of hereditary, metabolic, neoplastic, infectious, or immunological sources of osteolyses [4, 13, 16].

2. Case Description

A 77-year-old woman who complained accentuated rest pain in both shoulders 8 weeks after minor trauma was admitted to our clinic. Past medical history includes chronic bronchial asthma without steroid medication, hyperthyroidism (radiotherapy 2005), cerebrovascular event without residual neurologic deficiency (1998), and osteoporosis with three osteoporotic lumbar spine fractures (vertebroplasty 2006). Plain

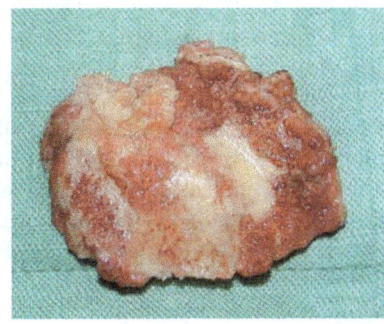

FIGURE 3: Macroscopic specimen of the humeral head showing massive osteolysis.

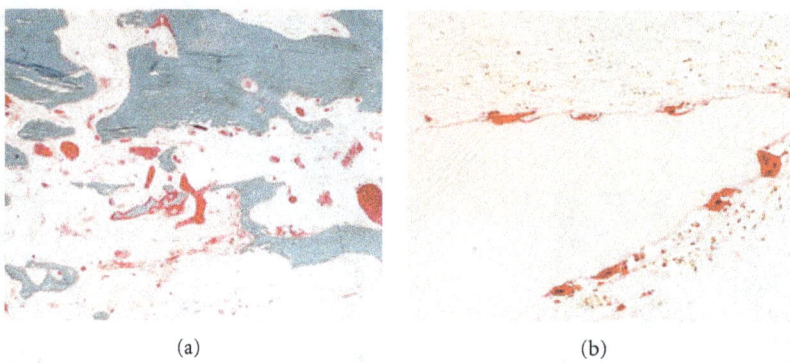

(a)   (b)

FIGURE 4: Histological stains showing altered osteoclastic resorption (acid phosphatase reaction 200x) (a); cortical and cancellous bone with stimulated turnover and marrow fibrosis (Goldner) (b).

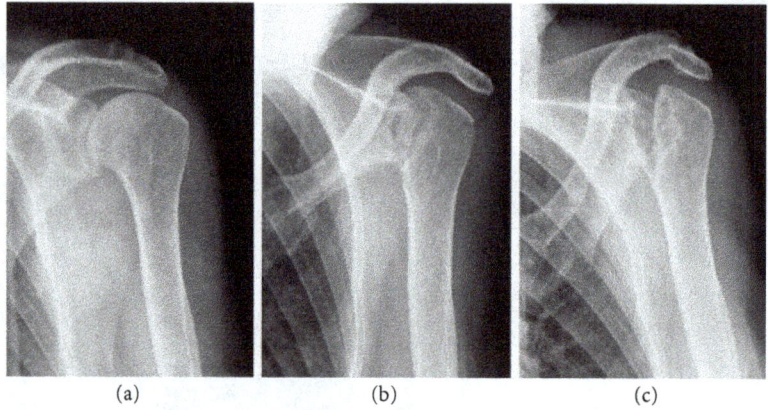

(a)   (b)   (c)

FIGURE 5: Plain true a.p. X-rays of the left shoulder in the same patient showing progressive osteolyses of the humeral head, the acromion, the lateral clavicle, and the glenoid in Gorham-Stout disease.

X-rays of both shoulders showed osteolyses of both humeral heads, glenoids, and lateral clavicles (Figures 1 and 2(a)). After ruling out of secondary osteolysis, we started the patient on bisphosphonates (alendronate 70 mg per week), calcium, and calcitonin. Early follow-up X-rays showed the termination of progressive osteolyses (Figure 2(b)). After clinical and radiological termination of the progressive disease after three months, the patient was readmitted with poor function and constant rest pain accentuated on the right side. After obtaining CT and MRI scans, we performed reconstruction on the right side by implantation of anatomical shoulder prosthesis (AFFINIS, Mathys Ltd., Switzerland). Intraoperative findings where massive synovitis with significant thickening of the capsule and massive osteolysis of the humeral head (Figure 3) and the glenoid. The rotator cuff was not affected. Pathological and microbiological specimens where taken and sent to a specialized laboratory. The cemented prosthesis was implanted in typical fashion; the glenoid was resurfaced with a polyethylene component. Microbiological specimens came back negative. Pathological findings confirmed macroscopic findings of a detritus-synovitis, massive osteoclastic resorption with stimulated osteoclastic resorption, edema, and fibroses of the bone marrow. These findings were consistent with Gorham-Stout syndrome (Figure 4).

On postoperative followup 1 year after surgery, the patient presented with significant improvement in function and pain. The ASES-Score [17] improved from 9.6 to 35, constant score [18] improved from 11% to 34%, and DASH score [14] improved from 81.6 to 59. Plain X-rays showed a correctly implanted prosthesis without signs of loosening; in the glenoid and the lateral clavicle we found minor progression of the osteolysis (Figure 2(d)).

3. Discussion

Our case is the first reported case of bilateral shoulder involvement in GSD. We were able to show the benefit of bisphosphonate therapy in disease control of Gorham Stout as the progression stopped about 3 month after initiation. The effectiveness of this therapy was described in detail before, and we can fully confirm these results [9, 12, 19]. Eventually, the osteolysis stopped in an early stage with limited bone loss. Because the patient complained of limited function and severe pain in both shoulders, we decided to do perform prosthetic replacement of the right glenohumeral joint. The left side showed comparable radiologic findings but the patient did not complain of severe pain and did not require surgical therapy (Figure 5). One year after surgery, the patient reported significant improvement in function and pain relief in the right shoulder represented in almost threefold enhancement in the shoulder scores as shown in results. For the timing of surgery, there is no clear guideline and surgeons are concerned about progression of the osteolysis resulting in loosening of the prosthesis. We performed a relatively early operation and achieved a good result without loosening of the prosthesis [20]. The histopathological specimens showed significant osteoclastic resorption with fibrosis and edema of the bone marrow. Even though the histological findings were not characteristic for the Gorham-Stout disease as they were described in the original paper, we made the diagnosis from the massive osteoclastic resorption without osteoblastic stimulation together with the classical clinical and radiological findings [1, 6, 15]. Histological specimens showed no ulcers; secondary osteonecrosis was ruled out by CT of the abdomen, laboratory tests, chest X-ray, and colonoscopy. Kawasaki et al. reported on an autopsy case of GSD and discussed our question—if angiomatosis is an intrinsic pathohistological feature of GSD—in detail [5]. They did not find any of the vascular changes in cases of GSD consistent with other authors before. They concluded that vascular proliferation might not always be associated with GSD but may be one of the results of disease rather than the cause [5].

Disclosure

The authors, or any member of their family, have not received any financial remuneration related to the subject of the paper.

References

[1] F. Hardegger, L. A. Simpson, and G. Segmueller, "The syndrome of idiopathic osteolysis. Classification, review, and case report," *Journal of Bone and Joint Surgery*, vol. 67, no. 1, pp. 89–93, 1985.

[2] D. V. Patel, "Gorham's disease or massive osteolysis," *Clinical Medicine & Research*, vol. 3, no. 2, pp. 65–74, 2005.

[3] L. W. Gorham and A. P. Stout, "Massive osteolysis (acute spontaneous absorption of bone, phantom bone, disappearing bone); its relation to hemangiomatosis," *The Journal of Bone and Joint Surgery*, vol. 37-A, no. 5, pp. 985–1004, 1955.

[4] D. Bruch-Gerharz, C. D. Gerharz, H. Stege et al., "Cutaneous Vascular Malformations in Disappearing Bone (Gorham-Stout) Disease," *JAMA*, vol. 289, no. 12, pp. 1479–1480, 2003.

[5] K. Kawasaki, T. Ito, T. Tsuchiya, and H. Takahashi, "Is angiomatosis an intrinsic pathohistological feature of massive osteolysis? Report of an autopsy case and a review of the literature," *Virchows Archiv*, vol. 442, no. 4, pp. 400–406, 2003.

[6] G. Möller, H. Gruber, M. Priemel, M. Werner, A. S. Kuhlmey, and G. Delling, "Gorham-Stout idiopathic osteolysis—a local osteoclastic hyperactivity?" *Pathologe*, vol. 20, no. 3, pp. 177–182, 1999.

[7] K. Radhakrishnan and S. G. Rockson, "Gorham's disease: an osseous disease of lymphangiogenesis?" *Annals of the New York Academy of Sciences*, vol. 1131, pp. 203–205, 2008.

[8] P. Boyer, P. Bourgeois, O. Boyer, Y. Catonné, and G. Saillant, "Massive Gorham-Stout syndrome of the pelvis," *Clinical Rheumatology*, vol. 24, no. 5, pp. 551–555, 2005.

[9] G. Lehmann, A. Pfeil, J. Böttcher et al., "Benefit of a 17-year long-term bisphosphonate therapy in a patient with Gorham-Stout syndrome," *Archives of Orthopaedic and Trauma Surgery*, vol. 129, no. 7, pp. 967–972, 2009.

[10] A. Pfleger, W. Schwinger, A. Maier, J. Tauss, H. H. Popper, and M. S. Zach, "Gorham-Stout syndrome in a male adolescent—case report and review of the literature," *Journal of Pediatric Hematology/Oncology*, vol. 28, no. 4, pp. 231–233, 2006.

[11] A. Takahashi, C. Ogawa, T. Kanazawa et al., "Remission induced by interferon alfa in a patient with massive osteolysis and extension of lymph-hemangiomatosis: a severe case of Gorham-Stout syndrome," *Journal of Pediatric Surgery*, vol. 40, no. 3, pp. E47–E50, 2005.

[12] F. Hammer, W. Kenn, U. Wesselmann et al., "Gorham-Stout disease—stabilization during bisphosphonate treatment," *Journal of Bone and Mineral Research*, vol. 20, no. 2, pp. 350–353, 2005.

[13] A. Florchinger, E. Bottger, F. Claass-Bottger, M. Georgi, and J. Harms, "Gorham-Stout syndrome of the spine. Case report and review of the literature," *Rofo*, vol. 168, no. 1, pp. 68–76, 1998.

[14] G. Germann, G. Wind, and A. Harth, "The DASH(Disability of Arm-Shoulder-Hand) Questionnaire—a new instrument for evaluating upper extremity treatment outcome," *Handchir Mikrochir Plast Chir*, vol. 31, no. 3, pp. 149–152, 1999.

[15] G. Moller, M. Priemel, M. Amling, M. Werner, A. S. Kuhlmey, and G. Delling, "The Gorham-Stout syndrome (Gorham's massive osteolysis). A report of six cases with histopathological findings," *Journal of Bone and Joint Surgery*, vol. 81, no. 3, pp. 501–506, 1999.

[16] D. Bruch-Gerharz, C. D. Gerharz, H. Stege et al., "Cutaneous lymphatic malformations in disappearing bone (Gorham-Stout) disease: a novel clue to the pathogenesis of a rare syndrome," *Journal of the American Academy of Dermatology*, vol. 56, supplement 2, pp. S21–S25, 2007.

[17] P. M. McClure and L. Michener, "Measures of adult shoulder function," *Arthritis & Rheumatism*, vol. 49, no. 5S, pp. 50–58, 2003.

[18] C. R. Constant and A. H. Murley, "A clinical method of functional assessment of the shoulder," *Clinical Orthopaedics and Related Research*, vol. 214, pp. 160–164, 1987.

[19] M. Lehnhardt, H. U. Steinau, H. H. Homann, L. Steinstraesser, and D. Druecke, "Gorham-Stout disease: report of a case affecting the right hand with a follow-up of 24 years," *Handchirurgie Mikrochirurgie Plastische Chirurgie*, vol. 36, no. 4, pp. 249–254, 2004.

[20] B. Sestan and D. Miletic, "Rapid idiopathic osteolysis of the humeral head and clavicle," *West Indian Medical Journal*, vol. 55, no. 5, pp. 354–357, 2006.

18

Bullous Systemic Lupus Erythematosus Associated with Esophagitis Dissecans Superficialis

Meera Yogarajah, Bhradeev Sivasambu, and Eric A. Jaffe

Department of Medicine, Interfaith Medical Center, Brooklyn, NY 11213, USA

Correspondence should be addressed to Meera Yogarajah; myogarajah@interfaithmedical.com

Academic Editor: Tsai-Ching Hsu

Bullous systemic lupus erythematosus is one of the rare autoantibody mediated skin manifestation of systemic lupus erythematosus (SLE) demonstrating subepidermal blistering with neutrophilic infiltrate histologically. We present a case of a 40-year-old Hispanic female who presented with a several months' history of multiple blistering pruritic skin lesions involving the face and trunk, a photosensitive rash over the face and neck, swelling of the right neck lymph node, and joint pain involving her elbows and wrist. Her malady was diagnosed as bullous systemic lupus erythematosus based on the immunological workup and biopsy of her skin lesions. The patient also complained of odynophagia and endoscopy revealed esophagitis dissecans superficialis which is a rare endoscopic finding characterized by sloughing of the esophageal mucosa. The bullous disorders typically associated with esophagitis dissecans superficialis are pemphigus and rarely bullous pemphigoid. However, this is the first reported case of bullous systemic lupus erythematosus associated with esophagitis dissecans superficialis.

1. Introduction

Bullous systemic lupus erythematosus is a subepidermal blistering disease mediated by autoantibodies that occurs in patients with SLE. The first case of bullous systemic lupus erythematosus was described in 1973. Esophagitis dissecans superficialis is a rare endoscopic finding characterized by sloughing of the entire length of the esophageal mucosal epithelium. Esophagitis dissecans superficialis has not been described with bullous systemic lupus erythematosus.

2. Case Report

A 40-year-old Hispanic woman with bronchial asthma and major depression was admitted complaining of a several months' history of multiple blistering pruritic skin lesions involving her face and trunk, a photosensitivity rash over her face and neck, swelling of a lymph node in her right neck, and joint pain involving her elbows and wrists. These symptoms were associated with hair loss. She also complained of painful swallowing of both solids and liquids. However, she denied symptoms of Raynaud's phenomenon, exertional dyspnea, hematuria, and proximal muscle weakness or pain.

On examination, she had pink conjunctiva, an erythematous malar rash, painless superficial oral ulcers, and a solitary nontender right-sided cervical lymph node. She also had vesicular lesions over her face and trunk with excoriations. Her elbows and wrist joints were tender but without swelling. Examination of her central nervous system was normal.

Our differential diagnosis included bullous systemic lupus erythematosus, epidermolysis bullosa acquisita, dermatitis herpetiformis, and bullous pemphigoid.

Initial workup revealed a normal complete blood count and comprehensive metabolic panel. Her autoimmune workup was significantly positive for anti-nuclear antibody (ANA) with a titer of 279 IU/mL (NR < 7.5), anti-double-stranded DNA antibody (ds-DNA) with a titer of 119 IU/mL (NR < 9), and anti-Smith antibody with a titer >8 AI (NR < 0.9). Tests for anti-ribonucleoprotein (anti-RNP) antibody, anti-centromere antibody, anti-topoisomerase-1 (anti-SCL-70), anti-Jo-1 antibody, anti-SSA antibody, and anti-SSB antibody were negative. Her erythrocyte sedimentation rate (ESR) was 18 and C-reactive protein (CRP) was 1.8 mg/L (normal 0–4.8) and complement levels were normal. Anti-neutrophil cytoplasmic antibody (ANCA) panel was

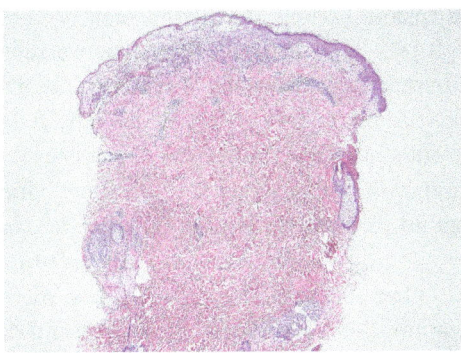

FIGURE 1: A low power (4x) skin H&E image reveals superficial band-like and perivascular inflammatory infiltrate with overlying epidermal necrosis and vesiculation.

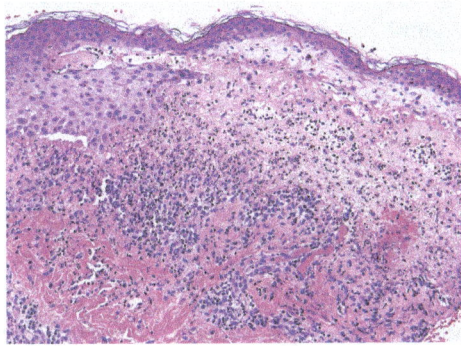

FIGURE 2: A higher power (20x) skin H&E image reveals abundant neutrophils and scattered eosinophils with a focal subepidermal split. Epidermal necrosis is again noted.

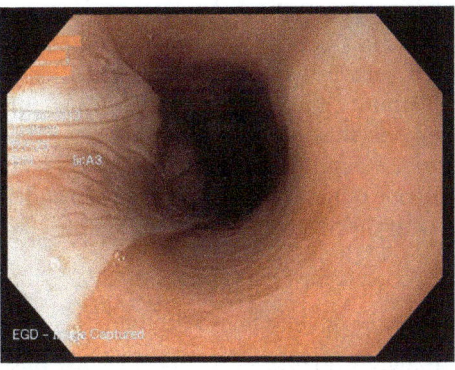

(a)

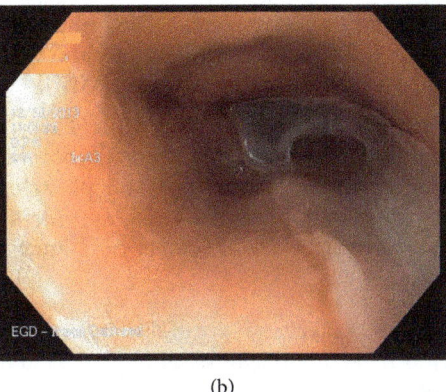

(b)

FIGURE 3: EGD showing vertical fissures in the distal esophagus with sloughing of the mucosa.

negative. Biopsy of her cervical lymph showed follicular hyperplasia.

Skin biopsy showed subepidermal vesicular dermatitis with overlying epidermal necrosis, predominantly neutrophilic infiltrate and focal interface changes (Figures 1 and 2). These findings suggested the presence of an immunoblistering process or a bullous drug eruption. Direct immunofluorescence did not show any abnormal deposits of IgG, IgM, IgA, C3, or fibrin in the epidermis or blood vessels but did reveal linear deposits of C3 and IgG and weak linear deposit of IgM in the basement membrane. No IgA or fibrin deposits were detected in the basement membrane.

These findings can be seen in bullous pemphigoid, epidermolysis bullosa acquisita, and bullous systemic lupus erythematosus. A direct immunofluorescence of the salt-split skin demonstrated linear deposit of C3 and IgG and weak linear deposit of IgM on the dermal floor side of the salt-split skin which was consistent with bullous systemic lupus erythematosus as the patient also fulfilled the ACR criteria for diagnosis of SLE.

However, as the patient also complained of painful swallowing, mixed connective tissue disease with dysphagia due to systemic sclerosis was a concern. Tests for anti-ribonucleoprotein (anti-RNP) antibody, anti-centromere antibody, anti-topoisomerase I (anti-SCL70), and anti-Jo-1

antibody were negative. Polymyositis was unlikely as patient did not have any muscle weakness and her creatine kinase and aldolase levels were normal.

She underwent endoscopy which showed sloughing of the esophageal mucosa suggestive of esophagitis dissecans superficialis (Figures 3(a) and 3(b)) and biopsy revealed chronic inflammatory changes with no evidence of yeast or pseudohyphae invasion.

We are presenting a case of bullous systemic lupus erythematosus associated with esophagitis dissecans superficialis. There have been reported cases of esophagitis dissecans superficialis associated with bullous autoimmune disorders mainly pemphigus. However, this is the first reported case of esophagitis dissecans superficialis associated with bullous systemic lupus erythematosus.

3. Discussion

Bullous systemic lupus erythematosus is an autoantibody mediated subepidermal blistering disease that occurs in patients with SLE [1]. The first case of bullous systemic lupus erythematosus was described by Pedro and Dahl in 1973 [2].

Severe cutaneous lupus erythematosus can present as vesiculobullous lesions due to extensive damage of epidermal basal layer. As all bullous lesions occurring in SLE patients are not bullous systemic lupus erythematosus, a criterion to diagnose bullous systemic lupus erythematosus was initially proposed by Camisa and Sharma [3]. Then Gammon and Briggaman [4] classified bullous systemic lupus erythematosus into two subtypes, type 1 with circulating antibodies and type 2 without circulating antibodies. Currently, bullous systemic lupus erythematosus is classified into 3 subtypes [5]. The diagnosis of bullous systemic lupus erythematosus type 1 requires all five of the following. But types 2 and 3 could be diagnosed with the first four criteria [5, 6]:

(i) ACR criteria for the diagnosis of SLE,

(ii) acquired vesiculobullous eruption,

(iii) histologic evidence of a subepidermal blister and a predominantly neutrophilic dermal infiltrate,

(iv) direct immunofluorescence (DIF) microscopy demonstrating IgG with or without IgA and IgM deposits at the basement membrane zone (BMZ),

(v) evidence of antibodies to type VII collagen via direct immunofluorescence (DIF) microscopy or indirect immunofluorescence (IIF) on salt-split skin, immunoblotting, immunoprecipitation, enzyme-linked immunosorbent assay (ELISA), or immunoelectron microscopy.

All of the above criteria were fulfilled in our patient and allowed us to make the diagnosis of bullous systemic lupus erythematosus type 1.

The differential diagnosis of blistering eruptions in patients with SLE includes dermatitis herpetiformis [5], bullous pemphigoid [7, 8], epidermolysis bullosa acquisita [9], and bullous systemic lupus erythematosus [10, 11]. Dermatitis herpetiformis [12] can be differentiated by light microscopy and direct immunofluorescence. Bullous pemphigoid, epidermolysis bullosa acquisita, and bullous systemic lupus erythematosus demonstrate similar direct immunofluorescence patterns. Salt-split skin test [13] demonstrates IgG antibodies on the epidermal side (roof pattern) of the split skin in bullous pemphigoid as opposed to epidermolysis bullosa acquisita [14] and bullous systemic lupus erythematosus [15] that demonstrate IgG antibodies on the dermal side (floor pattern) of the split skin and therefore is difficult to differentiate. Presence of ACR criteria for the diagnosis of SLE favors the diagnosis of bullous systemic lupus erythematosus.

Esophagitis dissecans superficialis is a rare endoscopic finding characterized by sloughing of the entire length of the esophageal mucosal epithelium. This was first described by Carmack [16]. It has been associated with bisphosphonates [17], nonsteroidal anti-inflammatory drugs [15], celiac disease [18], collagen disease [19], and autoimmune bullous disease typically pemphigus vulgaris [20]. There have been few reported cases associated with bullous pemphigoid [21]. However, there have been no reported cases of bullous systemic lupus erythematosus associated with esophagitis dissecans superficialis. It is very rare to get esophagitis dissecans superficialis with a subepidermal blistering disorder as it has antibodies against the epithelial basement membrane as in bullous systemic lupus erythematosus and the treatment of choice is steroids. Our patient was started on steroids and the odynophagia improved.

In conclusion, bullous skin lesions can be seen in SLE and though is a rare skin manifestation, warrants a skin biopsy with immunofluorescence studies to make a diagnosis of bullous systemic lupus erythematosus. The treatment of choice for bullous systemic lupus erythematosus is dapsone [22]. Steroid is the other alternative drug for patients who fail to respond to dapsone, have intolerance to dapsone, or have other systemic manifestations of SLE warranting steroid treatment. Other therapeutic options include methotrexate (MTX), azathioprine, mycophenolate mofetil, and rituximab.

This case highlights the importance of endoscopy in a patient with bullous systemic lupus erythematosus who complains of odynophagia as it is necessary to make the correct diagnosis since esophagitis dissecans superficialis and bullous systemic lupus erythematosus are treated differently.

References

[1] L. Uva, D. Miguel, C. Pinheiro, J. P. Freitas, M. Marques Gomes, and P. Filipe, "Cutaneous manifestations of systemic lupus erythematosus," *Autoimmune Diseases*, vol. 2012, Article ID 834291, 15 pages, 2012.

[2] S. D. Pedro and M. V. Dahl, "Direct immunofluorescence of bullous systemic lupus erythematosus," *Archives of Dermatology*, vol. 107, no. 1, pp. 118–120, 1973.

[3] C. Camisa and H. M. Sharma, "Vesiculobullous systemic lupus erythematosus. Report of two cases and a review of the literature," *Journal of the American Academy of Dermatology*, vol. 9, no. 6, pp. 924–933, 1983.

[4] W. R. Gammon and R. A. Briggaman, "Epidermolysis bullosa acquisita and bullous systemic lupus erythematosus: diseases of autoimmunity to type VII collagen," *Dermatologic Clinics*, vol. 11, no. 3, pp. 535–547, 1993.

[5] I. D. Camacho, H. D. Johnson-Jahangir, and J. V. Schaffer, Bullous Systemic Lupus Erythematosus, http://emedicine.medscape.com/article/1065402.

[6] P. Patrício, C. Ferreira, M. M. Gomes, and P. Filipe, "Autoimmune bullous dermatoses: a review," *Annals of the New York Academy of Sciences*, vol. 1173, pp. 203–210, 2009.

[7] R. E. Jordon, S. A. Muller, W. L. Hale, and E. H. Beutner, "Bullous pemphigoid associated with systemic lupus erythematosus," *Archives of Dermatology*, vol. 99, no. 1, pp. 17–25, 1969.

[8] V. Kumar, W. L. Binder, E. Schotland, E. H. Beutner, and T. P. Chorzelski, "Coexistence of bullous pemphigoid and systemic lupus erythematosus," *Archives of Dermatology*, vol. 114, no. 8, pp. 1187–1190, 1978.

[9] G. Obermoser, R. D. Sontheimer, and B. Zelger, "Overview of common, rare and atypical manifestations of cutaneous lupus erythematosus and histopathological correlates," *Lupus*, vol. 19, no. 9, pp. 1050–1070, 2010.

[10] S. Vassileva, "Bullous systemic lupus erythematosus," *Clinics in Dermatology*, vol. 22, no. 2, pp. 129–138, 2004.

[11] P. Bernard, L. Vaillant, B. Labeille et al., "Incidence and distribution of subepidermal autoimmune bullous skin diseases

in three French regions," *Archives of Dermatology*, vol. 131, no. 1, pp. 48–52, 1995.

[12] E. A. I. M. Freedberg, K. Wolff, S. I. Katz et al., *Dermatitis Herpetiformis. Fitzpatrick's Dermatology in General Medicine*, McGraw-Hill, Health Professions Division, New York, NY, USA, 5th edition, 1999.

[13] W. R. Gammon, J. D. Fine, M. Forbes, and R. A. Briggaman, "Immunofluorescence on split skin for the detection and differentiation of basement membrane zone autoantibodies," *Journal of the American Academy of Dermatology*, vol. 27, no. 1, pp. 79–87, 1992.

[14] D. T. Woodley, R. A. Briggaman, E. J. O'Keefe, A. O. Inman, L. L. Queen, and W. R. Gammon, "Identification of the skin basement-membrane autoantigen in epidermolysis bullosa acquisita," *The New England Journal of Medicine*, vol. 310, no. 16, pp. 1007–1013, 1984.

[15] L. S. Chan, J. C. Lapiere, M. Chen et al., "Bullous systemic lupus erythematosus with autoantibodies recognizing multiple skin basement membrane components, bullous pemphigoid antigen 1, laminin-5, laminin-6, and type VII collagen," *Archives of Dermatology*, vol. 135, no. 5, pp. 569–573, 1999.

[16] S. W. Carmack, R. Vemulapalli, S. J. Spechler, and R. M. Genta, "Esophagitis dissecans superficialis ('sloughing esophagitis'): a clinicopathologic study of 12 cases," *The American Journal of Surgical Pathology*, vol. 33, no. 12, pp. 1789–1794, 2009.

[17] A. Hokama, Y. Ihama, M. Nakamoto, N. Kinjo, F. Kinjo, and J. Fujita, "Esophagitis dissecans superficialis associated with bisphosphonates," *Endoscopy*, vol. 39, supplement 1, article E91, 2007.

[18] G. Hage-Nassar, H. Rotterdam, D. Frank, and P. H. R. Green, "Esophagitis dissecans superficialis associated with celiac disease," *Gastrointestinal Endoscopy*, vol. 57, no. 1, pp. 140–141, 2003.

[19] N. K. Patel, C. Salathé, C. Vu, and S. H. Anderson, "Esophagitis dissecans: a rare cause of odynophagia," *Endoscopy*, vol. 39, E127, 2007.

[20] R. P. Kaplan, J. Touloukian, A. R. Ahmed, and V. D. Newcomer, "Esophagitis dissecans superficialis associated with pemphigus vulgaris," *Journal of the American Academy of Dermatology*, vol. 4, no. 6, pp. 682–687, 1981.

[21] B. M. Tijjani, I. Masoodi, and S. N. Hassan, "Esophagitis dissecans superficialis presenting with massive haematemesis in a patient with bullous pemphigoid," *Nigerian Journal of Medicine*, vol. 22, no. 4, pp. 354–356, 2013.

[22] R. P. Hall, T. J. Lawley, H. R. Smith, and S. I. Katz, "Bullous eruption of systemic lupus erythematosus. Dramatic response to dapsone therapy," *Annals of Internal Medicine*, vol. 97, no. 2, pp. 165–170, 1982.

19

A Case of Docetaxel Induced Myositis and Review of the Literature

Alexandra Perel-Winkler,[1] Regina Belokovskaya,[1] Isabelle Amigues,[1] Melissa Larusso,[2] and Nazia Hussain[2]

[1]Department of Medicine, St. Luke's-Roosevelt Hospital Center, and Department of Medicine, Icahn School of Medicine at Mount Sinai, New York, NY 10025, USA
[2]Division of Rheumatology, Department of Medicine, St. Luke's-Roosevelt Hospital Center, and Department of Medicine, Icahn School of Medicine at Mount Sinai, New York, NY 10025, USA

Correspondence should be addressed to Alexandra Perel-Winkler; alexandracpw@gmail.com

Academic Editor: Toshiaki Takahashi

In phase I and II trials taxane chemotherapeutic agents reported side effects, including myelosuppression, peripheral edema, and fluid retention. With further use of these agents, studies in the late 1980s and early 1990s began to report peripheral neuropathy and proximal muscle weakness as common complaints, the later with unexplained pathophysiology. We report a 65-year-old Hispanic woman with estrogen receptor (ER) and progesterone receptor (PR) positive invasive ductal breast carcinoma who presented with right thigh pain and swelling eight days after her third infusion of docetaxel (a taxane chemotherapeutic) and cyclophosphamide. Laboratory findings were notable for elevation in creatine phosphokinase (CPK), aldolase, and erythrocyte sedimentation rate (ESR); a magnetic resonance imaging (MRI) of her lower extremities showed evidence of bilateral muscle edema involving the anterior compartment muscles of the thighs. A workup to rule out other causes of myositis was negative. Docetaxel was not reintroduced and the patient improved with corticosteroids. Since 2005 this is, to our knowledge, the fifth reported case of docetaxel related inflammatory myositis. Taxanes have been noted to cause disabling but transient arthralgias and myalgias; it is important to consider the possibility of inflammatory myopathy as a possible complication in patients undergoing treatment with these agents.

1. Introduction

Taxane drugs, paclitaxel and docetaxel, are chemotherapeutic agents which work by disrupting microtubule function to inhibit cell division. Docetaxel has become a frequently used agent, known for its efficacy in solid tumors, primarily breast cancer, metastatic prostate cancer, and non-small cell lung cancer. Breast cancer is the most common cancer and the second leading cause of cancer death in American women [1]. Medical advances have considerably improved survival, largely due to newer anticancer medications. With efficiency, these agents also come with new side effects which physicians should be made aware of. Both paclitaxel and docetaxel (the taxanes) are known to cause myalgias, arthralgias, and neuropathy; however, there are few studies describing direct muscle inflammation caused by these agents. Myositis, an inflammation of muscle, can be caused by injury, infection,

medications, toxins, exercise, or autoimmune disease. In this report we describe the case of a patient who developed a case of docetaxel induced myositis when undergoing treatment for invasive ductal breast cancer. We will also include a description of other inflammatory muscle reactions in the setting of taxane agents.

2. Case

A 65-year-old Hispanic female presented to our Emergency Department with one week of right thigh pain and swelling. Her past medical history includes asthma, peripheral vascular disease, coronary artery disease, seizure disorder, hypertension, and hyperlipidemia. She was diagnosed with poorly differentiated invasive ductal carcinoma, with estrogen and progesterone receptor (ER and PR) positivity and human epidermal growth receptor 2 (HER2) negative, of her right

TABLE 1: Home medications.

Medication	Dose
Amlodipine besylate	5 mg daily
Aspirin	81 mg daily
Nebivalol	5 mg daily
Dexamethasone	4 mg (2 tablets BID, only for 3 days starting 1 day before chemotherapy)
Docusate sodium	100 mg daily PRN
Ferrous sulfate	325 mg BID
Folic acid	1 mg daily
Hydrochlorothiazide	12.5 mg daily
Hydrocodone-acetaminophen	5–500 mg daily PRN
Levetiracetam	750 mg q 12 hours
Insulin glargine	45 units at bedtime
Linaclotide	145 mcg daily
Pregabalin	25 mg daily
Meclizine	12.5 mg 2 tablets daily
Memantine HCl	5 mg daily
Metoclopramide	10 mg q 6 hours PRN
Pegfilgrastim	6 mg once SubQ per chemotherapy cycle, beginning 24–72 hours after completion of chemotherapy
Esomeprazole	40 mg daily
Insulin aspart	12 units TIDAC
Ondansetron	8 mg TID for 2 days after chemotherapy
Prasugrel	5 mg daily
Ranitidine	150 mg daily
Rosuvastatin	10 mg daily
Trazodone	50 mg at bedtime
Vitamin C	500 mg 2 tabs. daily

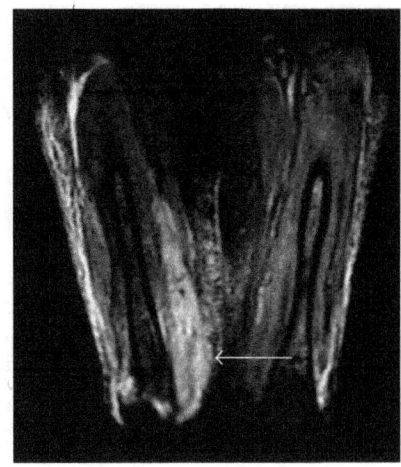

FIGURE 1: Axial T2-weighted FAT SAT image illustrating diffuse muscle edema involving the lower two-thirds of the anterior compartment muscles.

breast in July 2013. She underwent a right breast lumpectomy and was started on adjuvant chemotherapy with a plan for 4 cycles of docetaxel 75 mg/m^2 IV and cyclophosphamide 600 mg/m^2 IV every 3 weeks. She completed 3 cycles and had tolerated the treatment well with no notable side effects, until she presented to the ED eight days after the last infusion complaining of right thigh pain. Her medications at the time of presentation are listed in Table 1. No changes had been made to any of her medications in the last few months prior to this presentation.

The patient had begun to develop rapidly progressive pain and swelling of her right thigh, without complaints of weakness, eight days after her third infusion of docetaxel and cyclophosphamide. On examination, she was hemodynamically stable and afebrile. Her right thigh was erythematous and tender to light touch. She had decreased active range of motion of her right hip. There were no skin lesions. Her neurological examination was unremarkable; she had neither objective muscle weakness nor sensory deficit and

had normal deep tendon reflexes. There was no fasciculation or muscle wasting. Her distal pulses were palpable.

Basic laboratory values demonstrated a leukocytosis of 12×10^9/L. There were no electrolyte abnormalities. Her creatinine phosphokinase (CPK) was elevated to 341 (normal range: 30–135 U/L), her aldolase was 13.3 (normal range: ≤8.1 U/L), and her erythrocyte sedimentation rate (ESR) was 38 (normal range: 0–24 mm/hr). Autoantibodies including antinuclear antibody, double stranded DNA, anti-Smith, rheumatoid factor, cyclic citrullinated peptide, anti-Ro (SSA) and anti-La (SSB), ribonucleoprotein, and Scl 70 were all negative.

Initially, the unilateral thigh pain and swelling in a patient undergoing chemotherapy and on oral steroids raised suspicion for cellulitis. The patient was commenced on a 7-day treatment of IV Vancomycin and Cefepime and transitioned to oral Clindamycin and Augmentin after the first week of antibiotics. The patient's right thigh pain did not improve while on antibiotics. An MRI of the thighs was done (Figures 1 and 2), which demonstrated diffuse muscle edema involving the lower two-thirds of the anterior compartment muscles. There was also patchy edema of the posterior compartment muscles especially at the level of the mid belly of the semitendinosus. On postgadolinium injection images, there were patchy areas of nonenhancement in some of the anterior compartment muscles. Small patch of nonenhancement was also noted in the long head of the rectus femoris. Subcutaneous edematous changes were noted especially along the lateral aspect of the thigh. Partially visualized left thigh images also showed muscle edema along the superior aspect of the rectus femoris and inferior aspect of the posterior compartment muscles. Gadolinium injection enhancement images were suggestive of myonecrosis. The overall findings were consistent with nonspecific myositis.

Upon review of her diagnostic results, recent medications, and chemotherapy treatments, it was suspected that docetaxel was the offending agent causing the myositis.

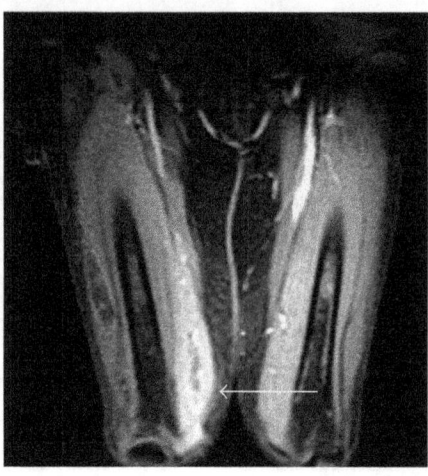

FIGURE 2: Coronal T2-weighted FAT SAT showing diffuse muscle edema involving the lower two-thirds of the anterior compartment muscles. The left thigh also shows muscle edema especially along the superior aspect of the rectus femoris and inferior aspect of the posterior compartment muscles.

Antibiotics were discontinued and the patient was commenced on prednisone 20 mg orally for 9 days and tapered down to 10 mg orally for another 5 days. The patient's symptoms improved significantly, including the erythema, tenderness, swelling, and range of motion. Her CPK normalized the day after prednisone was initiated.

Eight months after the last docetaxel treatment the patient remains asymptomatic without evidence of recurrent myositis. After her discharge the patient was treated with 4 months of radiation therapy. The patient is currently being treated with an aromatase inhibitor.

3. Discussion

Our case describes a patient with ER and PR + invasive ductal carcinoma presenting with unilateral thigh pain and swelling after her third cycle of docetaxel. Due to the asymmetric presentation the patient was initially treated for cellulitis without improvement. Further evaluation by MRI showed evidence of bilateral myositis, despite the unilateral symptoms. The MRI results alongside elevated CPK levels suggested acute myositis. The patient improved with a prednisone taper and symptoms did not recur after cessation of docetaxel treatment. It is important to note the rapid resolution of CPK, which is unusual for myositis. In this case, the presumed offending agent, docetaxel, had been held for almost two weeks at the point of diagnosis and an element of spontaneous resolution is to be expected.

Docetaxel is a taxane chemotherapeutic agent, which promotes the polymerization and inhibits depolymerization of microtubules causing interference of cell division. Docetaxel has been used with efficacy, usually in combination with another chemotherapeutic agent, in breast, ovarian, refractory prostate, head and neck, gastric, and non-small cell lung cancers [10]. The most commonly recorded side effects

of taxane agents are peripheral edema and fluid retention; however, the drug can cause dose dependent, severe myelosuppression, most commonly neutropenia. Myalgia and neuropathies were not noted as common taxane side effects in the early trials; however, studies in the late 1980s to mid-1990s began reporting frequent peripheral neuropathy [11–13] and myalgias [14–18] as side effects in patients receiving docetaxel. Neuropathy, paresthesia, myalgias, and arthralgias are now known to be common complications of these chemotherapeutic agents, recognized mostly by clinicians due to patient discomfort. These complaints, however, have not been considered significant by the research community, as they are not an indication for cessation of treatment. More recent research has shown that, despite the description of these side effects as "not significant" in most of phase II and subsequent trials, clinical experience and recent evidence are showing that up to 79% of patients develop toxicity leading to pain during treatment with taxanes [19]. While myositis has not been commonly attributed to these drugs, it is an important consideration in light of the large degree of patient who reported myalgias, weakness, and pain.

While Lipton et al. were the first to report taxane induced neuropathy in 1989 [20], in 1996 Freilich et al. described evidence of proximal muscle weakness in patients participating in phase II docetaxel trials. In this study 60 patients were prospectively followed as they were treated with docetaxel (fifty-four) or paclitaxel (six). The authors evaluated neurologic complications. Seven patients in the docetaxel group developed weakness, graded as "mild objective weakness without significant impairment of function." Other neurologic side effects were also reported including impairment of cutaneous sensation (two) and diminished reflexes (two). Interestingly, in 40% of patients treated with docetaxel who did not develop weakness, proximal myalgia was reported. In all patients, weakness abated after 1 to 2 months of drug cessation. The authors hypothesized that docetaxel may cause an idiosyncratic weakness that may occur at any stage of treatment and is associated with a predominantly proximal myopathy. The mechanism of the described proximal muscle weakness was unclear. Electrodiagnostic studies revealed a range of abnormalities including axonal sensorimotor neuropathy, multilevel radiculopathies, and absent lower limb motor and sensory responses. Of note, all patients had a reported CPK in normal range, suggesting a neuropathic etiology of weakness [21].

In 2005, two reports documented cases of acute inflammatory myositis developing in patients treated with docetaxel. Ardavanis et al. described the case of a 57-year-old man treated with a combination of gemcitabine and docetaxel for non-small cell lung cancer with positive results. After his fourth cycle of treatment the patient developed a symmetric proximal muscle weakness with elevations of CPK, lactate dehydrogenase (LDH), and aldolase. EMG and MRI investigation was not pursued due to the classic clinical picture and supportive lab results. The patient was treated with methylprednisolone and had resolution of muscle symptoms and normalization of enzymes within four weeks [2].

Hughes and Stuart-Harris described another case of docetaxel associated myositis in a 47-year-old woman with

ER and PR + metastatic breast carcinoma. The patient experienced bilateral foot pain during her first cycle of treatment, which resolved between treatment cycles, and recurred after her second cycle with spontaneous resolution. After her third cycle of treatment the patient experienced a recurrence of her bilateral pain associated with weakness of her proximal lower extremities. The weakness progressed over 10 days to the point of difficulty with ambulation and transferring. The patient was found to have a markedly elevated CPK and was started on dexamethasone. After 6 days of treatment the patient was discharged home with strength sufficient to mobilize safely. Again, in this case, the clinical features and elevated CPK were taken as sufficient evidence of myositis and EMG; MRI and muscle biopsy were not performed [3].

Two other cases of docetaxel induced myositis were documented in separate clinical trials in 2006. Myositis was listed as a toxic side effect without details of the specific cases or description of workup for the diagnosis. Kalmadi et al. reported results from a phase II trial using docetaxel and gemcitabine as first-line therapy for non-small cell lung cancer. Of the 49 patients who were treated with this regimen one patient was noted to require dose adjustment for myositis [6]. Fardet et al. described the use of docetaxel and paclitaxel for treatment of non-HIV related Kaposi sarcoma. Twelve patients were enrolled in this study and one patient experienced "diffuse myalgia with biologic myositis" after treatment with a taxane agent; however, the specific agent was not specified [5].

In 2014, Winkelmann et al. described a case of a 64-year-old woman who was treated with paclitaxel and carboplatin for metastatic, poorly differentiated, serous adenocarcinoma. Between her second and third treatments the patient developed diffuse muscular weakness, as well as Raynaud's phenomenon, skin tightness, and gastroesophageal reflux. Further investigation showed an elevation of ESR, liver function tests (LFTs), and a CPK of 1523 U/L. While her serum Scl70, ANA, and anticentromere were negative, a punch biopsy showed thickened collagen bundles consistent with sclerosis. After completion of chemotherapy and treatment with methotrexate and prednisone, the patient's sclerosis improved and CPK trended downwards; however, muscle weakness persisted. A muscle biopsy was only done at this time, which showed nonspecific inflammation. This case exhibits two rare taxane induced symptoms, sclerosis and myositis [8].

Other interesting cases linking polymyositis with taxane agents have been described by Sasaki et al. and Gidron et al. (see Table 2). In the case described by Sasaki's group, a 58-year-old man with a type B2 thymoma, unrelated to Myasthenia Gravis (MG), was treated with 2 cycles of carboplatin and paclitaxel. Eighteen days after this treatment the patient was admitted to the hospital with fevers, chills, and muscle weakness. The patient was found to have elevation of LFTs and a CPK of 7271 U/L. While polymyositis and myocarditis have been associated with thymomas, these tumors are exceptionally rare and usually in association with MG [7]. Gidron et al. described a similar case of a 32-year-old woman with hairy cell leukemia and a large malignant thymoma, also treated with carboplatin and paclitaxel, after which she developed terminal polymyositis and myocarditis [4].

Perel-Winkler and Derk describe another case of diffuse cutaneous mucinosis and dermatomyositis in a 57-year-old man who was treated with paclitaxel and carboplatin for non-small cell lung cancer. The patient had good response to the treatment but developed a progressive, erythematous, pruritic rash four months after completion of his treatment. No active cancer was found on full body PET-CT; muscle enzymes were normal; however, MRI showed hyperenhancement of quadriceps muscles bilaterally. The patient did not respond to steroids or methotrexate and required IVIG for symptomatic resolution [9].

In our case and in many of the other published cases of docetaxel and paclitaxel induced myopathic toxicity (Table 2), there is no biopsy to support the diagnosis of myositis. Temporal relationship with recent use of the chemotherapeutic agents, alongside the laboratory findings of elevated muscle enzymes and supportive imaging, was accepted as sufficient to make a diagnosis. For academic purposes a biopsy is preferable to definitively rule out all other differentials. Below we describe potential differential diagnoses and discuss why we feel docetaxel induced myositis is the best diagnosis for our case.

In the setting of active malignancy, dermatomyositis (DM) and polymyositis (PM) should be considered in a patient presenting with muscle weakness, pain, and evidence of inflammation. Our patient did not have any of the classic cutaneous signs of DM, such as heliotropic rash, Gottron's papules, shawl sign, and/or erythematous plaques. Furthermore, in both DM and PM, the presentation of muscle pathology usually occurs earlier in the course of the malignancy and improves with successful treatment [22, 23]. Hence, we feel secure in associating the presence of myositis with the taxane agent and not as a sequela of the cancer itself.

Sensorimotor polyneuropathy can occur as a paraneoplastic syndrome or as a complication of chemotherapy treatments, including taxane agents as described above. With cases associated as side effects of treatment, the provider will likely note a progressive time course to presentation of symptoms. In the case of a paraneoplastic syndrome, neuropathic symptoms more often precede detection of malignancy. Paraneoplastic neurologic symptoms have varied presentations, including motor, sensory, and autonomic changes; muscle enzymes will remain in normal range and swelling is not a common presenting complaint [24].

Another rare cause of muscle pain and swelling which should be considered in an immunocompromised host is pyomyositis. In this pathology, a deep muscular infection exists and signs of infection are present including fevers and leukocytosis. On imaging one may note obvious abscesses within the thigh and gluteal muscles. Bacterial pyomyositis has been reported in association with both hematologic and solid organ malignancies. There have also been reports of toxicity-related pyomyositis in the setting of taxane agents. Two such cases have been described in the setting of paclitaxel treatment for endometrial cancer. Both patients presented classically with fever, pain, and decreased range of motion, but due to the rarity of the diagnosis appropriate treatment

TABLE 2: Documented case reports of taxane related myopathies.

Case	Demographics	Taxane ± other agents	Cancer type	Onset of muscle pathology	Treatment	Effect
Ardavanis et al. 2005 [2]	57, male	Docetaxel, gemcitabine	NSCLC	Day 7 after 4th cycle	Prednisone	Myositis of bilateral thighs
Hughes and Stuart-Harris, 2005 [3]	47, female	Docetaxel, epirubicin, and cyclophosphamide	Breast cancer, ER/PR+, HER2−	Day 11 after 2nd cycle	Prednisone	Myositis of bilateral thighs
Gidron et al., 2006 [4]	32, female	Paclitaxel, carboplatin	Hairy cell leukemia and thymoma	Day 7 after second cycle	IV corticosteroids, IVIG	Polymyositis and myocarditis (terminal)
Fardet et al, 2006 [5]	Unknown	Docetaxel or paclitaxel, agent unknown	Kaposi sarcoma	Unknown	Unknown	Unknown
Kalmadi et al., 2006 [6]	Unknown	Docetaxel and gemcitabine	NSCLC	Unknown	Unknown	Unknown
Sasaki et al., 2012 [7]	58, male	Paclitaxel, carboplatin	B cell thymoma	Day 18 after 2nd cycle	Not reported	Polymyositis, myocarditis (terminal)
Winkelmann et al., 2014 [8]	64, female	Paclitaxel, carboplatin	Ovarian adenocarcinoma	After second cycle	Methotrexate, prednisone	Polymyositis, scleroderma, Raynaud's and GERD
Perel-Winkler and Derk, 2014 [9]	57, male	Paclitaxel and carboplatin	NSCLC	Months	Prednisone, plaquenil, methotrexate, and IVIG	Mucinous dermatomyositis
Current case: Perel-Winkler et al.	65, female	Docetaxel and cyclophosphamide	Breast cancer (ER/PR+, HER2−)	Day 8 after 3rd cycle	Prednisone	Bilateral proximal thigh myositis R > L

including drainage of the abscess collection was delayed [25, 26]. Our patient did not present with fever or leukocytosis; there was no evidence of abscesses which were noted on MRI and did not improve with antibiotics.

Diabetes can also cause both neurologic and myopathic complications. Diabetic lumbosacral radiculoplexus neuropathy (DLRPN), also known as diabetic amyotrophy, is a rare complication of diabetes causing a debilitating proximal diabetic neuropathy leading to weakness and pain of the pelvic girdle and proximal muscles of the lower extremities. DLRPN affects less than 1% of diabetic patients, and the risk of developing this disorder is unrelated to glycemic control. The first presentation of this syndrome is usually unilateral thigh pain leading to weakness and atrophy and may progress to bilateral and more distal weakness. Autonomic involvement may occur leading to bladder, bowel, and sexual disorder; sensory involvement is also reported in advanced cases. DLRPN is diagnosed by EMG and is often associated with nonspecific markers of inflammation and immune mediated disease markers such as a positive antinuclear antibody test or rheumatoid factor [27]. EMG results are usually suggestive of axonal degeneration. Biopsy reports show varied evidence of ischemic injury to nerves. The leading accepted theory of the pathophysiology of DLRPN is an immune mediated microvasculitis affecting the lumbar plexus. This disorder has an insidious presentation and is self-limiting; however, symptoms often persist from months to years [28]. In DLRPN patients often report symptoms in association with weight loss and good glycemic control and are not usually treated with insulin. In contrast, our patient's diabetic control was poor, with an HBA1c of 9.7%, and she was treated with insulin. The elevation in CPK and aldolase in our patient supports our diagnosis of myositis, whereas DLRPN's pathology is accepted as microvascular ischemia affecting nerves. Finally, our patient's quick recovery, within weeks, is not in line with the time course associated with DLRPN.

Diabetic myonecrosis must also be considered as a differential. This disorder is a rare complication of poorly controlled diabetes, usually occurring in patients with preexisting microvascular disease. Acute onset of pain and swelling of the thigh is the most common presenting complaint [29]. Laboratory workup in these patients is usually nondiagnostic, with normal white cell count and CPK, and moderately elevated ESR. Biopsies have been done, demonstrating muscle necrosis and edema; however, studies have shown that time to resolution doubled from 29 to 60 days after biopsy was performed. Biopsy, therefore, is not recommended for diagnosis. The modality of choice for further evaluation is MRI, which is claimed to be both sensitive and specific enough for diagnosis, although its specificity has been refuted [30]. Typical MRI features of diabetic myonecrosis include a hyperintense signal on T2-weighted images and an isointense to hypointense signal on T1-weighted images from the affected muscle, with associated marked edema and enhancement around irregular regions of muscle necrosis [31]. Our patient fits into the criteria of a poorly controlled diabetic, presenting with acute onset of thigh pain and swelling. The MRI images in our patient are more consistent with a diagnosis of an inflammatory myopathy, particularly the diffuse muscle edema and subcutaneous involvement. While diabetic myonecrosis cannot be completely ruled out without biopsy, the temporal relationship to docetaxel in our case makes this a more likely diagnosis.

Finally, drug-induced myopathy should also be considered in all cases of unexplained myalgias and weakness. Muscle toxicity can occur in association with many drugs. The large mass of muscle and its exposure to large amounts of blood flow make muscle a common source of adverse drug reactions. Drug-induced myopathy can be the cause of direct myotoxicity, most often associated with statins, colchicine, steroids, and antiretroviral agents [32]. Other mechanisms of drug-induced myopathy include inflammation, interference of neuromuscular transmission, or indirect metabolic causes, such as drug-induced hypokalemia, hypermagnesemia, or drug-induced hyperkinetic states [33].

Statin induced myopathy is a spectrum of disorders ranging from myalgias (muscle pain without CPK elevation) to myositis (muscle inflammation evidenced by CPK elevation) and rhabdomyolysis (debilitating muscle weakness with CPK > 10 times the normal range, often accompanied by kidney injury). While pain and muscle weakness are reported in 1–20% of patients taking statins, myositis and rhabdomyolysis reactions are rare and have been reported in less than 0.001% cases. Reactions to statins are related to dose but not time course, and drug-drug interactions are known to significantly affect the incidence of statin induced myopathies [34]. Most often drugs that increase the metabolism and systemic exposure of statins are implicated, such as gemfibrozil, nicotinic acid, macrolide antibiotics, azole antifungal agents, protease inhibitors, ranolazine, and calcium channel blockers [35]. Muscle related symptoms have been reported in simvastatin and atorvastatin more than other agents; however, severe rhabdomyolysis and myositis have not been reported in any agent more than another currently on the market. Biopsies of patients currently taking, or recently discontinued, statins with myopathy show extensive intracellular vacuolization in skeletal muscles. Visualization with electron microscopy indicated that intracellular vacuoles corresponded to membranous cavities in a distribution consistent with the T tubule system [36]. Our patient was taking a low dose of rosuvastatin concomitantly with a calcium channel blocker putting her at risk for statin associated myopathy. The statin and antihypertensive were stopped during her hospitalization and were not restarted as an outpatient. While statin induced myopathies can occur at any time, the temporal relationship with docetaxel is in line with the other reported cases of docetaxel induced myositis, favoring the later diagnosis. Further, amlodipine has been recognized to more often potentiate the myopathic toxicity of atorvastatin not rosuvastatin. Our diagnosis would be more convincing if there was a biopsy that differed from the findings of a statin induced myositis biopsy; however, as none of the reported cases of docetaxel induced myositis have a biopsy reported, there would not be strong comparison even if our patient had one.

In our case a docetaxel induced inflammatory myositis was the best diagnosis, in consideration of all the differentials. Diabetic myonecrosis and statin induced myopathy cannot be definitely ruled out without further investigation with muscle biopsy. We believe that, in comparing our case to another docetaxel related myositis and in consideration of the temporal relationship, it is highly likely that our patient's myositis was related to the taxane agent. Taxanes are known to cause disabling but transient arthralgias and myalgias in up to 75% of patients; these events typically occur 1 to 3 days after therapy and may significantly affect a patient's quality of life for several days [37]. It is important for practitioners to recognize that inflammatory myopathy is also a possible complication for patients when treated with these agents.

4. Conclusion

Neuromuscular side effects such as myalgia and neuropathy are now considered commonly known consequences of docetaxel treatment. Our case is the fifth documented case of inflammatory myositis in the setting of docetaxel treatment. A few other cases of myositis have been reported in association with the taxane agent, paclitaxel. Due to the small sample size, correlations between lengths of treatments, types of malignancy, or patient demographics cannot be made. It is important for clinicians to be aware that inflammatory myositis can be an adverse effect of docetaxel treatment. Myositis should be considered in the differential when managing a patient with muscle weakness after treatment with a taxane agent.

References

[1] American Cancer Society, *Cancer Facts and Figures 2014*, 2014, http://www.cancer.org/acs/groups/content/@research/documents/webcontent/acspc-042151.pdf.

[2] A. S. Ardavanis, G. N. Ioannidis, and G. A. Rigatos, "Acute myopathy in a patient with lung adenocarcinoma treated with gemcitabine and docetaxel," *Anticancer Research*, vol. 25, no. 1, pp. 523–525, 2005.

[3] B. G. M. Hughes and R. Stuart-Harris, "Docetaxel-induced myositis: report of a novel side-effect," *Internal Medicine Journal*, vol. 35, no. 6, pp. 369–370, 2005.

[4] A. Gidron, M. Quadrini, N. Dimov, and A. Argiris, "Malignant thymoma associated with fatal myocarditis and polymyositis in a 32-year-old woman with a history of hairy cell leukemia," *American Journal of Clinical Oncology*, vol. 29, no. 2, pp. 213–214, 2006.

[5] L. Fardet, P.-E. Stoebner, H. Bachelez et al., "Treatment with taxanes of refractory or life-threatening Kaposi sarcoma not associated with human immunodeficiency virus infection," *Cancer*, vol. 106, no. 8, pp. 1785–1789, 2006.

[6] S. Kalmadi, G. McNeill, M. Davis, D. Peereboom, D. Adelstein, and T. Mekhail, "Phase II trial of weekly docetaxel and gemcitabine as first-line therapy for patients with advanced non-small cell lung cancer," *Medical Oncology*, vol. 23, no. 4, pp. 507–513, 2006.

[7] H. Sasaki, M. Yano, O. Kawano, Y. Hikosaka, and Y. Fujii, "Thymoma associated with fatal myocarditis and polymyositis

[8] in a 58-year-old man following treatment with carboplatin and paclitaxel: a case report," *Oncology Letters*, vol. 3, no. 2, pp. 300–302, 2012.

[8] R. R. Winkelmann, J. A. Yiannias, D. J. Dicaudo et al., "Paclitaxel-induced diffuse cutaneous sclerosis: a case with associated esophageal dysmotility, Raynaud's phenomenon, and myositis," *The International Journal of Dermatology*, 2014.

[9] A. C. Perel-Winkler and C. T. Derk, "Diffuse cutaneous mucinosis in dermatomyositis: a case report and review of the literature," *Case Reports in Dermatological Medicine*, vol. 2014, Article ID 938414, 6 pages, 2014.

[10] L. S. Bachegowda, D. F. Makower, and J. A. Sparano, "Taxanes: impact on breast cancer therapy," *Anti-Cancer Drugs*, vol. 25, no. 5, pp. 512–521, 2014.

[11] P. H. E. Hilkens, J. Verweij, G. Stoter, C. J. Vecht, W. L. J. van Putten, and M. J. van den Bent, "Peripheral neurotoxicity induced by docetaxel," *Neurology*, vol. 46, no. 1, pp. 104–108, 1996.

[12] P. H. E. Hilkens, L. C. Pronk, J. Verweij, C. J. Vecht, W. L. J. Van Putten, and M. J. Van Den Bent, "Peripheral neuropathy induced by combination chemotherapy of docetaxel and cisplatin," *British Journal of Cancer*, vol. 75, no. 3, pp. 417–422, 1997.

[13] P. H. Wiernik, E. L. Schwartz, J. J. Strauman, J. P. Dutcher, R. B. Lipton, and E. Paietta, "Phase I clinical and pharmacokinetic study of taxol," *Cancer Research*, vol. 47, no. 9, pp. 2486–2493, 1987.

[14] R. C. Donehower, E. K. Rowinsky, L. B. Grochow, S. M. Longnecker, and D. S. Ettinger, "Phase I trial of taxol in patients with advanced cancer," *Cancer Treatment Reports*, vol. 71, no. 12, pp. 1171–1177, 1987.

[15] A. Sulkes, U. Beller, T. Peretz et al., "Taxol: initial Israeli experience with a novel anticancer agent," *Israel Journal of Medical Sciences*, vol. 30, no. 1, pp. 70–78, 1994.

[16] V. Valero, F. A. Holmes, R. S. Walters et al., "Phase II trial of docetaxel: a new, highly effective antineoplastic agent in the management of patients with anthracycline resistant metastatic breast cancer," *Journal of Clinical Oncology*, vol. 13, no. 12, pp. 2886–2894, 1995.

[17] G. Giaccone, M. Huizing, W. T. B. Huinink et al., "Preliminary results of two dose-finding studies of paclitaxel (taxol) and carboplatin in non-small cell lung and ovarian cancer: a European Cancer Center effort," *Seminars in Oncology*, vol. 21, no. 5, pp. 34–38, 1994.

[18] E. K. Rowinsky, P. J. Burke, J. E. Karp, R. W. Tucker, D. S. Ettinger, and R. C. Donehower, "Phase I and pharmacodynamics study of taxol in refractory acute leukemias," *Cancer Research*, vol. 49, no. 16, pp. 4640–4647, 1989.

[19] S. Saibil, B. Fitzgerald, O. C. Freedman et al., "Incidence of taxane-induced pain and distress in patients receiving chemotherapy for early-stage breast cancer: a retrospective, outcomes-based survey," *Current Oncology*, vol. 17, no. 4, pp. 42–47, 2010.

[20] R. B. Lipton, S. C. Apfel, J. P. Dutcher et al., "Taxol produces a predominantly sensory neuropathy," *Neurology*, vol. 39, no. 3, pp. 368–373, 1989.

[21] R. J. Freilich, C. Balmaceda, A. D. Seidman, M. Rubin, and L. M. DeAngelis, "Motor neuropathy due to docetaxel and paclitaxel," *Neurology*, vol. 47, no. 1, pp. 115–118, 1996.

[22] J. P. Callen, "Myositis and malignancy," *Current Opinion in Rheumatology*, vol. 6, no. 6, pp. 590–594, 1994.

[23] Z. A. Zahr and A. N. Baer, "Malignancy in myositis," *Current Rheumatology Reports*, vol. 13, no. 3, pp. 208–215, 2011.

[24] H. Koike, F. Tanaka, and G. Sobue, "Paraneoplastic neuropathy: wide-ranging clinicopathological manifestations," *Current Opinion in Neurology*, vol. 24, no. 5, pp. 504–510, 2011.

[25] Y. Nakao, M. Yokoyama, S. Nishiyama et al., "Pyomyositis associated with chemotherapy for endometrial cancer: a case report," *World Journal of Surgical Oncology*, vol. 11, article 45, 2013.

[26] P. Singh, W. Chan, P. Blomfield, and R. McIntosh, "Pyomyositis after chemotherapy for endometrial cancer," *International Journal of Gynecological Cancer*, vol. 20, no. 7, pp. 1256–1258, 2010.

[27] J. W. Albers and R. Pop-Busui, "Diabetic neuropathy: mechanisms, emerging treatments, and subtypes," *Current Neurology and Neuroscience Reports*, vol. 14, no. 8, article 473, 2014.

[28] P. J. B. Dyck and A. J. Windebank, "Diabetic and nondiabetic lumbosacral radiculoplexus neuropathies: new insights into pathophysiology and treatment," *Muscle & Nerve*, vol. 25, no. 4, pp. 477–491, 2002.

[29] B. Choudhury, U. Saikia, D. Sarma, M. Saikia, S. D. Choudhury, and D. Bhuyan, "Diabetic myonecrosis: an underreported complication of diabetes mellitus," *Indian Journal of Endocrinology and Metabolism*, vol. 15, no. 5, pp. S58–S61, 2011.

[30] W. B. Horton, J. S. Taylor, T. J. Ragland, and A. R. Subauste, "Diabetic muscle infarction: a systematic review," *BMJ Open Diabetes Research & Care*, vol. 3, no. 1, 2015.

[31] M. Schulze, I. Kotter, U. Ernemann et al., "MRI findings in inflammatory muscle diseases and their noninflammatory mimics," *American Journal of Roentgenology*, vol. 192, no. 6, pp. 1708–1716, 2009.

[32] T. Klopstock, "Drug-induced myopathies," *Current Opinion in Neurology*, vol. 21, no. 5, pp. 590–595, 2008.

[33] R. M. Pascuzzi, "Drugs and toxins associated with myopathies," *Current Opinion in Rheumatology*, vol. 10, no. 6, pp. 511–520, 1998.

[34] A. L. Catapano, "Statin-induced myotoxicity: pharmacokinetic differences among statins and the risk of rhabdomyolysis, with particular reference to pitavastatin," *Current Vascular Pharmacology*, vol. 10, no. 2, pp. 257–267, 2012.

[35] P. D. Thompson, P. Clarkson, and R. H. Karas, "Statin-associated myopathy," *Journal of the American Medical Association*, vol. 289, no. 13, pp. 1681–1690, 2003.

[36] M. G. Mohaupt, R. H. Karas, E. B. Babiychuk et al., "Association between statin-associated myopathy and skeletal muscle damage," *Canadian Medical Association Journal*, vol. 181, no. 1-2, pp. 11–18, 2009.

[37] E. K. Rowinsky, V. Chaudhry, A. A. Forastiere et al., "Phase I and pharmacologic study of paclitaxel and cisplatin with granulocyte colony-stimulating factor: neuromuscular toxicity is dose-limiting," *Journal of Clinical Oncology*, vol. 11, no. 10, pp. 2010–2020, 1993.

20

A Case of Subacute Cutaneous Lupus Erythematosus in a Patient with Mixed Connective Tissue Disease: Successful Treatment with Plasmapheresis and Rituximab

M. Fantò,[1] S. Salemi,[1] F. Socciarelli,[2] A. Bartolazzi,[2] G. A. Natale,[3] I. Casorelli,[3] A. Pavan,[3] S. Vaglio,[3] R. Di Rosa,[1] and R. D'Amelio[1]

[1] *Department of Allergy, Clinical Immunology and Rheumatology, S. Andrea Hospital, Sapienza University of Rome, Italy*
[2] *Department of Pathology, S. Andrea Hospital, Sapienza University of Rome, Italy*
[3] *Department of Immunohematology and Transfusion Unit, S. Andrea Hospital, Sapienza University of Rome, Italy*

Correspondence should be addressed to M. Fantò; martafanto@gmail.com

Academic Editors: L.-P. Erwig, M. A. Hunt, and M. Soy

A 30-year-old woman affected by Mixed Connective Tissue Disease with scleroderma spectrum developed a facial eruption, a clinical and histological characteristic of subacute cutaneous lupus erythematosus (SCLE). Speckled anti-nuclear antibodies, high-titer anti-ribonucleoprotein1, anti-Sm, anti-Cardiolipin (aCL) IgG/IgM, and anti-Ro/SSA antibodies were positive. SCLE was resistant to Azathioprine, Hydroxychloroquine, and Methotrexate while Mycophenolate Mofetil was suspended due to side effects. Subsequently, the patient was treated with three cycles of therapeutic plasma exchange (TPE) followed, one month after the last TPE, by the anti-CD20 antibody Rituximab (RTX) (375 mg/m^2 weekly for 4 weeks). Eight and 16 months later the patient received other two TPE and RTX cycles, respectively. This therapeutic approach has allowed to obtain a complete skin healing persistent even after 8-month follow-up. Moreover, mitigation of Raynaud's phenomenon, resolution of alopecia, and a decline of aCL IgG/IgM and anti-Ro/SSA antibodies were observed.

1. Introduction

Mixed Connective Tissue Disease (MCTD) is currently defined as an overlapping syndrome with clinical features of Systemic Sclerosis (SSc), Systemic Lupus Erythematosus (SLE), Rheumatoid arthritis (RA), and Polymyositis/Dermatomyositis (PM/DM); the presence of high-titer anti-ribonucleoprotein1 (U1RNP) or speckled anti-nuclear antibodies (ANA) at titer $\geq 1 : 2,000$ is necessary for the diagnosis. The disease affects mainly women in the third decade of life (from 80 to 90%) but it has been also reported in children and in over-80-year-old people [1].

The most frequent clinical manifestations are Raynaud's phenomenon (RP), swollen hands, sclerodactyly, arthritis, myalgias, and oesophageal dysmotility, and also alopecia, malar rash, lymphadenopathy, or kidney damage can be present. Rarely, subacute cutaneous lupus erythematosus (SCLE), characterized by annular or papulosquamous lesions, photosensitivity, and presence of anti-Ro/SSA and anti-La/SSB antibodies, has been described in MCTD patients [2, 3]. MCTD therapy should be identified for each patient depending on the affected organ, but generally there is a good response to steroids, different types of vasodilators, and immunosuppressive agents such as Hydroxychloroquine (HCQ), Azathioprine (AZA), Methotrexate (MTX), or Cyclophosphamide (CYC) [1].

2. Case Presentation

A case of a thirty-year-old woman affected by MCTD with scleroderma spectrum and epilepsy since she was fifteen is here reported. At the beginning she presented fever up to

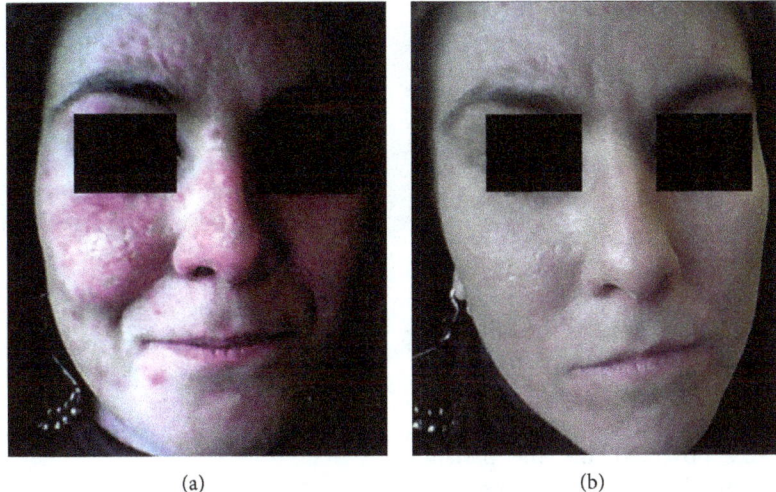

(a)   (b)

Figure 1: (a) SCLE: cutaneous eruption which infiltrates forehead, cheeks, and chin. (b) Disappearance of facial SCLE after the third cycle of TPE plus RTX.

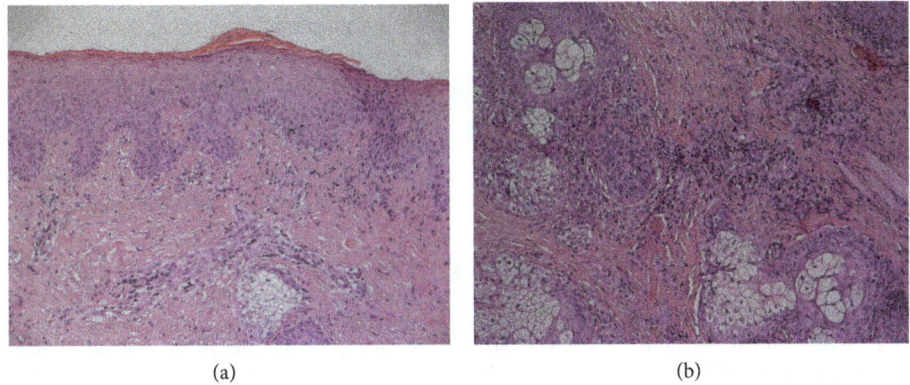

(a)   (b)

Figure 2: (a) The epidermal layer is characterized by a mild degree of papillomatosis, acanthosis, and focal mixed orthokeratotic and parakeratotic hyperkeratoses. The underlying papillary and reticular dermis shows a marked fibrotic change associated with a chronic mononuclear perivascular inflammatory infiltrate (H&E, 100x magnification). (b) A moderate mononuclear chronic infiltrate is present around adnexal structures (H&E, 100x magnification).

40°C, arthalgias mainly at knees, wrists, and shoulders, and increased levels of erythrocyte sedimentation rate (ESR) and C-reactive protein (CRP). She also had speckled type of ANA up to 1 : 2,560, anti-U1RNP, anti-Sm, anti-Cardiolipin (aCl) IgG and IgM positivity, hypergammaglobulinemia, myositis, lymphopenia, RP, cutaneous calcinosis, and scleroderma. She started treatment with Cyclosporine A (CYA), corticosteroids (CCS), and nifedipine in 1998. The following year myositis worsened with an increase of Creatinphosphokinase (CPK) up to 8,000; thus she received pulse steroid therapy, 800 mg/die methylprednisolone, monthly for six months; four years later, in 2001, because of exacerbation of arthralgias she started HCQ, with satisfying improvement. In August 2003 a grade C esophagitis and a diffuse bilateral interstitial lung disease with severe decrease of carbon monoxide diffusing capacity (DLCO) were detected. Irregular urticarial lesions in her arms and chest and purpura in her legs and alopecia also arose. Thus she started AZA, with lung and cutaneous improvement. In 2007 CYA was suspended after

a blood pressure increase. Subsequently, a facial eruption appeared in correspondence of forehead, cheeks, and chin (Figure 1(a)). Histopathological examination of a skin biopsy revealed "a skin characterized by modest papillomatosis, acanthosis, and focal hyperkeratosis of the epidermis. The superficial and deep dermis showed marked sclerosis associated with lymphomononuclear perivascular and periadnexal cellular infiltrate" (Figures 2(a)-2(b)).

Direct immunofluorescence on frozen skin biopsy ("lupus band test") demonstrated "a dust-like IgG particles staining pattern consisting of fine granular Ig deposition scattered through the epidermis." This picture has been reported to be specific for SCLE [4]. Taking into account the clinical and histological features and anti/Ro antibodies positivity, a diagnosis of subacute cutaneous lupus erythematosus (SCLE) associated to dermal sclerosis was made. In 2008 MTX and the subsequent year Mycophenolate Mofetil (MMF) were able to induce a slight skin improvement but they were stopped due to inefficacy and excessive weight loss, respectively. Therefore, in December 2010, therapeutic plasma exchange (TPE) was performed, every other day for a total of five exchanges, using albumin to replace the plasma removed. The same cycle was repeated in February and in March 2011 followed, one month after, by Rituximab (RTX) (375 mg/m^2 weekly for 4 weeks). Eight and 16 months later the patient received other two TPE procedures followed by RTX (375 mg/m^2 weekly for 4 weeks), respectively. After the first 3 TPE cycles there was a slight improvement of SCLE and the addition of RTX has allowed for obtaining a further clearing of facial eruption, while 8 weeks after the last RTX infusion a complete skin healing was reached and is still persistent after 8-month follow-up (Figure 1(b)). Mitigation of RP and resolution of alopecia were also observed. During this period no flares-up were observed and the patient assumed only HCQ and a low-dose of CCS (5 mg/die). Interestingly, aCl-IgG/IgM and anti-Ro/SSA antibodies disappeared after the first TPE and RTX treatment, whereas they showed a slight increase before the third cycle at the end of which they became definitively negative for the next 8 months.

3. Discussion

Successful off-label use of RTX in SLE manifestations as cytopenia, diffuse erythematosus lesions, and alopecia or as rescue therapy in life-threatening complications of several autoimmune diseases has been sometimes reported [5, 6]; in addition, the anti-CD20 therapy has even been employed in dermatologic field including blistering diseases, graft versus host disease, and DM/PM but, to our knowledge, only one case of refractory SCLE treated with RTX has been described [7]. Recently, the role of B cells in the pathogenesis of SSc has been underlined, and the RTX efficacy to improve skin fibrosis and pulmonary function has been reported [8, 9].

Regarding MCTD, a successful treatment with RTX (in combination with CCS, CYC, and iloprost) has been reported in a case of severe, refractory RP [10], while on the contrary, Dunkley et al. reported a case of MCTD with scleroderma spectrum in which RTX was not able to control RP [11]. Moreover two MCTD cases in which TPE was able to treat visceral RP with multiple organ damage (treated with combination with CYA and CCS) [12] and acute renal failure (in combination with CYC and captopril) [13] have been described.

Plasmapheresis, in association with RTX, has been used in only one case of MCTD patient, in whom were observed RP resolution, ANA, anti-centromere (CENP-B) antibodies, and decrease of serum IgG-IgM [14].

A case of MCTD patient with scleroderma spectrum, in whom therapy-resistant facial SCLE was completely resolved after combination of TPE and RTX (375 mg/m^2 weekly for 4 weeks), is here reported. Moreover, we observed RP improvement and alopecia, aCl, and anti-Ro/SSA serum antibodies disappearance. Anti-Ro/SSA antibodies are closely associated with SCLE, and the resolution of clinical features accompanied by the disappearance of these antibodies from

serum strongly suggests a primary role of anti-Ro/SSA autoantibodies in the pathogenesis of SCLE.

Before starting this new approach, in order to exclude a iatrogenic cause in SCLE induction, carbamazepine and nifedipine were replaced with similar noninducing drugs, but no clinical effects on SCLE were observed [15].

In conclusion, association of TPE and RTX should be considered as a valid and safe therapeutic tool for controlling SCLE in therapy-resistant MCTD. Moreover, despite the relative short follow-up, the intriguing observation of the beneficial effects that this treatment could exert also on cutaneous sclerosis occurring in MCTD patients makes this therapeutic approach very promising.

References

[1] O.-D. Ortega-Hernandez and Y. Shoenfeld, "Mixed connective tissue disease: an overview of clinical manifestations, diagnosis and treatment," *Best Practice and Research*, vol. 26, no. 1, pp. 61–72, 2012.

[2] A. Parodi, M. Caproni, C. Cardinali et al., "Clinical, histological and immunopathological features of 58 patients with subacute cutaneous lupus erythematosus. A review by the Italian Group of Immunodermatology," *Dermatology*, vol. 200, no. 1, pp. 6–10, 2000.

[3] D. Lipsker, M.-P. Di Cesare, B. Cribier, E. Grosshans, and E. Heid, "The significance of the "dust-like particles" pattern of immunofluorescence. A study of 66 cases," *British Journal of Dermatology*, vol. 138, no. 6, pp. 1039–1042, 1998.

[4] K. M. David-Bajar, S. D. Bennion, J. D. DeSpain, L. E. Golitz, and L. A. Lee, "Clinical, histologic, and immunofluorescent distinctions between subacute cutaneous lupus erythematosus and discoid lupus erythematosus," *Journal of Investigative Dermatology*, vol. 99, no. 3, pp. 251–257, 1992.

[5] M. Ramos-Casals, M. J. Soto, M. J. Cuadrado, and M. A. Khamashta, "Rituximab in systemic lupus erythematosus: a systematic review of off-label use in 188 cases," *Lupus*, vol. 18, no. 9, pp. 767–776, 2009.

[6] Y. Braun-Moscovici, Y. Butbul-Aviel, L. Guralnik et al., "Rituximab: rescue therapy in life-threatening complications or refractory autoimmune diseases: a single center experience," *Rheumatology International*, vol. 33, no. 6, pp. 1495–1504, 2013.

[7] V. Kieu, T. O'Brien, L.-M. Yap et al., "Refractory subacute cutaneous lupus erythematosus successfully treated with rituximab," *Australasian Journal of Dermatology*, vol. 50, no. 3, pp. 202–206, 2009.

[8] V. Smith, Y. Piette, J. T. van Praet et al., "Two-year results of an open pilot study of a 2-treatment course with rituximab in patients with early systemic sclerosis with diffuse skin involvement," *The Journal of Rheumatology*, vol. 40, pp. 52–57, 2013.

[9] D. Daoussis, S. N. Liossis, A. C. Tsamandas et al., "Effect of long-term treatment with rituximab on pulmonary function and skin fibrosis in patients with diffuse systemic sclerosis," *Clinical and Experimental Rheumatology*, vol. 30, no. 2, supplement 71, pp. S17–S22, 2012.

[10] M. Haroon, D. O'Gradaigh, and D. Foley-Nolan, "A case of Raynaud's phenomenon in mixed connective tissue disease responding to rituximab therapy," *Rheumatology*, vol. 46, no. 4, pp. 718–719, 2007.

[11] L. Dunkley, M. Green, and A. Gough, "Comment on: a case of Raynaud's phenomenon in mixed connective tissue disease responding to Rituximab therapy—response," *Rheumatology*, vol. 46, no. 10, pp. 1628–1629, 2007.

[12] M. Seguchi, Y. Soejima, A. Tateishi et al., "Mixed connective tissue disease with multiple organ damage: successful treatment with plasmapheresis," *Internal Medicine*, vol. 39, no. 12, pp. 1119–1122, 2000.

[13] R. M. Crapper, J. P. Dowling, I. R. Mackay, and J. A. Whitworth, "Acute scleroderma in stable mixed connective tissue disease: treatment by plasmapheresis," *Australian and New Zealand Journal of Medicine*, vol. 17, no. 3, pp. 327–329, 1987.

[14] J. Rech, S. Kallert, A. J. Hueber, C. Requadt, J. R. Kalden, and H. Schulze-Koops, "Combination of immunoadsorption and CD20 antibody therapy in a patient with mixed connective tissue disease," *Rheumatology*, vol. 45, no. 4, pp. 490–491, 2006.

[15] G. Lowe, C. L. Henderson, R. H. Grau, C. B. Hansen, and R. D. Sontheimer, "A systematic review of drug-induced subacute cutaneous lupus erythematosus," *British Journal of Dermatology*, vol. 164, no. 3, pp. 465–472, 2011.

21

Severe Rhabdomyolysis without Systemic Involvement: A Rare Case of Idiopathic Eosinophilic Polymyositis

Ayesha Farooq, Vivek Choksi, Andrew Chu, Dhruti Mankodi, Sameer Shaharyar, Keith O'Brien, and Uday Shankar

Aventura Hospital and Medical Center Internal Medicine Department, Aventura, FL 33180, USA

Correspondence should be addressed to Ayesha Farooq; afarooq912@gmail.com

Academic Editor: Mario Salazar-Paramo

Introduction. Eosinophilic polymyositis (EPM) is a rare cause of rhabdomyolysis characterized by eosinophilic infiltrates in the muscle. We describe the case of a young patient with eosinophilic polymyositis causing isolated severe rhabdomyolysis without systemic involvement. *Case Presentation.* A 22-year-old Haitian female with no past medical history presented with progressive generalized muscle aches without precipitating factors. Examination of the extremities revealed diffuse muscle tenderness. Laboratory findings demonstrated peripheral eosinophilia and high creatinine phosphokinase (CPK) and transaminase levels. Workup for the common causes of rhabdomyolysis were negative. Her CPK continued to rise to greater than 100,000 units/L so a muscle biopsy was performed which showed widespread eosinophilic infiltrate consistent with eosinophilic polymyositis. She was started on high dose systemic corticosteroids with improvement of her symptoms, eosinophilia, and CPK level. *Discussion.* This case illustrates a systematic workup of rhabdomyolysis in the presence of peripheral eosinophilia. Many differential diagnoses must be considered before establishing a diagnosis of idiopathic eosinophilic polymyositis. To our knowledge, our case of eosinophilic polymyositis is unique as it presented with severe rhabdomyolysis without another organ involvement. Clinicians should maintain a high index of suspicion for this physically debilitating disease to aid in prompt diagnosis.

1. Introduction

Rhabdomyolysis is a common condition with multiple causes including physical exertion, trauma, and inflammation. Among the less common etiologies of this finding is eosinophilic polymyositis (EPM). Eosinophilic polymyositis is a rare disease with only a handful of cases [1–16] reported in the literature, mostly in the setting of malignancy [11], autoimmune disease [5], genetic abnormalities [8], hypereosinophilic syndrome (HES) [17], and even medications [1, 4, 7]. When no etiologic factor can be identified, idiopathic eosinophilic polymyositis is diagnosed. It appears that only two cases of idiopathic eosinophilic polymyositis without systemic involvement have been reported [2, 10]. We present the rare case of a young woman with idiopathic eosinophilic polymyositis presenting with muscle pain without involvement of other organ systems. This will be followed by a discussion of the approach to this condition, from clinical presentation to therapy.

2. Case Presentation

A 22-year-old Haitian female with no significant prior history presented to the emergency department with severe and generalized muscle aches for the past week mainly involving the shoulder and thigh muscles. Two days prior to presentation, her muscle aches had progressed to the point that they were limiting her mobility. She denied fever, chills, chest pain, palpitations, shortness of breath, skin rashes, or joint pain. She denied recent illness, trauma, physical exertion, excessive heat exposure, or use of medications. The patient had been sluggish and was gaining weight over the past 2 months but she denied cold intolerance, menstrual abnormalities, or peripheral edema. One month ago, she developed a 2-3 cm nodule in her anterior neck that spontaneously resolved within a few days.

On initial examination her vital signs were temperature of 36.8°C, pulse rate of 90/minute, respiratory rate of 16/minute, blood pressure of 116/66 mm Hg, and oxygen saturation of 99%. Her body mass index was 23.03 kg/m^2. Physical examination revealed a female in mild distress due to muscle pain. Head and neck exam was normal with no thyroid or anterior neck swelling. No lymphadenopathy was appreciated. Her cardiac, pulmonary, and abdominal exams were unremarkable. Exam of the extremities revealed diffuse muscle tenderness with limited flexion/extension and abduction/adduction of the upper and lower extremities due to bilateral pain. She had no peripheral edema.

A complete blood count showed a white blood cell count of 5,700/μL with 13.7% eosinophils (780/μL) and hemoglobin of 12.8 g/dL. A complete metabolic panel revealed normal sodium, potassium, and creatinine with an elevated AST level of 1248 units/L and ALT level of 481 units/L. Alkaline phosphatase and bilirubin were within normal limits. Creatinine phosphokinase (CPK) was 14,913 units/L (26–192 units/L), C-reactive protein was 1.69 mg/dL (0.000–0.300 mg/dL), and erythrocyte sedimentation rate was 9 mm/hr (0–12 mm/hr). An initial urinalysis showed large blood and 15–25 RBCs/HPF but the urine sample was contaminated with menstrual blood. Urine toxicology screen was negative. L-tryptophan ingestion was considered but the patient denied use of any supplements. Toxic oil syndrome was considered unlikely as she denied recent travel history or unusual food ingestion. We started treatment for rhabdomyolysis with aggressive intravenous fluid hydration. A liver ultrasound was negative for cirrhosis, biliary obstruction, or gallstones. Over the next 2 weeks, her CPK continued to increase to levels greater than 100,000 units/L despite aggressive hydration with intravenous fluids at rates of up to 300cc per hour. Bicarbonate was also added to maintain alkalinized urine. Her renal function remained stable with a BUN ranging from 3 to 13 mg/dL and creatinine ranging from 0.15 to 0.43 mg/dL. A repeat urinalysis at this time showed large blood, 0–2 RBCs/HPF, protein, and amorphous sediment.

Further diagnostic workup to elucidate the cause of rhabdomyolysis was unrevealing, with normal levels of thyroid-stimulating hormone, cortisol, aldolase, ANA, C-ANCA, P-ANCA, anti-Jo-1, anti-Ro, anti-La, anti-Sm, anti-RNP, dsDNA, and C3 and C4. Cardiac echogram and troponins revealed no cardiac involvement. Tests for infective causes including viruses (coxsackie, CMV, EBV, viral hepatitis, HSV, HIV, and influenza) and parasites (*Schistosoma*, *Giardia*, *Toxocara*, *Trichinella*, and *Strongyloides*) were negative, with the exception of influenza A and B antibody titers, which were 1 : 64 and 1 : 8, respectively. However, she did not report any upper respiratory tract symptoms that would have suggested influenza. A muscle biopsy was attained, as the etiology for rhabdomyolysis remained unclear. While awaiting the pathology report, she was started on steroids 10 days after admission for suspected inflammatory myopathy leading to a gradual improvement in her symptoms, CPK level, liver function tests, and peripheral eosinophilia.

Her muscle biopsy demonstrated widespread eosinophilic infiltrate consistent with eosinophilic polymyositis as well as numerous plasma cells (Figure 1). There were no parasites like *Toxoplasma* or *Trichinella* seen on H&E stain. There were no hydatid cysts seen on biopsy making

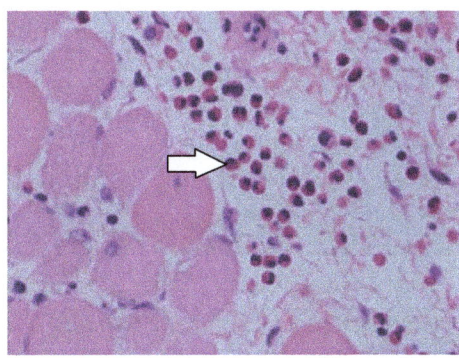

FIGURE 1: Cross section of skeletal muscle biopsy using H&E stain showing generalized myofiber atrophy with eosinophilic infiltrates (arrow) in the endomysium.

Echinococcus unlikely. While *Toxoplasma* and *Taenia solium* were not specifically tested for by serology, our patient did not display gastrointestinal or neurological symptoms to support these pathologies. SPEP and UPEP were normal making multiple myeloma unlikely. We did not suspect a hematological malignancy warranting a bone marrow biopsy. This biopsy result was not consistent with rhabdomyolysis caused by influenza based on review of the literature. Given significant improvement with steroids, this treatment was continued and the patient was advised to follow up with a neuromuscular disease specialist. She was seen in our internal medicine clinic after discharge and a slow steroid taper was continued for 6 months with successful remission of symptoms and normalization of CPK and liver enzyme levels, which would not be expected if an infectious entity were the cause.

3. Discussion

The present case illustrates an unusual cause of rhabdomyolysis. The etiologies of rhabdomyolysis are subdivided into four categories: exertional, nontraumatic exertional normal muscle, nontraumatic exertional abnormal muscle, and nonexertional. Our patient had an inflammatory myopathy, which is a nonexertional subtype. The inflammatory myopathies can be further divided into the rare eosinophilic myopathies (EM) and the more common noneosinophilic myopathies (NEM) like noneosinophilic polymyositis, dermatomyositis, and inclusion body myositis [19]. There are different classification systems to help diagnose these inflammatory myopathies but without biopsy and positive autoantibodies, identification remains a challenge [20].

Eosinophilic myositis (EM) usually presents between the ages of 14 and 70 and is twice as common in females compared to males [19]. The most common presenting symptoms include a gradual onset of muscle pain, edema of the upper and/or lower extremities, muscle weakness, and joint pains [19]. Other signs, symptoms, and lab findings of EM are listed in Tables 1 and 2. This slowly progressive myopathy mostly causes proximal muscle weakness with a marked increase in creatinine kinase.

TABLE 1: Signs and symptoms of eosinophilic myositis [18].

Clinical features	Percentage
Muscle pain, cramping, or tenderness	68%
Upper or lower extremity swelling edema	45%
Muscle weakness	16%
Arthralgias/arthritis	10%
Myocarditis/pericarditis	10%
Vasculitis	6%
Inflammatory eye disease	6%
Raynaud's phenomenon	6%
Eosinophilic pneumonia	3%
Angioedema	3%

*Permission for reuse in a journal was acquired from Elsevier.

TABLE 2: Laboratory findings of eosinophilic myositis [18].

Laboratory findings	Percentage
Peripheral eosinophilia (eosinophil count $>4.5 \times 10^8$)	77%
Inflammatory markers	
Elevated ESR	77%
Muscle markers	
Elevated CPK	68%
Elevated aldolase	44%
Autoimmune markers	
Rheumatoid factor	33%
ANA	6%

*Permission for reuse in a journal was acquired from Elsevier. Table formatting was modified for clarification of content.

Myositis with eosinophilic infiltrates most commonly involves parasites [17, 21] (*Trichinella*, *Echinococcus*, *Taenia solium*, and *Toxoplasma gondii*), viruses (EBV and coxsackie), inflammatory myopathies (dermatomyositis, polymyositis), and systemic diseases (Churg-Strauss syndrome) [13]. Other less common etiologies like muscular dystrophies (calpainopathy [8] and Becker Disease [14]), toxic exposures to L-tryptophan [7], toxic oil syndrome, malignancy, and EM as a component of idiopathic hypereosinophilic syndrome (HES) can also have eosinophilic predominant myositis [13]. Other drugs associated with myopathy and eosinophilia include cimetidine, phenytoin, and penicillamine [19]. Once all the above etiologies have been considered, and no cause has been identified, idiopathic eosinophilic myositis can be diagnosed as in our case.

Eosinophilia associated myopathy is categorized into 3 subtypes: focal eosinophilic myositis, eosinophilic perimyositis, and eosinophilic polymyositis (Table 3). Focal EM usually causes lower extremity pain and calf swelling. Eosinophilic perimyositis generally causes myalgias and mild proximal muscle weakness. Labs may show normal creatinine kinase levels. Eosinophilic polymyositis is more commonly a systemic disease with frequent cardiac, lung, or gut involvement [6, 13]. Interestingly, peripheral eosinophilia is not needed to diagnose any of the above entities [2, 15]. Clinically, our

patient had severe muscle weakness, elevated CPK levels, a high degree of peripheral eosinophilia, and the need for steroids for symptomatic involvement. Histologically, her muscle biopsy revealed widespread eosinophilic infiltration consistent with a diagnosis of eosinophilic polymyositis.

The overall prognosis of EM is good and is most favorable in the localized form. As is shown in Table 2, eosinophilic polymyositis is the only subtype of EM that almost always requires prednisone for symptomatic improvement. However, the role of disease modifying drugs in eosinophilic polymyositis is yet to be determined. In some cases, IVIG [3, 10] and azathioprine have led to successful remission of the disease [3].

To the best of our knowledge, only two other cases of idiopathic eosinophilic polymyositis have been described in the English literature. In 1992, Behari et al. [2] described the case of a 24-year-old male who had muscle pain that gradually progressed for 2.5 years prior to presentation. Two months after treatment with steroids, his CPK levels remained elevated. In 1994, Mancias et al. [10] reported the case of an 8-year-old girl who had muscle weakness that progressed to myalgias. She also had an asthma exacerbation a few months prior to presentation. They initiated treatment with steroids but the patient's CPK levels remained elevated. They attempted intravenous immunoglobulins but a repeat muscle biopsy showed persistent eosinophilic infiltrate. However, no systemic involvement was noted in either case, including ours. Our patient presented with an acute onset of muscle pain with no prior complaints of weakness or myalgias, in contrast to the more insidious course described in the above two cases. Additionally, our patient responded well to 2 months of steroid therapy, with CPK levels returning to normal. Six months later her CPK levels remain within normal limits on a long steroid taper.

4. Conclusion

Myositis with eosinophilic infiltrates has a broad differential. This case report introduces an unusual presentation of an unusual illness and illustrates a systematic workup for rhabdomyolysis in the presence of peripheral eosinophilia. Before a diagnosis of eosinophilic myositis can be made, a wide array of diagnostic tests has to be completed. In order to determine the best treatment for a patient with EM, further defining the extent of eosinophilic infiltrate by a biopsy is of utmost importance. This case of idiopathic eosinophilic polymyositis, to our knowledge, is unique because it is a rare cause of severe rhabdomyolysis without another organ involvement. Clinicians should maintain a high index of suspicion for this physically debilitating disease to aid in prompt diagnosis.

Abbreviations

AST: Aspartate aminotransferase
ALT: Alanine aminotransferase
HPF: High powered field
ANA: Antinuclear antibody

TABLE 3: Proposed criteria for diagnosis for eosinophilic myositis [13].

	Focal eosinophilic myositis[a]	Eosinophilic polymyositis[b]	Eosinophilic perimyositis[c]
Major	(1) Pain and calf swelling (other muscles can be affected) (2) Deep eosinophilic infiltration with muscle fiber invasion and necrosis on muscle biopsy	(1) Proximal weakness affecting limb girdle muscles (may be severe) (2) Widespread deep infiltration of eosinophil into muscles, with eosinophilic cuffing, on histology. Myonecrosis and endomysium inflammation usually +ve. If −ve deposition of MBP should be demonstrated by immunostain	(1) Myalgia, proximal mild weakness (2) Eosinophilic infiltrate confined to fascia and superficial perimysium, absence of myofiber necrosis
Minor	(1) ↑ CPK and aldolase (2) MRI or EMG evidence of focal myositis (3) Absence of systemic illness (4) Eosinophilia $>0.5 \times 10^9$/L	(1) ↑ CPK and aldolase (2) Eosinophilia $>0.5 \times 10^9$/L (3) Systemic illness with frequent cardiac involvement (4) Steroids are needed	(1) Absence of systemic manifestations (2) Normal CK and aldolase levels (3) Eosinophilia $>0.5 \times 10^9$/L
Exclude	DVT, cellulitis, parasitic infection	HES, cell T clonality, DM, vasculitis (CSS), drugs, calpainopathy, parasitic infections	Toxic oil syndrome, myalgia-eosinophilia, exposure to inorganic or organic substances
Treatment	No steroid treatment required. Symptoms resolve spontaneously	Prednisone 0.5–1 mg/kg/day is the treatment of choice	Rarely requires steroid treatment for symptom resolution

[a]2 major or 1 major and 3 minor criteria establish the diagnosis.
[b]Both major criteria or one major and two minor criteria establish the diagnosis.
[c]Both major criteria and major criteria number 2 plus two minor criteria enable the diagnosis.
* Permission for reuse in a journal was acquired from Elsevier. The treatment section is an addition to the original table.

C-ANCA:	Cytoplasmic anti-neutrophil cytoplasmic antibody
P-ANCA:	Perinuclear anti-neutrophil cytoplasmic antibody
Anti-dsDNA:	Anti-double stranded DNA
Anti-Sm Ab:	Anti-Smith antibodies
C3:	Complement 3
C4:	Complement 4
CMV:	Cytomegalovirus
EBV:	Epstein-Barr virus
HSV:	Herpes simplex virus
HIV:	Human immunodeficiency virus
H&E:	Hematoxylin and eosin
SPEP:	Serum electrophoresis
UPEP:	Urine electrophoresis.

References

[1] S. Arase, S. Kato, H. Nakanishi et al., "Eosinophilic polymyositis induced by Tranilast," *Journal of Dermatology*, vol. 17, no. 3, pp. 182–186, 1990.

[2] M. Behari, P. Saha, A. Dinda, K. Prasad, and G. K. Ahuja, "Eosinophilic polymyositis without peripheral eosinophilia," *Journal of the Association of Physicians of India*, vol. 40, no. 2, p. 132, 1992.

[3] E. J. de Kruijf, J. Rothbarth, S. G. van Duinen, P. H. de Meijer, and A. E. Meinders, "Patient with eosinophilic polymyositis," *Nederlands Tijdschrift voor Geneeskunde*, vol. 144, no. 42, pp. 2019–2023, 2000.

[4] L. Ellman, L. Miller, and J. Rappeport, "Leukopheresis therapy of a hypereosinophilic disorder," *Journal of the American Medical Association*, vol. 230, no. 7, pp. 1004–1005, 1974.

[5] Y. Ikeda, M. Tanaka, K. Mizushima, and K. Okamoto, "A case of eosinophilic polymyositis complicated by myasthenia gravis," *Muscle and Nerve*, vol. 21, no. 10, pp. 1356–1358, 1998.

[6] K. Ishizawa, D. Adachi, K. Kuboi et al., "Multiple organ involvement in eosinophilic polymyositis: an autopsy report," *Human Pathology*, vol. 37, no. 2, pp. 231–235, 2006.

[7] M. Ivey, M. S. Eichenhorn, M. R. Glasberg, and R. C. Hyzy, "Hypercapnic respiratory failure due to L-tryptophan-induced eosinophilic polymyositis," *Chest*, vol. 99, no. 3, pp. 756–757, 1991.

[8] M. Krahn, A. L. de Munain, N. Streichenberger et al., "CAPN3 mutations in patients with idiopathic eosinophilic myositis," *Annals of Neurology*, vol. 59, no. 6, pp. 905–911, 2006.

[9] E. Maeshima, T. Nishimoto, M. Yamashita, M. Mune, and S. Yukawa, "Progressive systemic sclerosis-polymyositis overlap syndrome with eosinophilic pleural effusion," *Rheumatology International*, vol. 23, no. 5, pp. 252–254, 2003.

[10] P. Mancias, T. P. Bohan, I. J. Butler, and M. B. Bhattacharjee, "Treatment-resistant eosinophilic polymyositis in a child," *Journal of Child Neurology*, vol. 9, no. 4, pp. 446–448, 1994.

[11] J.-I. Onodera, T. Hayashi, K. Chida, Y. Shiga, H. Mochizuki, and Y. Itoyama, "A case of Ki-1 lymphoma-associated eosinophilic

polymyositis," *Rinsho Shinkeigaku*, vol. 37, no. 4, pp. 314–318, 1997.

[12] A. Saito and I. Higuchi, "Eosinophilic polymyositis," *Ryoikibetsu Shokogun Shirizu*, no. 35, pp. 350–353, 2001.

[13] A. Selva-O'Callaghan, E. Trallero-Araguás, and J. M. Grau, "Eosinophilic myositis: an updated review," *Autoimmunity Reviews*, vol. 13, no. 4-5, pp. 375–378, 2014.

[14] G. Serratrice, J. F. Pellissier, H. Roux, and P. Quilichini, "Fasciitis, perimyositis, myositis, polymyositis, and eosinophilia," *Muscle and Nerve*, vol. 13, no. 5, pp. 385–395, 1990.

[15] R. J. Stark, "Eosinophilic polymyositis," *Archives of Neurology*, vol. 36, no. 11, pp. 721–722, 1979.

[16] A. Zurn, E. Domine, J. N. Cox, and J.-H. Saurat, "Eosinophilia and eosinophilic polymyositis," *Revue Medicale de la Suisse Romande*, vol. 111, no. 2, pp. 141–149, 1991.

[17] R. B. Layzer, M. A. Shearn, and S. Satya-Murti, "Eosinophilic polymyositis," *Annals of Neurology*, vol. 1, no. 1, pp. 65–71, 1977.

[18] A. Selva O'Callaghan and J. M. Grau, "Eosinophlic myositis," in *Diagnostic Criteria in Autoimmune Diseases*, pp. 179–182, Springer, 2008.

[19] L. D. Kaufman, G. M. Kephart, R. J. Seidman et al., "The spectrum of eosinophilic myositis: clinical and immunopathogenic studies of three patients, and review of the literature," *Arthritis and Rheumatism*, vol. 36, no. 7, pp. 1014–1024, 1993.

[20] I. N. Lazarou and P.-A. Guerne, "Classification, diagnosis, and management of idiopathic inflammatory myopathies," *Journal of Rheumatology*, vol. 40, no. 5, pp. 550–564, 2013.

[21] S. N. El-Beshbishi, N. N. Ahmed, S. H. Mostafa, and G. A. El-Ganainy, "Parasitic infections and myositis," *Parasitology Research*, vol. 110, no. 1, pp. 1–18, 2012.

22

Intestinal Infarction and Portal Vein Thrombosis in a Patient with Henoch Schonlein Purpura

Mekdess Abebe,[1] **Asha Patnaik,**[2] **Frederick Miller,**[3] **Heidi Roppelt,**[2]
Nand K. Wadhwa,[1] **Mersema Abate,**[1] **and Edward P. Nord**[1]

[1] Division of Nephrology, Department of Medicine, School of Medicine, State University of New York at Stony Brook,
  Stony Brook, NY 11794, USA
[2] Division of Rheumatology, Department of Medicine, School of Medicine, State University of New York at Stony Brook,
  Stony Brook, NY 11794, USA
[3] Department of Pathology, School of Medicine, State University of New York at Stony Brook, Stony Brook, NY 11794, USA

Correspondence should be addressed to Mekdess Abebe, mekdess2003@yahoo.com

Academic Editors: D. Aeberli, D. R. Alpert, R. Cevik, A. Chalmers, A. Giusti, and C. Schubert

Henoch Schonlein purpura is a systemic vasculitis that commonly affects children and teenagers but also affects adults of all ages. In most instances it has a benign course. Organ involvement, particularly in adults, and notably the kidneys and gastrointestinal tract may require therapeutic intervention and may have a less favorable outcome. We report a case of a 58-year-old man who presented with purpura and who rapidly developed catastrophic intestinal vasculitis, leading to his demise.

1. Introduction

Henoch Schonlein purpura (HSP) is a systemic vasculitis characterized by involvement of the skin, joints, kidney, and gastrointestinal tract [1–3]. It is primarily a disease of children but can occur at any age [2, 3]. In most cases, especially in children, it is a benign self-limiting disorder, but adults may require immunosuppressive therapy for complete recovery [2]. Gastrointestinal (GI) manifestations occur in 55–75% of adult HSP patients [1]. The most common GI symptoms include colicky abdominal pain, GI bleeding, and vomiting. Rarely, intussusception, bowel infarction and hemorrhagic ascites can complicate HSP [4–7]. Complete recovery with or without treatment usually occurs, and fatal complications are rare. We report an adult patient with HSP complicated by extensive infarction of the intestine, intraperitoneal hemorrhage, and portal vein thrombosis with a fatal outcome.

2. Case Report

A 58-year-old white man was referred to the outpatient nephrology office by his gastroenterologist because of microscopic hematuria and proteinuria in the setting of an evolving purpuric rash. The rash had progressed proximally from both feet to his thighs, upper extremities and abdomen over the past two weeks. He complained of nausea, and vomiting for one day but denied hematemesis, melanotic stools, or arthralgia. His significant comorbidities included hypertension, untreated hepatitis C, and alcohol abuse. He took no medications.

On physical examination blood pressure was 105/62 mmHg, pulse was 84 beats/minute and regular, and temperature 37.7°C. The skin showed nontender, palpable purpuric lesions involving both upper and lower extremities and the abdominal wall. Lungs were clear to auscultation and the cardiovascular exam was unremarkable. On abdominal examination no organomegaly was appreciated. There was no pedal edema.

Laboratory tests revealed a white blood cell count of 13.1×10^3/mcL, hemoglobin 14.7 g/dL, hematocrit 42.9%, and platelet count of 234×10^3/mcL. Serum chemistry showed sodium 136 mEq/L, potassium 4.2 mEq/L, chloride 101 mEq/L, bicarbonate 24 mEq/L, blood urea nitrogen (BUN) 34 mg/dL and serum creatinine 2.0 mg/dL. Liver

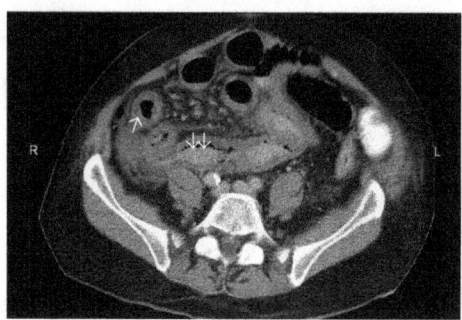

FIGURE 1: Computed tomography (CT) of the abdomen and pelvis with IV contrast showing marked thickening of the terminal ileum.

function tests revealed a total bilirubin of 1.3 mg/dL, direct bilirubin 0.5 mg/dL, ALT 75 units/L, AST 93 units/L, alkaline phosphatase 75 units/L, total protein 7.6 g/dL and albumin 3.7 g/dL. Hepatitis B core antibody, hepatitis B surface antibody and hepatitis C antibody were all positive. Urinalysis demonstrated trace hematuria and proteinuria. He was sent to the emergency room for further evaluation.

On admission the patient was started on intravenous fluids and additional tests were obtained. Antinuclear antibody (ANA) and serum complements (C_3 and C_4) were normal and antineutrophil cytoplasmic antibody (ANCA) and cryoglobulins were negative. The serum creatinine improved to 0.75 mg/dL on hydration alone. Two days later he complained of diffuse abdominal pain and dark stool followed by hematochezia. He remained afebrile with a blood pressure of 120/50 mmHg. On physical examination he had significant right upper abdominal quadrant and epigastric tenderness. Esophagogastroduodenoscopy (EGD) was performed that failed to reveal a lesion that could account for his symptoms. A biopsy of the stomach mucosa demonstrated mild chronic inflammation. Computerized tomography (CT) scan of the abdomen was next performed and showed marked thickening of the terminal ileum (Figure 1). Abdominal pain intensified, and the patient became tachycardic and tachypneic with a leukocytosis of 23×10^3/mcL, with deteriorating renal function (BUN 54 mg/dL, serum creatinine of 2.0 mg/dL) and evolving acidosis (bicarbonate 17 mEq/L). An emergency exploratory laparotomy was performed which revealed gangrenous bowel from the beginning of the ileum to the transverse colon. Small bowel resection (90 cm of ileum) and right hemicolectomy (including appendix which was involved) with end jejunostomy were performed.

Histopathologic examination of the resected intestinal tissue demonstrated an extensive necrotizing vasculitis with IgA deposition characteristic of HSP (Figure 2). Of particular note was the very widespread (perhaps 50%) involvement of medium sized vessels, particularly arteries, with extensive necrosis and secondary ischemic injury to the intestines. Small arteries, arterioles, and venules were also involved. Heavy granular IgA deposition was seen with no staining for IgG or IgM. Lesser amounts of C_3 paralleled the IgA deposition.

Intravenous methylprednisolone 1 g daily for three days was administered and then 30 mg every 12 hours. Postoperatively he continued to have an elevated white blood cell count and persistent fever, but his renal function improved. A repeat CT scan of the abdomen revealed persistent small bowel wall thickening. A second exploratory laparotomy was performed, but no additional ischemic bowel was identified. The patient was continued on broad-spectrum antibiotics and maintained on a ventilator due to respiratory failure. Eight days after the second laparotomy he developed severe lactic acidosis, right upper abdominal quadrant tenderness jaundice and worsening renal function. Ultrasound of the right upper quadrant showed findings compatible with portal vein thrombosis and cholelithiasis. Repeat CT scan of the abdomen showed increased ascites with intraperitoneal hemorrhage. Hemodialysis was initiated due to worsening oliguric acute kidney injury. His condition continued to deteriorate, and he died one day later, a total of 27 days after admission.

3. Discussion

HSP is a systemic small-vessel vasculitis that is mainly a disease of early childhood [1–3, 10]. Overall prognosis is good in both children and adults, with one study showing complete recovery occurring in 94% of children and 89% of adults [2]. In this regard, recovery is usually spontaneous in children, whereas in adults immunosuppressive therapy may be required in up to 63% of cases [2]. We present a case of a middle-aged man who developed extensive gangrenous bowel and intraperitoneal hemorrhage due to HSP vasculitis, with a fatal outcome.

GI symptoms are one of the commonest manifestations of HSP in adults, involving 55–75% of individuals [1]. In a retrospective analysis of 115 adults with the diagnosis of HSP, GI symptoms were reported in 90 patients (78.2%), abdominal pain being the most common (89%) followed by vomiting and GI bleeding [4]. Furthermore, 24% of patients had GI symptoms prior to the development of a cutaneous rash [4]. In another retrospective study involving 116 children and 46 adults, adults had a lower frequency of GI involvement (5%) at disease onset, but during the clinical course GI involvement was the same in both age groups (56.5% of adults versus 63.8% of children) [2]. In a retrospective analysis of 250 adults with HSP, GI involvement was observed in 48%. In 13 of these cases (11%) serious GI complication developed requiring transfusion or surgery or leading to death [3]. The small intestine is the most common site involved, terminal ileum (60%) and the second portion of the duodenum (53%). The rectum (80%) is the most frequently affected areas in the lower GI tract [4, 8]. Endoscopic findings include mucosal congestion, redness, petechiae, multiple ulcers, and hemorrhagic erosions [4, 8, 9]. Rarely, severe GI complication such as bowel infarction, perforation, fistula, intussusceptions (ileoileal), hemorrhagic ascites, and pancreatitis can occur [4–7, 10].

A number of inciting antigens have been implicated in the causation of HSP. These include bacterial and viral infections, vaccinations, drugs, malignancy, and autoimmune

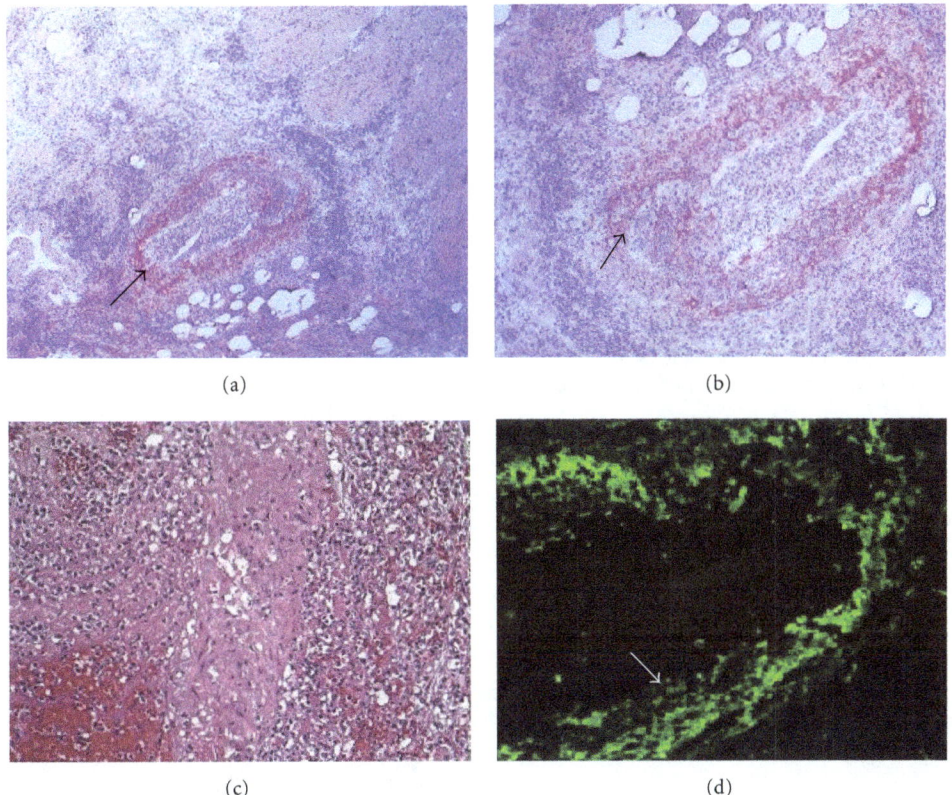

FIGURE 2: (a) A small artery in the intestinal submucosa showing necrotizing arteritis (H&E). (b) A higher power view of the same vessel showing early fibrin formation in the lumen (arrow). (c) A high power view of another vessel emphasizing the necrosis and the largely neutrophil reaction (H&E). (d) A randomly selected artery illustrating the heavy deposition of IgA (immunofluorescence with an alpha chain-specific antibody).

phenomena. The pathogenic mechanism of organ involvement in HSP is thought to be due to the deposition of antigen antibody complexes in the small vessel walls. This leads to activation of the alternate complement pathway leading to neutrophil accumulation resulting in inflammation and vasculitis [9, 10]. IgA is the antibody class most often seen in the immune complex [10]. The presence of hepatitis C virus could have been a triggering factor in our patient as has been suggested by others [10].

To the best of our knowledge, the extensive small and large intestine infarction with gangrene that led to a fatal outcome in our patient is rarely seen in HSP. In this case, in contrast to the majority of those reported, the arteritis was extensive and involved medium sized vessels (0.3–0.5 cm) in many areas as well as the small arteries, arterioles, and venules. The involvement of the transverse colon and appendix as seen in our patient is also rare in HSP. An additional complicating factor in this case was the occurrence of portal vein thrombosis. In reviewing the literature, there is only one reported case of portal vein thrombosis complicating HSP [11]. However, in the patient presented here, we are unable to conclude whether the portal vein thrombosis was associated with underlying hepatitis C or was a complication of HSP. Hepatitis C, without cirrhosis would be unlikely to cause portal vein thrombosis.

The mainstay of therapy in HSP with severe organ involvement has been high-dose steroids. Other immunosuppressive agents such as cyclophosphamide, azathioprine, and mycophenolate mofetil have also been used [12, 13]. There has been only one prospective randomized trial comparing steroid therapy with and without cyclophosphamide in cases of severe visceral HSP [14]. The results of that study showed that addition of cyclophosphamide to steroids did not improve the outcome of the disease as compared to steroids alone. Our patient was treated with pulse steroids alone, with no significant improvement.

In conclusion, given the potential severity and fatal outcome of HSP involving the intestines in adults, prompt and early recognition of this entity is crucial. The mainstay of therapy remains high-dose steroids, with little evidence to support the use of other immunosuppressive agents. In catastrophic circumstances as described in this instance, even high-dose steroids may not alter the course of events.

References

[1] F. T. Saulsbury, "Clinical update: Henoch-Schönlein purpura," Lancet, vol. 369, no. 9566, pp. 976–978, 2007.

[2] R. Blanco, V. M. Martínez-Taboada, V. Rodríguez-Valverde, M. García-Fuentes, and M. A. González-Gay, "Henoch-Schonlein purpura in adulthood and childhood: two different

expressions of the same syndrome," *Arthritis and Rheumatism*, vol. 40, no. 5, pp. 859–864, 1997.

[3] E. Pillebout, E. Thervet, G. Hill, C. Alberti, P. Vanhille, and D. Nochy, "Henoch-Schönlein Purpura in adults: outcome and prognostic factors," *Journal of the American Society of Nephrology*, vol. 13, no. 5, pp. 1271–1278, 2002.

[4] Y. Zhang and X. Huang, "Gastrointestinal involvement in Henoch-Schönlein purpura," *Scandinavian Journal of Gastroenterology*, vol. 43, no. 9, pp. 1038–1043, 2008.

[5] D. H. Akbar, "Fatal complication of Henoch-Schonlein purpura: case report and literature review," *Saudi Journal of Gastroenterology*, vol. 6, no. 3, pp. 165–168, 2000.

[6] E. C. Ebert, "Gastrointestinal manifestations of Henoch-Schonlein purpura," *Digestive Diseases and Sciences*, vol. 53, no. 8, pp. 2011–2019, 2008.

[7] P. Carmichael, E. Brun, S. Jayawardene, A. Abdulkadir, and P. J. O'Donnell, "A fatal case of bowel and cardiac involvement in Henoch-Schönlein purpura," *Nephrology Dialysis Transplantation*, vol. 17, no. 3, pp. 497–499, 2002.

[8] A. Hamzaoui, W. Melki, O. Harzallah, L. Njim, R. Klii, and S. Mahjoub, "Gastrointestinal involvement revealing Henoch Schonlein purpura in adults: report of three cases and review of the literature," *International Archives of Medicine*, vol. 4, no. 1, Article ID Article number31, 2011.

[9] S. Kato, K. Ebina, H. Naganuma, S. I. Sato, S. I. Maisawa, and H. Nakagawa, "Intestinal IgA deposition in Henoch-Schönlein purpura with severe gastro-intestinal manifestations," *European Journal of Pediatrics*, vol. 155, no. 2, pp. 91–95, 1996.

[10] A. B. Sohagia, S. G. Gunturu, T. R. Tong, and H. I. Hertan, "Henoch-schonlein purpura—a case report and review of the literature," *Gastroenterology Research and Practice*, vol. 2010, Article ID 597648, 7 pages, 2010.

[11] S. J. Choi, S. K. Park, W. S. Uhm et al., "A case of refractory Henoch-Schönlein purpura treated with thalidomide," *The Korean Journal of Internal Medicine*, vol. 17, no. 4, pp. 270–273, 2002.

[12] P. S. Kellerman, "Henoch-Schönlein purpura in adults," *American Journal of Kidney Diseases*, vol. 48, no. 6, pp. 1009–1016, 2006.

[13] A. A. Nikibakhsh, H. Mahmoodzadeh, M. Karamyyar et al., "Treatment of complicated henoch-schnlein purpura with mycophenolate mofetil: a retrospective case series report," *International Journal of Rheumatology*, vol. 2010, Article ID 254316, 2010.

[14] E. Pillebout, C. Alberti, L. Guillevin, A. Ouslimani, and E. Thervet, "Addition of cyclophosphamide to steroids provides no benefit compared with steroids alone in treating adult patients with severe Henoch Schönlein Purpura," *Kidney International*, vol. 78, no. 5, pp. 495–502, 2010.

23

Successful Discontinuation of Infliximab in a Refractory Case of Vasculo-Behçet Disease

Akihiro Nakamura,[1,2] **Tomoya Miyamura,**[1] **and Eiichi Suematsu**[1]

[1]*Department of Internal Medicine and Rheumatology, Clinical Research Institute, National Hospital Organization,*
Kyushu Medical Center, Fukuoka 810-8563, Japan
[2]*Department of Genetics and Development, Krembil Research Institute, University Health Network, Toronto, ON, Canada M5T 2S8*

Correspondence should be addressed to Akihiro Nakamura; anakamur@uhnresearch.ca

Academic Editor: Suleyman Serdar Koca

Reports have shown that antitumor necrosis factor alpha (anti-TNF-α) agents including infliximab (IFX) can dramatically suppress the disease activity of refractory vasculo-Behçet disease (vasculo-BD). However, it is completely unknown whether we can discontinue anti-TNF-α agents under clinical remission. A 31-year-old patient with vasculo-BD was initially treated with a high dose of steroid and intravenous cyclophosphamide therapy. Six months later, however, the disease recurred. IFX was administered and immediately the disease activity was reduced. Fortunately, we could discontinue IFX after 18-month remission and no recurrence has been observed. Based on previous reports and our patient, all patients who could discontinue IFX sustained clinical remission for at least one year, continued taking immunosuppressive agents such as methotrexate and azathioprine, and had vascular involvements only in non-life-threatening major vessels such as leg or arm arteries/veins. This is a report suggesting the possibility of discontinuation of IFX in vasculo-BD.

1. Introduction

Vasculo-Behçet disease (vasculo-BD) is one of the most severe and life-threatening facets of BD which predominantly appears in large blood vessels [1]. Furthermore, unpredictable recurrence is not uncommon even under strict immunosuppressive treatment. However, since there are no control studies for the management of vasculo-BD, specific guidelines and recommendations for treatments are unavailable excluding the usage of strong immunosuppressive agents [2]. This deficiency of strong evidence leads to ambiguity and difficulty when determining therapeutic strategies.

Recent reports reveal inhibition of tumor necrosis factor alpha (TNF-α) has dramatic efficacy for the successful treatment of various types of BD, including vasculo-BD, through controlling inflammation [3–6]. In Japan, usage of infliximab (IFX), a chimeric mouse-human anti-TNF-α monoclonal antibody, has recently been covered by national health insurance in refractory cases of specific types of BD including entero-BD, neuro-BD, and vasculo-BD. However, it is completely unknown whether we can discontinue anti-

TNF-α agents for patients with vasculo-BD under clinical remission. We herein report a suggestive case of successful discontinued IFX treatment and sustained long-term remission in a patient with refractory vasculo-BD.

2. Case Presentation

A 31-year-old previously healthy male was admitted for evaluation for persistent low grade fever and gradual onset of swelling and claudication on his left arm. Further detailed medical history revealed that the patient had a history of recurrent oral aphthae which started 7 years ago. Physical examination on admission determined swelling on his left upper arm, erythema nodosum on his left forearm, and purpura on his left wrist indicating insufficient blood supply (Figures 1(a)–1(c)). Left radial artery pulse was palpable and Allen's test was negative. Joint tenderness was also identified on bilateral knee and ankle joints, suggesting the existence of arthritis. Laboratory studies showed leukocytosis (14,200/μL) with 88.0% of neutrophil, increased levels of serum inflammatory markers such as C-reactive protein

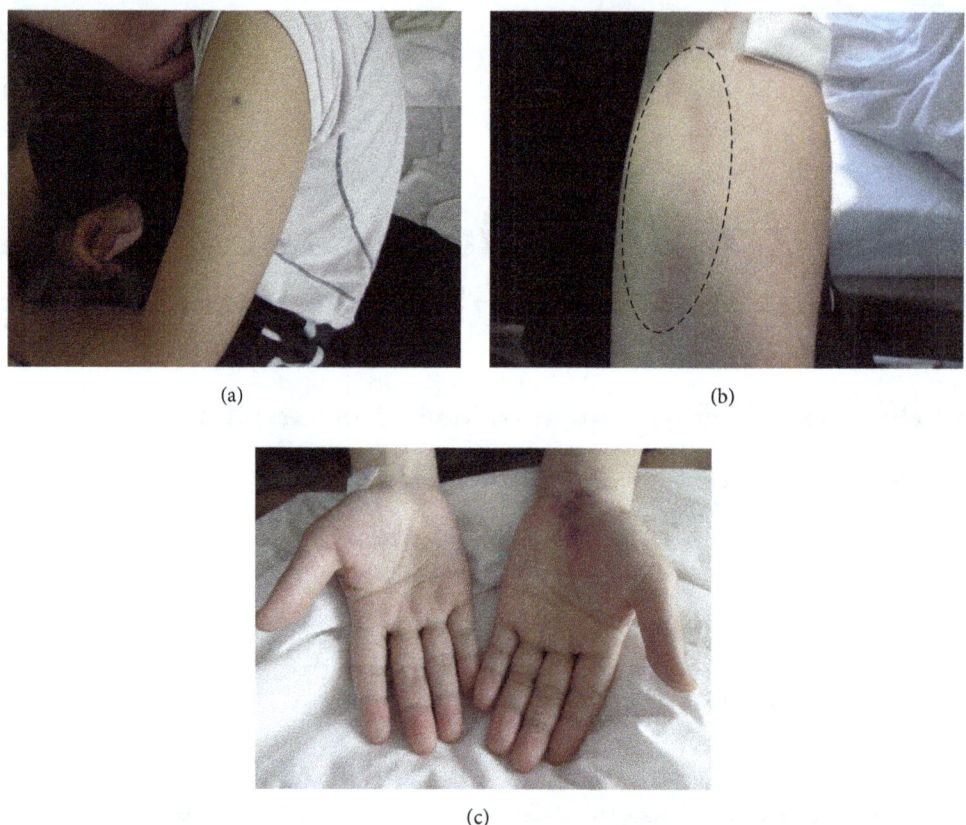

(a)

(b)

(c)

FIGURE 1: Clinical manifestations on admission. Physical examination identified swollen left upper arm (a), erythema nodosum on the left forearm (b), and purpura on the left wrist joint (c), suggesting a deficiency of blood supply on the left arm.

(CRP) (12.4 mg/dL), and erythrocyte sedimentation rate (ESR) (50 mm/h). Normal results of protein C, protein S, antithrombin, activated partial thromboplastin time (aPTT), anticardiolipin antibody, anti-β2GPI antibody, and lupus anticoagulants excluded the possibility of prothrombotic disorders and antiphospholipid syndrome. Antineutrophil cytoplasmic antibodies (ANCA), including proteinase 3- (PR3-) ANCA and myeloperoxidase- (MPO-) ANCA, were negative and hepatitis B virus (HBV) antigen (HBs antigen) and antibody (HBs antibody) which suggest the possibility of polyarteritis nodosa were also not detected. Result of HLA-B51, a well-known allele as BD preposition, was positive. Computed Tomography (CT) demonstrated inflammation of perivascular tissue around left axial artery and CT Angiography (CTA) clearly showed left brachial and radial artery stenosis, suggesting the diagnosis of arteritis from left axial to radial artery. According to the criteria for BD from Ministry of Health, Labor and Welfare in Japan, the patient was diagnosed with BD, specifically vasculo-BD based on prominent vascular manifestations.

Intravenous methylprednisolone (mPSL) (1000 mg/day for consequent three days) and cyclophosphamide (IVCY) pulse therapy (1000 mg/month) were initiated followed by oral prednisolone (PSL) (60 mg/day) according to the European League Against Rheumatism (EULAR) recommendations for the management of BD [2]. Anticoagulation therapies such as anticoagulants, antiplatelet, or antifibrinolytic agents were not considered based on no control studies as well as no evidence of benefit from them as stated in EULAR recommendations [2]. After the immunosuppressive therapy was initiated, clinical symptoms seemed to gradually subside.

Six months later, however, left arm pain and claudication recurred and levels of serum inflammatory markers such as CRP and ESR were elevated. At this time, the fifth time of IVCY had ended and the patient was taking 20 mg of PSL. After confirming the diagnosis with recurrent vasculo-BD based on severe stenosis of left brachial and radial artery on CTA (Figures 2(a) and 2(c)), IFX was started (5 mg/kg, 0, 2, and 6 weeks followed by every 8 weeks) in combination with oral methotrexate (MTX) (16 mg/week). Since the induction of IFX and MTX treatment, the symptoms including pain were alleviated within four weeks along with the rapid improvement of serum inflammatory markers. Additionally, the artery stenosis assessed by a repeated CTA was dramatically resolved (Figures 2(b) and 2(d)). Since then, the patient sustained a good response to IFX resulting in clinical remission (no clinical symptoms and normal ranges of serum inflammatory markers) with no remarkable drug side effects. Therefore, we planned to continue IFX. However, IFX was discontinued after 18 months by the patient due to the medical cost. Considering (i) sustained clinical remission of 18 months, (ii) limited artery involvement (only left brachial and radial artery), and (iii) continuation of taking MTX and PSL, we decided to discontinue IFX. Fortunately, no

Before IFX   After IFX (12 months)

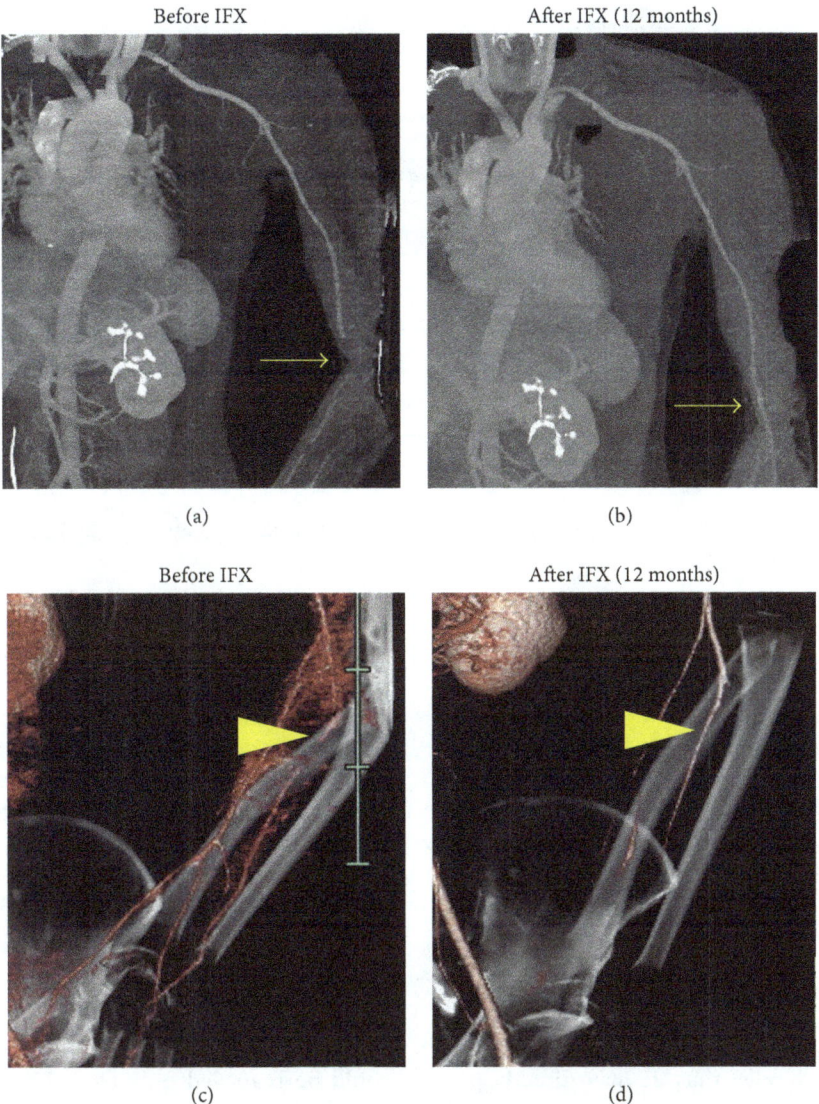

(a)   (b)

Before IFX   After IFX (12 months)

(c)   (d)

FIGURE 2: Computed Tomography Angiography showed severe stenosis of left brachial (a) and radial (c) arteries before infliximab (IFX) induction. After IFX therapy, the artery stenosis was immediately resolved and sustained clinical remission ((b) and (d) at 12 months since IFX was introduced).

recurrence has been observed for 24 months, with PSL (5 mg/day) and MTX (16 mg/week) as a maintenance therapy (Figure 3).

3. Discussion

Vasculo-BD is one of the most severe conditions that predominantly affect young men [1]. Given inflammation of all sizes (small, medium, and large) of blood vessels (both venous and arteries), most clinical manifestations observed in BD can be explained by vasculitis. Furthermore, even in patients without obvious vascular involvements of BD, endothelial and microvascular functions are compromised the same as patients with vascular involvements [7]. However, when specifically describing the term of vasculo-BD, involvements of large blood vessels predominantly appear among clinical manifestations. Superficial venous thrombophlebitis (SVT)

or deep venous thrombosis (DVT) has been reported as the most common manifestations in vasculo-BD [8], but arterial lesions including pulmonary artery aneurysms that can result in high mortality are also observed, suggesting early diagnosis and rapid induction of appropriate treatments are crucial. Conventional therapies including glucocorticoid and other immunosuppressive agents such as cyclophosphamide, azathioprine (AZA), and cyclosporine A may suppress the inflammation in both affected venous and arteries, resulting in downregulation of disease activity [9]. However, unpredictable recurrence of vascular events is not uncommon. Additionally, no specific biomarkers for BD hamper the judgment of opportune time for tapering the dose of glucocorticoid and immunosuppressive agents, leading to multiple burdensome side effects.

Usage of TNF-α inhibitors for BD has firstly been established as an optimal drug in cases of ocular BD [10] and then

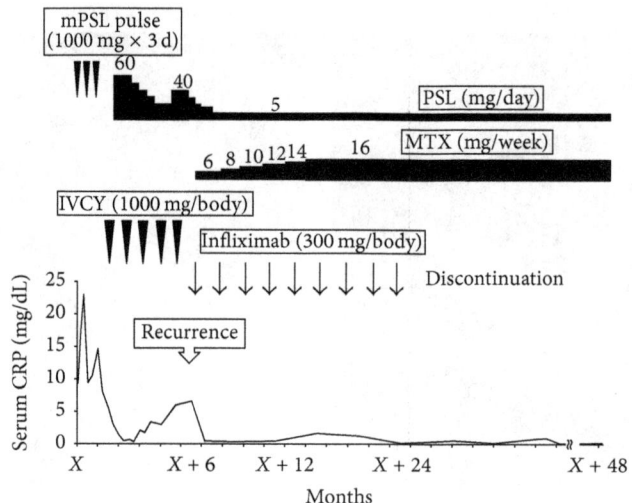

FIGURE 3: Patient's clinical time course. *mPSL* methylprednisolone, *PSL* prednisolone, *IVCY* intravenous cyclophosphamide, and *MTX* methotrexate.

the application has been extended to other types of BD, especially in refractory cases showing resistance to steroid and other conventional immunosuppressant therapies. Although the exact mechanism of vasculo-BD is not fully understood, since immunological cells including neutrophils and mononuclear cells (predominantly CD3+CD4+ T lymphocytes and NK cells) infiltrate into the media and adventitia of arterial wall, dysregulated expression of proinflammatory mediators such as TNF-α, interleukin- (IL-) 1β, IL-6, and IL-17 may be involved in the pathogenesis of vasculo-BD [11]. TNF-α produced primarily by cells of the macrophage-monocyte lineage showed biologic effects including adhesion molecule expression, synthesis of proinflammatory cytokines and chemokines, activation of immune system cells, and inhibition of regulatory T-cells; thus, it may directly participate in vascular inflammation as well as endothelial cell damage [7]. Previous reports suggested that anti-TNF-α agents show not only the dramatic efficacy on vasculo-BD but also their safety throughout the period of treatment [3–6]. Additionally, it has also been reported that switching drugs between anti-TNF-α agents are effective in refractory cases of BD [12]. However, it is a crucial problem for any autoimmune diseases including BD whether biologic agents can be discontinued after achievement of clinical remission to minimize drug side effects, complications, and medical costs. Recent studies on rheumatoid arthritis (RA) demonstrate that discontinuation of biologic agents, including anti-TNF-α agents, could be feasible for maintaining low disease activity without any additional therapies, suggesting potential of providing clinical benefits for patients with RA [13].

The patient initially seemed to respond to a high dose of steroid therapy followed by IVCY, but vasculo-BD involved in left brachial and radial arteries recurred. We decided to use IFX for this patient based on a number of reports showing the efficacy of IFX for refractory vasculo-BD and thus the disease activity was eventually reduced [3–6]. Furthermore, it is noted that we were fortunate to be able to discontinue IFX after sustaining 18-month remission with no recurrence

for 24 months. However, to date there are no indications for cessation of IFX in vasculo-BD.

To our knowledge, the only report published by Adler et al. showed two BD patients with leg artery and venous thrombosis or iliac vein thrombosis successfully discontinuing IFX after sustaining clinical remission for 3 years and 13 months, respectively. Similar to our patient, MTX or AZA was continued as a maintenance therapy after IFX discontinuation. Although the efficacy of MTX on vasculo-BD has not been established, the combination therapy with anti-TNF-α agents seemed to be effective in other BD-related vasculitis including retinal and entero-vasculitis [14], suggesting MTX can also be a reasonable immunosuppressive agent for vasculo-BD. It might be possible that our patient could be managed only by MTX at the recurrence, but it is well-known that the anti-inflammatory effect of MTX appears relatively slow compared to anti-TNF-α agents. Furthermore, in Japan the starting dose of MTX is usually low dose (from 6 to 8 mg/week) with concern about side effects such as gastrointestinal symptoms, which means only using low dose MTX would not be enough treatment as a rapid induction therapy for patients with refractory vasculo-BD.

While it is impossible to determine the criteria for IFX discontinuation based only on these patients, we can still identify some tendencies. All patients sustained clinical remission for at least one year, continued taking immunosuppressive agents such as MTX and AZA, and had vascular involvements only in non-life-threatening major vessels such as leg or arm arteries/veins.

Note that this report does not recommend discontinuing IFX in vasculo-BD. Magro-Checa et al. reported that life-threatening vasculo-BD emerged right after discontinuation of IFX even after 3 years of clinical remission [15]. Moreover, in the clinical trial for uveitis in BD, ocular attacks recurred in all patients after interruption of the therapy [10], presumably because concomitant use of immunosuppressive agents was prohibited in the trial. According to these reports, very careful judgement is necessary in deciding whether IFX can be discontinued or not; otherwise disease recurrence resulting in severe condition may occur.

Conclusively, this is a report to suggest the possibility of discontinuing IFX for vasculo-BD to date. Although further investigation and large cohort studies are necessary, this report could provide some clues about the discontinuation to prevent the implications of unnecessary treatment such as bothersome side effects and numerous medical costs.

Additional Points

It is controversial how to discontinue biologic agents in any diseases, because postdiscontinuation relapses are common. The consensus has not been shown even in RA in which a large number of patients receive biologics including IFX. In the clinical trial for uveitis in BD, ocular attacks recurred in all patients after interruption of the therapy [10], presumably because concomitant use of immunosuppressive agents was prohibited in the trial. Moreover, a recent case report showed that vascular involvement developed 4 months after discontinuation of IFX which maintained remission for 3 years [15], suggesting that decision making of the discontinuation is maybe more difficult in multiorgan diseases such as BD than single-organ diseases. However, this case report demonstrated the possibility of discontinuation of IFX in vasculo-BD. Based on previous reports and our patient, all patients who could discontinue IFX sustained clinical remission for at least one year, continued taking immunosuppressive agents such as MTX and AZA, and had vascular involvements only in non-life-threatening major vessels such as leg or arm arteries/veins. We believe this suggestive case would provide us with some clues about discontinuation of biologic agents including anti-TNF-α agents, resulting in keeping patients from huge medical costs, drug side effects, and complications.

Competing Interests

The authors declare that they have no competing interests.

References

[1] D. Saadoun, B. Wechsler, K. Desseaux et al., "Mortality in Behçet's disease," *Arthritis and Rheumatism*, vol. 62, no. 9, pp. 2806–2812, 2010.

[2] G. Hatemi, A. Silman, D. Bang et al., "EULAR recommendations for the management of Behçet disease," *Annals of the Rheumatic Diseases*, vol. 67, no. 12, pp. 1656–1662, 2008.

[3] P. P. Sfikakis, P. H. Kaklamanis, A. Elezoglou et al., "Infliximab for recurrent, sight-threatening ocular inflammation in adamantiades-behçet disease," *Annals of Internal Medicine*, vol. 140, no. 5, pp. 404–406, 2004.

[4] M. Melikoglu, I. Fresko, C. Mat et al., "Short-term trial of etanercept in Behçet's disease: a double blind, placebo controlled study," *Journal of Rheumatology*, vol. 32, no. 1, pp. 98–105, 2005.

[5] D. Perra, M. A. Alba, J. L. Callejas et al., "Adalimumab for the treatment of Behçet's disease: experience in 19 patients," *Rheumatology*, vol. 51, no. 10, Article ID kes130, pp. 1825–1831, 2012.

[6] S. Adler, I. Baumgartner, and P. M. Villiger, "Behçet's disease: successful treatment with infliximab in 7 patients with severe vascular manifestations. A retrospective analysis," *Arthritis Care & Research*, vol. 64, no. 4, pp. 607–611, 2012.

[7] M. Caliskan, H. Gullu, S. Yilmaz et al., "Cardiovascular prognostic value of vascular involvement in Behcet's disease," *International Journal of Cardiology*, vol. 125, no. 3, pp. 428–430, 2008.

[8] K. Tascilar, M. Melikoglu, S. Ugurlu, N. Sut, E. Caglar, and H. Yazici, "Vascular involvement in Behçet's syndrome: aretrospective analysis of associations and the time course," *Rheumatology*, vol. 53, no. 11, Article ID keu233, pp. 2018–2021, 2014.

[9] C. Comarmond, B. Wechsler, P. Cacoub, and D. Saadoun, "Approaches to immunosuppression in Behçet's disease," *Immunotherapy*, vol. 5, no. 7, pp. 743–754, 2013.

[10] S. Ohno, S. Nakamura, S. Hori et al., "Efficacy, safety, and pharmacokinetics of multiple administration of infliximab in Behçet's disease with refractory uveoretinitis," *Journal of Rheumatology*, vol. 31, no. 7, pp. 1362–1368, 2004.

[11] M. Kobayashi, M. Ito, A. Nakagawa et al., "Neutrophil and endothelial cell activation in the vasa vasorum in vasculo-Behçet disease," *Histopathology*, vol. 36, no. 4, pp. 362–371, 2000.

[12] P. Leccese, L. Latanza, S. D'Angelo, A. Padula, and I. Olivieri, "Efficacy of switching to adalimumab in a patient with refractory uveitis of Behçet's disease to infliximab," *Clinical and Experimental Rheumatology*, vol. 29, no. 4, p. S93, 2011.

[13] A. Kavanaugh, S. J. Lee, J. R. Curtis et al., "Discontinuation of tumour necrosis factor inhibitors in patients with rheumatoid arthritis in low-disease activity: persistent benefits. Data from the Corrona registry," *Annals of the Rheumatic Diseases*, vol. 74, no. 6, pp. 1150–1155, 2015.

[14] S. Iwata, K. Saito, K. Yamaoka et al., "Efficacy of combination therapy of anti-TNF-α antibody infliximab and methotrexate in refractory entero-Behçet's disease," *Modern Rheumatology*, vol. 21, no. 2, pp. 184–191, 2011.

[15] C. Magro-Checa, J. Salvatierra, J. L. Rosales-Alexander, J. Orgaz-Molina, and E. Raya-Álvarez, "Life-threatening vasculo-Behçet following discontinuation of infliximab after three years of complete remission," *Clinical and Experimental Rheumatology*, vol. 31, no. 77, pp. 96–98, 2013.

24

Piriformis Syndrome in Fibromyalgia: Clinical Diagnosis and Successful Treatment

Md Abu Bakar Siddiq,[1] Moshiur Rahman Khasru,[2] and Johannes J. Rasker[3]

[1] Physical Medicine and Rehabilitation Department, Feni Diabetes Hospital (FDH), Feni 3900, Bangladesh
[2] Physical Medicine and Rehabilitation Department, BSMMU, Dhaka 1000, Bangladesh
[3] Rheumatology Department, Faculty of Behavioral Sciences, University of Twente, P.O. Box 217, 7500 AE Enschede, The Netherlands

Correspondence should be addressed to Md Abu Bakar Siddiq; abusiddiq37@yahoo.com

Academic Editor: Remzi Cevik

Piriformis syndrome is an underdiagnosed extraspinal association of sciatica. Patients usually complain of deep seated gluteal pain. In severe cases the clinical features of piriformis syndrome are primarily due to spasm of the piriformis muscle and irritation of the underlying sciatic nerve but this mysterious clinical scenario is also described in lumbar spinal canal stenosis, leg length discrepancy, piriformis myofascial pain syndrome, following vaginal delivery, and anomalous piriformis muscle or sciatic nerve. In this paper, we describe piriformis and fibromyalgia syndrome in a 30-year-old young lady, an often missed diagnosis. We also focus on management of the piriformis syndrome.

1. Introduction

The piriformis, a "pear shaped" (Latin piriformis means pear shape) skeletal muscle underneath the gluteal muscles originates in the pelvic cavity (anterior to sacrum, sacroiliac joint capsule, superior margin of greater sciatic notch, and sacrotuberous ligament), runs through the greater sciatic notch, and inserts outside the pelvic cavity (top of greater trochanter of the femur). During its passage it divides the greater sciatic notch into two compartments: superior and inferior. The muscle externally rotates the corresponding femur in hip extension and abducts the femur in hip flexion [1]. The piriformis syndrome (PS) is a clinical entity related to piriformis muscle where patients usually present with localized buttock and radiating pain in thigh and or leg. The typical physical examination findings include tenderness on the buttocks from the sacrum to greater trochanter, piriformis tenderness on pelvic/rectal examination, or pain provocation by FAIR (flexion, adduction, and internal rotation) test, Pace sign, Freiberg test, and so forth [2]. Fibromyalgia (FMS) is an idiopathic, chronic, nonarticular pain syndrome defined by widespread musculoskeletal pain but is believed to involve genetic, psychological, and environmental factors [3].

Patients usually complain of widespread body ache with associated fatigue, anxiety, sleep disturbance, morning stiffness, headache, tingling/numbness, cognitive disturbance, and so forth [3]. Along with these clinical features there should be generalized tender points on palpation to satisfy American College of Rheumatology (ACR) 1990 criteria for fibromyalgia [4]. FMS and PS are predominant in women [2, 4]. We could not find any literature describing both these conditions in the same patient. In this paper we describe the occurrence of both piriformis and fibromyalgia syndrome in a patient, with the intention to increase awareness among physicians of this combination. Stress is also given on management of the piriformis syndrome.

2. Case Report

A 30-year-old Asian women, housewife, presented with complaints of multiple body area pain for the last few months, in left and right side of the body and upper and lower parts, hardly improving with traditional NSAIDs (like naproxen, etoricoxib, diclofenac) and analgesics (paracetamol, tramadol). She also complained of pain in multiple large and small joints with morning stiffness that lasted for more than half an hour. There was associated fatigability. She had no joint swelling or limitation of joint movements. There was no history of significant hair loss, oral ulceration, altered bowel/bladder habits, headache, and so forth. Her menstrual and obstetric history was uneventful. General and systemic examination was unremarkable except that 14 out of 18 ACR fibromyalgia tender points were extremely painful. Laboratory tests were normal including complete blood count; Hb-12 g/dL, ESR –20 mm 1st hr, TC-4500/cmm; C-reactive protein negative; anti-CCP and ANA negative. Serum lipids, thyroid, and viral profile for hepatitis B and C also were normal. After interpreting both clinical and laboratory information she was classified as fibromyalgia. The patient was treated with amitriptyline (10 mg) (at night) and fluoxetine (20 mg) (at morning). Aerobic exercise in the form of swimming was also encouraged. After 3 weeks of follow-up, she reported significant improvement of fatigue and body ache except a deep seated right gluteal pain and discomfort. The pain was also radiating in her right thigh and leg with tingling in the same distribution. The pain was aggravated on sitting, lying on her right side, forward bending, and walking. Sometimes sitting was so disturbing that she could not sit more than 30 minutes on a chair. She could not memorize any recent/previous trauma over the gluteal region, significant history of fall, or traffic accidents that did impact on her lower back. She had no history of vaginal delivery in her recent past.

On physical examination, tenderness was elicited over the right gluteal region mostly at the greater sciatic notch. The pain was provoked by FAIR test, Pace sign, and digital rectal examination. Nervous system examination of the lower limbs revealed no abnormalities. MRI lumbosacral spine revealed only discs bulging at L4-5-S1 levels. There was no disc degeneration or nerve roots compression. Ultrasonography (USG) (Siemens Acuson X300 premium edition, transducer: CH 5-2, Germany) of the gluteal region revealed asymmetry of the piriformis muscle thickness (right 12.2 and left 9.4 mm) (Figure 1). At that time her pain was quantified as 9/10 on a visual analogue scale (VAS, 0–10 cm) for pain. Along with oral medications she was taught how to do piriformis muscle stretching exercise. After 3 weeks of follow-up, the patient still had the same complaints but with less intensity and her pain was 4/10 on the VAS. Finally, we decided to put intralesional (IL) methylprednisolone 40 mg at the right piriformis muscle (Figure 2) and counseling was done accordingly. After that treatment, her buttock pain was found to be improved and it was felt only after sitting for longer than two hours.

2.1. Technique of Piriformis Muscle Injection (Figures 2(a)–2(d)). After obtaining informed consent the patient with PS is placed in the prone position. The buttock area on the right side is sterilized with povidone-iodine USP (10%) and draped in a sterile fashion. Using surface anatomy the lower one-third of the right sacroiliac joint is identified [5]: at the level of dimple is the middle of the sacroiliac joint and just inferior to the dimple, close to the greater sciatic notch is the lower part of sacroiliac joint. The skin over the gluteal region 1.5 cm lateral and 1.2 cm inferior to the lower sacroiliac joint is marked as the site of needle insertion. After skin infiltration

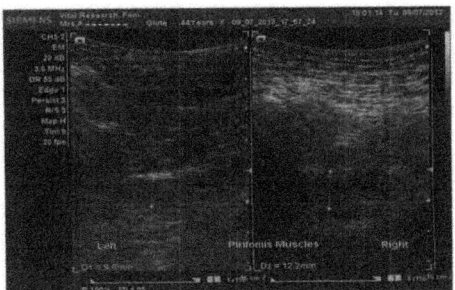

FIGURE 1: High frequency diagnostic ultrasonogram of both gluteal regions illustrates piriformis muscle thickness (right 12.2 and left 9.4 mm).

with 1 mL of 1% lidocaine, a 22-gauge, 10 cm insulated needle is inserted perpendicular to the right piriformis muscle until it touches the ilium and is then withdrawn 1-2 mm to relocate it in the piriformis muscle. At this point, the patient is asked whether she experiences any buttock pain and whether it coincides with her usual pain. A 10 mL disposable syringe is prepared with methylprednisolone (40 mg/mL), 1% lidocaine (4 mL), and 0.25% bupivacaine (3 mL) and injected in the desired place (Figures 2(a)–2(d)). After the procedure, the patient is brought to the recovery room for one hour or until any leg numbness has subsided, or for a longer period when necessary.

3. Discussion

The piriformis syndrome is an elusive medical condition [6], one of the most common extraspinal causes of sciatica. The reported incidence rates for PS among patients with low back pain vary widely from 5% to 36%. It is more common in females than in males [2, 7]. Symptoms and clinical signs relate either directly or indirectly to muscle spasm and resulting sciatic nerve compression. Pain originating from the trochanteric bursa, sacroiliac joint, or facet joint may also be confused with this clinical scenario. Patients usually present with low back pain mostly over the buttock that aggravates on sitting more than 20–30 minutes. Some patients may present with sudden severe low back pain causing difficulty in bodily movements, others give a history of deep seated gluteal pain for longer periods of time that interfere with daily activities. There may be an associated tingling sensation in the lower limb or subjective heaviness of the same extremity. Patients also complain of difficulty when walking, rising from sitting position, cross-legged sitting, or ambulation [2, 8]. Though there is no single test specific for PS, the following tests are generally used to diagnose PS [2]: the Freiberg test, the FAIR test, the Pace sign, the Beatty test, and straight leg raising (SLR). Tenderness with palpation over the piriformis muscle is common. Patients may also experience tenderness in the sacroiliac joints and greater sciatic notch. Some patients have a palpable sausage shaped mass in the buttock caused by contracted piriformis muscle [2]. Findings with straight leg raising are variable in PS [2, 9].

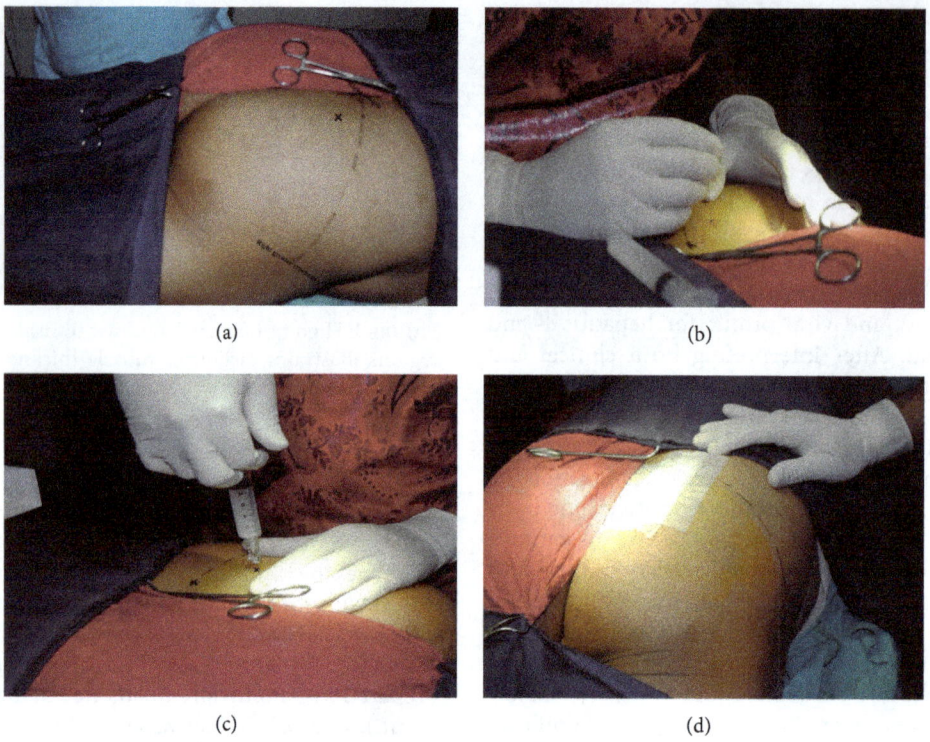

FIGURE 2: Intralesional steroid injection in right piriformis muscle. (a) **x** indicates point of needle entry at 1.5 cm lateral and 1.2 cm caudal to the lower 3rd of right sacroiliac joint and dotted line from right dimple of Venus to right greater trochanter runs parallel with superior margin of the right piriformis muscle; (b) after infiltration with 1% lidocaine spinal needle is placed; (c) 10 cc disposable syringe with injection methylprednisolone (40 mg/mL), 3 mL 1% lidocaine, and 2 mL 0.25% bupivacaine is in situ; (d) local gauze bandage after the procedure.

The following medical conditions are frequently associated with complaints of the piriformis syndrome: (1) preceding fall, (2) direct gluteal trauma, (3) overuse of piriformis muscle, (4) LLD (leg length discrepancy), (5) lumbar spinal stenosis, (6) myofascial pain syndrome (MPS), (7) piriformis muscle infection, and (8) local invasion of piriformis muscle by cervical cancer [2, 6, 10–16]. After a fall or direct gluteal blow there may be localized hematoma followed by scarring in between sciatic nerve and small hip extensors. Sometimes piriformis muscle spasm may irritate the underlying sciatic nerve [6]. LLD can be subdivided into two etiological groups: a structural LLD defined as those associated with a shortening of bony structures and a functional LLD defined as those that are a result of altered mechanics of the lower extremities or spine. The most controversial musculoskeletal disorder associated with leg length discrepancy is low back pain [14]. Gait pattern may be altered or remain unchanged in leg length inequality. Sustained stress on piriformis muscle with resultant impact on both stance and swing phases can produce altered gait pattern in LLD [6]. Overuse of piriformis muscle can occur following unaccustomed long distance walking, running, repeated squatting, kneeling, cycling, and so forth [2]. Piriformis pyomyositis is an infective condition involving the piriformis muscle, a clinical scenario that may report following vaginal delivery and usually is associated with fever and raised inflammatory biochemical markers [10]. Association of piriformis syndrome and lumbar stenosis can be explained by double crush hypothesis [16].

Sometimes PS is due to myofascial pain syndrome involving piriformis muscle with taut band and trigger points (TrPs). Primary MPS often regards the typical overuse syndrome that is named for the structures involved or the common conditions that produce it. PS is an example of primary MPS due to existing TrPs in the contracted piriformis muscle. Although the myofascial pain syndrome is a localized painful muscle condition, sometimes it may present as widespread body pain due to spread of TrPs: (i) through axial kinetic chain; (ii) through the activation of TrPs in the overloaded or mechanically stressed muscle compensating for the dysfunction of other muscles in the functional muscle units. Sometimes the clinical picture of widespread MPS may be confused with FMS [13]. MPS and FMS may also coexist in the same patient and may share common pathophysiology [13, 15]. Central sensitization is important in the genesis of both FMS and MPS. It could explain both the physical findings and biomechanical changes that have been documented in fibromyalgia [13]. According to Gerwin 75% of FMS may have significant MPS at one or more times during the course of their illness. In MPS an increase in TrPs Ach release could result in sustained depolarization of the postjunctional membrane of the muscle fiber and produce sustained sarcomere shortening and contracture with increased local energy consumption and reduction of local circulation, producing local ischemia and hypoxia. The localized muscle ischemia stimulates the release of prostaglandins, substance P, bradykinin, capsaicin, serotonin, and histamine that sensitize afferent nerve fibers in muscle. Under pathologic conditions, convergent connections from deep afferent nociceptors to dorsal horn neurons are facilitated and amplified in the spinal cord with pain referral beyond the initial nociceptive region owing to spreading of central sensitization to adjacent spinal segments. At the level of the central nervous system, spinal neuroplastic changes in the second order neuron pool produce a long lasting increase in the excitability of nociceptor pathways. Neurotransmitters involved in the process of central sensitization include substance P, N-methyl-D-aspartate, glutamate, and nitric oxide. In addition, there may be impairments in supraspinal inhibitory descending pain control pathways. Like MPS, there is no significant peripheral pathology in FMS. Central sensitization is the most important CNS aberration in FMS with altered neurotransmitters in serum (decrease serotonin) and CSF (increase substance P) [2, 13].

Since our patient had none of the cited risk factors for PS, another possibility might be sought. Although both conditions may be present in a single individual, unrecognized and poorly managed MPS of piriformis muscle appears to be the causative agent of FMS in our case. Longstanding nociceptive stimuli in piriformis muscle could cause sensitization in the central nervous system which is a manifestation of neuroplasticity or the remodeling of central processes produced generalized body ache in our patient. Along with widespread body ache and generalized tender areas, the patient also had fibromyalgia symptoms; morning stiffness and fatigability. Pain was provoked in favor of piriformis syndrome using FAIR test, Pace sign, and localized tenderness over the right gluteal region. On digital rectal examination piriformis tenderness was also elicited during finger gliding over the right lateral pelvic wall. Right piriformis muscle was found to be thicker than the left one using high frequency ultrasonography of gluteal region that indicated some sorts of muscle spasm.

NSAIDs, analgesics, and muscle relaxants are being used for the management of PS. Nonpharmacological approaches may also be efficacious in managing this painful condition like therapeutic deep heating, piriformis muscle stretching, and therapeutic manipulation. According to Fishman et al. 79% patients with PS had symptom reduction with conservative approaches. When all these approaches have failed, intralesional (IL) injection lidocaine and corticosteroid or botulinum toxin (A/B) under high resolution USG or fluoroscope can be an alternative to manage this condition [2]. Where high resolution ultrasonogram/fluoroscope are not available, motor stimulation guided piriformis muscle injection using surface anatomy can be another option [2]. In a cadaveric study by Gonzalez et al. it was described that needle positioning at a distance of approximately 1.5 cm lateral and 1.2 cm caudal to the lower border of the sacroiliac joint can be used successfully for piriformis muscle injection [17]. To accelerate pain relief, along with oral medications our patient was successfully treated with intralesional steroid using surface anatomy followed by gradual graded stretching exercises for the piriformis muscle.

In conclusion, PS may be associated with fibromyalgia and this case report should make physicians aware of neurological aspects of fibromyalgia in which the piriformis muscle is involved. Coexistence of FMS and MPS is not uncommon, but to our best knowledge this is the first clinical report describing MPS as piriformis syndrome in a patient with fibromyalgia. We strongly believe that a case study is not enough for establishing etiological association between PS and FMS. So, we recommend further prospective multicenter studies to measure prevalence, association of piriformis syndrome in fibromyalgia.

Acknowledgments

The authors are thankful to Akbar Ali, in charge of computing and information technology division of Feni Diabetes Hospital, Feni, Bangladesh, for his hard work with full of enthusiasm during preparation of this report. They also thank all the reviewers who were involved with the review process of this paper.

References

[1] G. Windisch, E. M. Braun, and F. Anderhuber, "Piriformis muscle: clinical anatomy and consideration of the piriformis syndrome," *Surgical and Radiologic Anatomy*, vol. 29, no. 1, pp. 37–45, 2007.

[2] L. A. Boyajian-O'Neill, R. L. McClain, M. K. Coleman, and P. P. Thomas, "Diagnosis and management of piriformis syndrome: an osteopathic approach," *The Journal of the American Osteopathic Association*, vol. 108, no. 11, pp. 657–664, 2008.

[3] F. Wolfe and J. J. Rasker, "Fibromyalgia," in *Kelley's Textbook of Rheumatology*, G. S. Firestein, R. C. Budd, S. Gabriel, I. B. McInnes, and J. R. O'Dell, Eds., 752, p. 733, Elsevier, Philadelphia, Pa, USA, 9th edition, 2012.

[4] F. Wolfe, H. A. Smythe, M. B. Yunus et al., "The American College of rheumatology 1990. criteria for the classification of fibromyalgia. Report of the multicenter criteria committee," *Arthritis and Rheumatism*, vol. 33, no. 2, pp. 160–172, 1990.

[5] K. L. Moore, A. F. Dalley, and A. M. Agur, *Clinically Oriented Anatomy*, Lippincott Williams & Wilkins, Philadelphia, Pa, USA, 6th edition, 2010.

[6] J. W. T. Byrd, "Piriformis syndrome," *Operative Techniques in Sports Medicine*, vol. 13, no. 1, pp. 71–79, 2005.

[7] K. Hopayian, F. Song, R. Riera, and S. Sambandan, "The clinical features of the piriformis syndrome: a systematic review," *European Spine Journal*, vol. 19, no. 12, pp. 2095–2109, 2010.

[8] R. A. Beatty, R. H. Patterson Jr., and D. G. Kline, "The piriformis muscle syndrome: a simple diagnostic maneuver," *Neurosurgery*, vol. 34, no. 3, pp. 512–514, 1994.

[9] L. M. Fishman, G. W. Dombi, C. Michaelsen et al., "Piriformis syndrome: diagnosis, treatment, and outcome—a 10-year study," *Archives of Physical Medicine and Rehabilitation*, vol. 83, no. 3, pp. 295–301, 2002.

[10] K. W. Chong and B. K. Tay, "Piriformis pyomyositis: a rare cause of sciatica," *Singapore Medical Journal*, vol. 45, no. 5, pp. 229–231, 2004.

[11] K. Dere, M. Akbas, and N. Luleci, "A rare cause of a piriformis syndrome," *Journal of Back and Musculoskeletal Rehabilitation*, vol. 22, no. 1, pp. 55–58, 2009.

[12] S. Y. Jeon, H. S. Moon, Y. J. Han, and C. H. Sung, "Post-radiation piriformis syndrome in a cervical cancer patient—a case report," *The Korean Journal of Pain*, vol. 23, no. 1, pp. 88–91, 2010.

[13] R. D. Gerwin, "Classification, epidemiology, and natural history of myofascial pain syndrome," *Current Pain and Headache Reports*, vol. 5, no. 5, pp. 412–420, 2001.

[14] B. Gurney, "Leg length discrepancy," *Gait & Posture*, vol. 15, no. 2, pp. 195–206, 2002.

[15] J. Borg-Stein, "Treatment of fibromyalgia, myofascial pain, and related disorders," *Physical Medicine and Rehabilitation Clinics of North Ameria*, vol. 17, no. 2, pp. 491–510, 2006.

[16] A. L. Dellon and S. E. Mackinnon, "Chronic nerve compression model for the double crush hypothesis," *Annals of Plastic Surgery*, vol. 26, no. 3, pp. 259–264, 1991.

[17] P. Gonzalez, M. Pepper, W. Sullivan, and V. Akuthota, "Confirmation of needle placement within the piriformis muscle of a cadaveric specimen using anatomic landmarks and fluoroscopic guidance," *Pain Physician*, vol. 11, no. 3, pp. 327–331, 2008.

25

SLE and Non-Hodgkin's Lymphoma

Prajwal Boddu,[1] **Abdul S. Mohammed,**[1] **Chandrahasa Annem,**[2] **and Winston Sequeira**[2]

[1]*Department of Internal Medicine, Advocate Illinois Masonic Medical Center, 836 W. Wellington Avenue, Chicago, IL 60657, USA*
[2]*Department of Rheumatology, Rush University Medical Center, 1725 West Harrison Street, Chicago, IL 60612, USA*

Correspondence should be addressed to Abdul S. Mohammed; mabdulsalman@gmail.com

Academic Editor: Ruben Burgos-Vargas

Systemic lupus erythematosus (SLE) is a multisystem autoimmune disorder punctuated by varied multiorgan complications all along the course of its natural history. Lymphoma represents a relatively well-recognized malignant phenomenon associated with lupus. The cause and effect relationships of lymphoma in SLE have been subject to extensive scrutiny with several studies reporting on clinic-pathologic characteristics and risk factors predicting lymphoma development in SLE. However, the pathogenic role of immunosuppressives in SLE-related lymphoma still remains unclear, and indices to help guide diagnosis, prognostication, therapy, and posttreatment monitoring are yet to be established. In this review, we describe 3 SLE patients who developed non-Hodgkin's lymphoma at different time points of their disease. Through a careful dissection of the aforementioned cases, we intend to apprise readers of the currently available literature surrounding risk factors, management, and prognosis in SLE-related lymphoma. We will also review and discuss the implications of immunosuppressives in SLE-related lymphoma and the role of mycophenolate mofetil in SLE-related primary CNS lymphoma development.

1. Introduction

Systemic lupus erythematosus (SLE) is an autoimmune disease with myriad presentations and multisystem complications arising from both underlying disease activity and therapy-related side effects. SLE's association with lymphoma is a well-established phenomenon. A number of studies have reported a higher incidence of lymphoma in the SLE population compared with healthy cohorts [1–3]. The effects of lymphoma development in SLE and its impact on modifying the disease's natural history are a matter of great interest amongst both clinicians and researchers. This has spawned a proliferation of studies examining predictors of lymphoma development, its effect on SLE prognosis, and optimal treatment strategies in its management. In this article, we describe 3 SLE patients who developed lymphoma at different time points of their disease. Of note, all these patients were diagnosed with SLE based on fulfilling the 1997 American College of Rheumatology (ACR) criteria. We will attempt to understand potential factors that may have contributed to disease development in each of the three patients, rationalize treatment strategies that they had received, and identify clinicopathological indices predicting lymphoma development by reviewing the currently updated literature.

2. Case #1

A 36-year-old Asian female presented to our hospital with complaints of one month of progressive back pain and two weeks of left lower extremity numbness, cramps, and weakness. She endorsed a two-week history of bowel and bladder retention. She was diagnosed with SLE, over 10 years ago, and was on hydroxychloroquine with reasonable control of her symptoms until a month prior to hospitalization. Her past medical history was also significant for intermittent autoimmune neutropenia. Physical exam at initial evaluation was remarkable for 4/5 strength in both lower extremities with an associated left foot drop. Labs including blood counts and routine serum chemistries were unremarkable at presentation. An MRI of lumbar spine was performed and revealed two peripherally enhancing extradural/subdural masses in the lumbar spinal canal at the L2 and L3-L4 level with additional nodular and linear enhancement of cauda equina nerve roots. A lumbar puncture performed revealed normal CSF cell count, protein 227 mg/dL, and glucose 24 mg/dL; cytopathology was positive for atypical mononuclear cells confirming leptomeningeal involvement. The patient was treated over three days with emergent radiation therapy along with intravenous dexamethasone (10 mg followed by 16 mg daily in divided doses) without further tissue confirmation. Flow cytometry on repeat lumbar puncture, postradiation therapy, showed no diagnostic abnormalities. A L3-vertebral tissue biopsy was performed a day later and showed chronic inflammatory cells and CD20+ necrotic cells consistent with a vanishing lymphoma. Staging with PET and bone marrow biopsy was negative for disseminated lymphomatous involvement. Given the severity of presentation, the patient was treated further with 5 cycles of high dose methotrexate, alternating with rituximab and intrathecal methotrexate. She was started on entecavir, for positive hepatitis B antibody serologies, to prevent possible reactivation of hepatitis while receiving Rituxan. The patient improved clinically over her three-month chemotherapy course after which a restaging PET was performed that showed mild hyper enhancement in the L2 vertebral region. The hyperenhancement on PET was deemed to be postsurgical, based on a preceding core biopsy that was negative for malignancy, and hence an open biopsy was deferred. She completed her localized radiation therapy sessions and proceeded to receive two cycles of consolidation chemotherapy with cytarabine three months later. Six months after her last Rituxan dose, repeat hepatitis B quantitative titers and liver enzymes were negative/normal and entecavir was discontinued. On her most recent follow-up, she continues to make progress and is planned for surveillance monitoring with regular lab work and MRI every 6 months to monitor for disease status and treatment related toxicities.

3. Case #2

A 57-year-old African American female presented to the hospital with complaints of headache, fevers, dysarthria, and tremors. She had a 19-year long history of SLE complicated by Class IIIA + Class V lupus nephritis requiring treatment with cyclophosphamide and mycophenolate (MMF). She was also on hydroxychloroquine and had a prolonged course of prednisone (5–10 mg/day). Her other past medical history included anemia of chronic disease, hypertension, hypothyroidism, and listeria meningitis (five months prior to this hospital presentation). Her other relevant medications included trimethoprim sulfa for PJP prophylaxis. Labs at presentation were significant for a Hgb 9 gm/dL, normal WBC and platelet counts, creatinine 2.12 mg/dL, albumin 3.6 mg/dL, bilirubin 0.21 mg/dL, ALP 71 IU/L, ALT 32 IU/L, AST 31 IU/L, LDH 772 IU/L, and uric acid 6.6 mg/dL. Brain MRI was performed for her neurological symptoms and revealed T2-hyperintensive periventricular lesions extending into the corona radiata and internal capsule. A stereotactic brain biopsy was performed which showed large discohesive neoplastic lymphoid cells forming characteristic perivascular cuffing which stained positive for CD20 suggestive of diffuse large B cell lymphoma (DLBCL). Staging PET/CT showed

hyper metabolic mediastinal nodes and nodules in the left lower lobe, lesions that were biopsied and showed *Cryptococcus neoformans*. There was no evidence of lymphoma on bone marrow biopsies. A repeat MRI, one month later, demonstrated interval increase in the size of periventricular lesions. A lumbar puncture at this time showed normal cell count with no abnormal cell morphology or flow cytometry. She was started on allopurinol for tumor lysis prophylaxis and fluconazole for recently diagnosed cryptococcosis. She received adjusted high dose intravenous methotrexate for her DLBCL. Her neurological symptoms began to improve after her first session of treatment. At the time of this writing, she is planned to receive further cycles of methotrexate treatment.

4. Case #3

A 50-year-old African American male presented to the emergency department with complaints of fever and progressive fatigue over a month. He reported fevers, night sweats, and 17-pound weight loss over this period. His past medical history was significant for SLE with Class II lupus glomerulonephritis and chronic lupus interstitial nephritis for which he was being treated with azathioprine and hydroxychloroquine. Labs at presentation revealed pancytopenia, Hgb 5.6 gm/dL, WBC 3700/mm^3, and platelets 90000/mm^3. CT scans of the chest, abdomen, and pelvis demonstrated diffuse lymphadenopathy above and below the diaphragm with no evidence of involvement of extranodal sites. A bone marrow biopsy was performed which showed a hypocellular (30%) marrow with 15–20% of involvement of marrow cells by large CD5, CD19, CD20 positive; Cyclin D1, BCL6 negative B cells with lambda light chain restriction consistent with diffuse large B cell lymphoma. Azathioprine was promptly discontinued. He was determined to have a good prognostic, revised international prognostic index category (R-IPI) Stage IVB DLBCL and treated with 6 cycles of R-CHOP regimen. First chemotherapy cycle was complicated by neutropenic fevers (requiring broad spectrum antibiotics) and progression of kidney disease to end-stage renal disease (ESRD) requiring hemodialysis. Fortunately, he completed the other five cycles without incident. Interim CTs and post-chemo-CT scans with bone marrow biopsy showed complete response with no evidence of residual disease. On repeat evaluation during her follow-up visit, a month after completing treatment, she is asymptomatic with a good recovery of her peripheral blood counts (Hgb 10.2 gm/dL, platelets 195 K/microL, and WBC 3470/mm^3).

5. Summary of the Cases

In summary, patient #1, with a 10-year history of SLE and chronic hepatitis B, presented with primary CNS lymphoma (PCNSL) of leptomeningeal/spinal type and was treated successfully with high dose methotrexate and rituximab. Patient #2 had a 19-year long history of SLE and also presented with a localized CNS lymphoma. Importantly, she was on mycophenolate mofetil (MMF) and cyclophosphamide at the time of her presentation. Mycophenolate therapy was discontinued soon after diagnosis. She was treated with high dose intravenous methotrexate. Patient #3 presented with DLBCL while he was being treated with azathioprine which was later discontinued. He showed good clinical response to chemotherapy and was in complete remission at the end of his R-CHOP regimen. Two of our patients presented with a primary CNS lymphoma, a rare and unusual presentation in SLE patients. Of note, all patients were diagnosed with SLE based on the 1997 ACR criteria.

6. Discussion

6.1. Incidence and Epidemiology. The association between lymphoma and SLE has been examined in varied detail and studies have reported an increased incidence of lymphoma in SLE [1–3]. Immune dysregulation coupled with the use of immunosuppression may account for the increased incidence of cancer (and lymphoma) in SLE. A recent meta-analysis which included 16 observational studies showed a mildly increased risk of overall cancer in SLE compared with the general population [1]. This risk is most pronounced in SLE-related non-Hodgkin's lymphoma with reported relative risk estimates ranging widely from 4.39 to 44.4 in various studies [1–3].

Based on two studies with a total of 37 patients, SLE patients presenting with lymphoma typically age between 57 and 61 years with the majority of them being women [10, 13]. In a study involving 11 SLE-NHL patients, the mean duration of SLE at the time of NHL diagnosis was found to be 18 years, but cases of NHL occurring prior to concurrently with a diagnosis of SLE have also been reported [5, 7]. Unlike the increased overall cancer risk which is generally confined to Caucasian SLE patients, lymphoma risk in SLE is uniformly higher across all ethnicities [14].

6.2. Pathology. The most common histological type of NHL in SLE is the DLBCL type constituting 50–65% of the SLE-lymphoma cases [5, 10, 13]. Gene expression profiling in DLBCL has revealed at least three different subgroups, each driven by different pathophysiological mechanisms and characterized by different responses to therapy. Of these, the "activated B-cell-like DLBCL" type is derived from postgerminal center B cells while the "germinal center B-cell-like DLBCL" type originates from germinal center B cells. DLBCL of the activated B cell type carries a worse prognosis compared with DLBCL of the germinal type (GCB) [10, 15]. Importantly, DLBCL arising in patients with a history of SLE showed an enrichment of non-GCB subtype, and this has potential implications on therapy and prognosis.

6.3. Clinical and Laboratory Features. Signs and symptoms like fever and adenopathy are shared clinical features in SLE-related lymphoma and infections complicating SLE. However, a thorough assessment of the duration of lymphadenopathy and chronicity of symptoms, exhaustive exclusion of potential infectious etiologies, and examination of tissue and bone marrow biopsies are essential in arriving at the right diagnosis [16, 17]. Though NHL in SLE is predominantly nodal, extranodal involvement may also occur. Prognosis of NHL in SLE is heavily weighted upon the stage of the disease,

with a higher stage predicting for a worsened outcome [18, 19]. Early stage lymphoma can share similar clinical and hematological findings observed in SLE. In addition, lymphadenopathy is very common in SLE, occurring in up to 67% of patients [20]. Hence, the diagnosis often hinges upon a lymph node biopsy or peripheral blood sampling for immunophenotyping to detect a monoclonal cell expansion consistent with lymphoma.

A study examining predictors of increased lymphoma risk in systemic lupus suggested a potential role of cyclophosphamide and high cumulative steroid use [21]. In their sample, disease activity was found to be associated with increased lymphoma risk. A study on Sjogren's syndrome patients with lymphoma identified simple hematological factors such as neutropenia, low complement, and cryoglobulinemia as highly predictive factors in the development of NHL [21]. Of note, we observed our three study patients to have either bicytopenia or pancytopenia for a brief time period just prior to the diagnosis of lymphoma.

6.4. Role of Immunosuppressives. Most SLE patients are on potent immunosuppressives for the management of lupus and its complications. Pertinent concerns have been raised against the plausible role of immunosuppressives in lymphomagenesis. The potential association between cyclophosphamide and azathioprine use and lymphoma in SLE has been widely studied in literature. Most of the evidence suggests that immunosuppressives do not increase the incidence of lymphoma [4–12]. Studies, in fact, have shown conflicting results and failed to demonstrate a significant risk of lymphoma with use of cyclophosphamide and azathioprine (see Table 1). The role of other agents like MMF is detailed in the following sections.

6.5. Pathophysiology. Biological mechanisms behind lymphomagenesis in SLE remain to be better defined. Constitutive immune activation from prolonged antigen stimulation may result in active lymphocyte proliferation which can eventually terminate into a lymphoma. Bone marrow derived naïve B cells ingress into the lymph node and enter a germinal center reaction, after antigen stimulation, where they proliferate rapidly and undergo class switching and somatic hypermutation [22]. DLBCL subtype is derived from activated B cells suggesting that an increased incidence of lymphoma may be a secondary effect of chronic inflammation in this subgroup [23]. Activating mutations in multi-proto-oncogenes have been reported in DLBCL [24]. It is noteworthy to mention that chromosomal translocation break points in SLE DLBCL have been shown to occur in the very same regions as non-SLE DLBCL [25–27].

Epstein Barr virus (EBV) infection is being increasingly recognized as a potential pathogenetic link to lymphomagenesis. It has been observed that EBV antigens share structural similarities with certain SLE antigens. Additionally, SLE patients tend to have frequent viral reactivations as suggested by higher EBV seroconversion rates [28]. These reactivations are partly the effect of defective EBV-specific T cell suppression allowing enhanced expression of viral genes [28, 29] in SLE patients. It is also interesting to note that EBV

TABLE 1: Studies on the role of cyclophosphamide and azathioprine on SLE-related lymphomagenesis.

Ref.	Study design	Pt follow-up	Number of patients with lymphoma/hematological malignancies	Drugs studied	Comments	Outcomes
[4]	Prospective observational	68592 patient months	3	Azathioprine & cyclophosphamide	3/914 patients had lymphoma. 1 was on AZT, 1 on CYP, and 1 on both. 348/911 were on AZT, 188/911 on CYP	No association
[5]	Retrospective	2020	11	Azathioprine & CYP	1 on CYP; 0 on AZT	No association
[6]	Retrospective	219	1	Azathioprine & CYP	0 on immunosuppressives	No association
[7]	Retrospective	784 246 cancer cases and 538 controls without cancer	46	Azathioprine & CYP	Cyclophosphamide: 17.5% of 538 cancer free patients, 7.4% of 246 cancer patients; azathioprine: 34.9% of 538 cancer free patients, 25.0% of 246 cancer patients	No association Cyclophosphamide 2.09 (0.69–6.30) Azathioprine 1.19 (0.48–2.92)
[8]	Retrospective	864	8	Azathioprine & CYP	11 of 28 cancer patients on CYP, 12 of 28 cancer patients on AZP	No association
[9]	Retrospective	5036	75	Azathioprine, CYP, MMF, and prednisone	75 lymphoma cases, only 15 had prior exposure to CYP, 19 to AZA, 9 to methotrexate, and 6 to MMF	No association Cyclophosphamide ever used 2.80 (0.87 to 8.98) Azathioprine (AZA) ever used fully adjusted 0.84 (0.32 to 2.25)
[10]	Retrospective	6438	16	Azathioprine, CYP	Cyclophosphamide: 2/16 in patients with NHL, 3/26 in patients without NHL Azathioprine: 5/16 in patients with NHL, 9/26 in patients without NHL	No association CYP (RR 0.3–3.3) AZP RR 0.9 [0.4–2.1]
[11]	Prospective	5976 patient years	1	CYP	1/49 on CYP developed NHL	No association
[12]	Prospective	17376 patient years	3	AZT, CYP	None on CYP or AZT	No association

infection of B cells upregulates the expression of enzymes like cytidine deaminase expression, an essential mediator in the process of somatic hypermutation [30].

6.6. Primary CNS Lymphoma.

Primary CNS lymphoma (PCNSL) is a regional type of non-Hodgkin lymphoma and is defined by central nervous system involvement without evidence of concomitant systemic disease. The diagnosis of PCNSL carries a worse prognosis compared with its systemic counterpart [31]. Histologically, about 95% of PCNSL is $CD20^+$ DLBCL type [32]. Immunodeficiency predisposes to PCNSL development; however, it has also been associated independently with the presence of autoimmune diseases [33]. Almost all cases of PCSNL reported in SLE patients are associated with the use of immunosuppressives [33–38]. As alluded above, patient #1 was treated with endeavor to prevent hepatitis B reactivation, a potential complication while receiving rituximab [39]. Hepatitis B independently associates with increased PCSNL risk and may be due to HBV causing chronic antigenic stimulation [40, 41]. However, our patient was HBsAg negative and anti-HBs Ab positive, an association not likely associated with an increased risk of PCSNL [40]. This patient was only on hydroxychloroquine, a weak immunosuppressant, when she presented with PCSNL. It is worth mentioning that the use of hydroxychloroquine may actually positively influence the cancer risk in SLE patients [42]. An observational prospective study involving 235 SLE patients with a median 10-year follow-up (156 on hydroxychloroquine) determined a decreased cancer incidence while on hydroxychloroquine [adjusted hazard ratio 0.15 (95% CI 0.02 to 0.99)]. Finally, it currently remains unknown if SLE has an immunosuppressive-independent association with primary CNS lymphoma.

PCNSL in SLE is being diagnosed more frequently since the introduction of MMF in the management of lupus nephritis and post-transplant [35–38]. All case studies including ours were treated long term with mycophenolate indicating that prolonged immunosuppression may be one of the prerequisites for PCNSL development [23, 36–38]. All reported patients had at least 5 years of autoimmune disease. All patients were on mycophenolate 1 gram twice daily dosing for 8 months to 46 months prior to diagnosis. Of the five patients, including ours, three were diagnosed with DLBCL and two had polymorphous B cell lymphoproliferative disorder. Three patients went into complete remission after steroid/rituximab regimen; one patient had progressive disease on the same. Our patient was not assessed for CD20 marker status. MMF induces a compromise in T cell immune function thereby likely causing dysregulated B cell proliferation in the setting of chronic antigen stimulation. In all the reports mentioned above, patients had tumors which were positive for EBV, a factor which may well have contributed to chronic antigen stimulation. The EBV status of our patient's tumor was not evaluated. In this context, EBV episomes tend to be absent in immunocompetent PCNSL patients, and other mechanisms of disease induction might be responsible for lymphomagenesis [43]. Finally, PCNSL in SLE without mycophenolate has also been rarely described [34].

All patients were diagnosed with PCNSL within 1–3 months of onset of neurological symptoms. Rapid onset of neurological symptoms in SLE patients on long term immunosuppressives, especially MMF, should raise concern for PCNSL.

6.7. Management and Prognosis.

Diffuse large B cell lymphoma is highly aggressive but responds well to the traditional CHOP regimen (cyclophosphamide, doxorubicin, vincristine, and prednisone) [44]. Addition of rituximab to CHOP improves response rates and survival outcomes [45]. The optimal regimen for PCSNL is unestablished, with the traditional CHOP regimens generally proving ineffective due to poor penetrance through the blood brain barrier. Hence intrathecal chemotherapy involving high dose methotrexate and rituximab now forms the standard first line regimen in PCSNL [46]. Patient #1 responded well to the combined high dose methotrexate and rituximab regimen with complete response after completion of his chemotherapy.

Course of these patients has not been well studied and may be poor given the relatively higher proportion of DLBCL non-GCB types and higher disease stage at presenting diagnosis. Rossi et al. reported on the outcomes of 5 patients, who on attaining complete remission after treatment with high dose chemotherapy found that 3 of the 4 patients continued to have persistent autoantibody elevation with frequent lupus flares [19]. The potential of stem cell transplantation in serving a potentially curative role not only in the management of DLBCL but also in inducing prolonged serological remissions of autoimmune disease should be explored in future studies [19, 47, 48].

7. Conclusion

There has been a wealth of progress in the understanding of SLE-related lymphoma in the past two decades. The availability of simple hematological/laboratory indices predicting lymphoma development can facilitate early identification of disease and warrant further evaluation in future studies. Although immunosuppressives have no clear role in the pathogenesis of SLE-related lymphoma, reports including ours suggest an etiological role of mycophenolate in PCNSL development. The therapeutic role of allogenic stem cell transplant in curing both lymphoma and SLE holds promise and prognostic risk stratification studies are required to identify patients who best benefit from this therapeutic approach.

References

[1] L. Cao, H. Tong, G. Xu et al., "Systemic lupus erythematous and malignancy risk: a meta-analysis," *PLoS ONE*, vol. 10, no. 4, Article ID e0122964, 2015.

[2] S. Bernatsky, R. Ramsey-Goldman, J. Labrecque et al., "Cancer risk in systemic lupus: an updated international multi-centre

cohort study," *Journal of Autoimmunity*, vol. 42, pp. 130–135, 2013.

[3] T. Pettersson, E. Pukkala, L. Teppo, and C. Friman, "Increased risk of cancer in patients with systemic lupus erythematosus," *Annals of the Rheumatic Diseases*, vol. 51, no. 4, pp. 437–439, 1992.

[4] K. Y. Kang, H. O. Kim, H. S. Yoon et al., "Incidence of cancer among female patients with systemic lupus erythematosus in Korea," *Clinical Rheumatology*, vol. 29, no. 4, pp. 381–388, 2010.

[5] J. K. King and K. H. Costenbader, "Characteristics of patients with systemic lupus erythematosus (SLE) and non-Hodgkin's lymphoma (NHL)," *Clinical Rheumatology*, vol. 26, no. 9, pp. 1491–1494, 2007.

[6] D. M. Sweeney, S. Manzi, J. Janosky et al., "Risk of malignancy in women with systemic lupus erythematosus," *Journal of Rheumatology*, vol. 22, no. 8, pp. 1478–1482, 1995.

[7] S. Bernatsky, L. Joseph, J.-F. Boivin et al., "The relationship between cancer and medication exposures in systemic lupus erythaematosus: a case-cohort study," *Annals of the Rheumatic Diseases*, vol. 67, no. 1, pp. 74–79, 2008.

[8] T. Tarr, B. Gyorfy, É. Szekanecz et al., "Occurrence of malignancies in Hungarian patients with systemic lupus erythematosus: results from a single center," *Annals of the New York Academy of Sciences*, vol. 1108, pp. 76–82, 2007.

[9] S. Bernatsky, R. Ramsey-Goldman, and A. E. Clarke, "Malignancy in systemic lupus erythematosus: what have we learned?" *Best Practice and Research: Clinical Rheumatology*, vol. 23, no. 4, pp. 539–547, 2009.

[10] B. Löfström, C. Backlin, C. Sundström, A. Ekbom, and I. E. Lundberg, "A closer look at non-Hodgkin's lymphoma cases in a national Swedish systemic lupus erythematosus cohort: a nested case-control study," *Annals of the Rheumatic Diseases*, vol. 66, no. 12, pp. 1627–1632, 2007.

[11] S. M. Sultan, Y. Ioannou, and D. A. Isenberg, "Is there an association of malignancy with systemic lupus erythematosus? An analysis of 276 patients under long-term review," *Rheumatology*, vol. 39, no. 10, pp. 1147–1152, 2000.

[12] M. Abu-Shakra, D. D. Gladman, and M. B. Urowitz, "Malignancy in systemic lupus erythematosus," *Arthritis & Rheumatism*, vol. 39, no. 6, pp. 1050–1054, 1996.

[13] S. Bernatsky, R. Ramsey-Goldman, R. Rajan et al., "Non-Hodgkin's lymphoma in systemic lupus erythematosus," *Annals of the Rheumatic Diseases*, vol. 64, no. 10, pp. 1507–1509, 2005.

[14] S. Bernatsky, J. F. Boivin, L. Joseph et al., "Race/ethnicity and cancer occurrence in systemic lupus erythematosus," *Arthritis Care and Research*, vol. 53, no. 5, pp. 781–784, 2005.

[15] U. Hassan, S. Mushtaq, N. Mamoon, A. Hussain Asghar, and S. Ishtiaq, "Prognostic sub-grouping of diffuse large B-cell lymphomas into germinal centre and post germinal centre groups by immunohistochemistry after 6 cycles of chemotherapy," *Asian Pacific Journal of Cancer Prevention*, vol. 13, no. 4, pp. 1341–1347, 2012.

[16] R. Gillmore and W. Y. Sin, "Systemic lupus erythematosus mimicking lymphoma: the relevance of the clinical background in interpreting imaging studies," *BMJ Case Reports*, 2014.

[17] S. Bernatsky, R. Ramsey-Goldman, S. Lachance, C. A. Pineau, and A. E. Clarke, "Lymphoma in a patient with systemic lupus erythematosus," *Nature Clinical Practice Rheumatology*, vol. 2, no. 10, pp. 570–574, 2006.

[18] R. I. Fisher, "Overview of non-Hodgkin's lymphoma: biology, staging, and treatment," *Seminars in Oncology*, vol. 30, no. 2, supplement 4, pp. 3–9, 2003.

[19] E. Rossi, G. Catania, M. Truini, G. L. Ravetti, L. Grassia, and A. M. Marmont, "Patients with systemic lupus erythematosus (SLE) having developed malignant lymphomas. Complete remission of lymphoma following high-dose chemotherapy, but not of SLE," *Clinical and Experimental Rheumatology*, vol. 29, no. 3, pp. 555–559, 2011.

[20] J. R. Brown and A. T. Skarin, "Clinical mimics of lymphoma," *The Oncologist*, vol. 9, no. 4, pp. 406–416, 2004.

[21] S. Bernatsky, R. Ramsey-Goldman, L. Joseph et al., "Lymphoma risk in systemic lupus: effects of disease activity versus treatment," *Annals of the Rheumatic Diseases*, vol. 73, no. 1, pp. 138–142, 2014.

[22] J. L. Browning, "B cells move to centre stage: novel opportunities for autoimmune disease treatment," *Nature Reviews Drug Discovery*, vol. 5, no. 7, pp. 564–576, 2006.

[23] E. S. Jaffe, N. L. Harris, H. Stein, and J. W. Vardiman, Eds., *Pathology and Genetics of Tumours of Haematopoietic and Lymphoid Tissues*, IARC Press, Lyon, France, 2001.

[24] L. Pasqualucci, P. Neumeister, T. Goossens et al., "Hypermutation of multiple proto-oncogenes in B-cell diffuse large-cell lymphomas," *Nature*, vol. 412, no. 6844, pp. 341–346, 2001.

[25] F. N. Papavasiliou and D. G. Schatz, "Somatic hypermutation of immunoglobulin genes: merging mechanisms for genetic diversity," *Cell*, vol. 109, no. 2, supplement 1, pp. S35–S44, 2002.

[26] M. Montesinos-Rongen, D. Van Roost, C. Schaller, O. D. Wiestler, and M. Deckert, "Primary diffuse large B-cell lymphomas of the central nervous system are targeted by aberrant somatic hypermutation," *Blood*, vol. 103, no. 5, pp. 1869–1875, 2004.

[27] R. Küppers, U. Klein, M.-L. Hansmann, and K. Rajewsky, "Cellular origin of human B-cell lymphomas," *New England Journal of Medicine*, vol. 341, no. 20, pp. 1520–1529, 1999.

[28] J. A. James and J. M. Robertson, "Lupus and epstein-barr," *Current Opinion in Rheumatology*, vol. 24, no. 4, pp. 383–388, 2012.

[29] A. H. Draborg, K. Duus, and G. Houen, "Epstein-barr virus and systemic lupus erythematosus," *Clinical and Developmental Immunology*, vol. 2012, Article ID 370516, 2012.

[30] M. Epeldegui, Y. P. Hung, A. McQuay, R. F. Ambinder, and O. Martínez-Maza, "Infection of human B cells with Epstein-Barr virus results in the expression of somatic hypermutation-inducing molecules and in the accrual of oncogene mutations," *Molecular Immunology*, vol. 44, no. 5, pp. 934–942, 2007.

[31] P. Bailey, "Intracranial sarcomatous tumors of leptomeningeal origin," *Archives of Surgery*, vol. 18, no. 4, pp. 1359–1402, 1929.

[32] T. N. Shenkier, J.-Y. Blay, B. P. O'Neill et al., "Primary CNS lymphoma of T-cell origin: a descriptive analysis from the international primary CNS lymphoma collaborative group," *Journal of Clinical Oncology*, vol. 23, no. 10, pp. 2233–2239, 2005.

[33] F. H. Hochberg and D. C. Miller, "Primary central nervous system lymphoma," *Journal of Neurosurgery*, vol. 68, no. 6, pp. 835–853, 1988.

[34] C. N. Pisoni, A. R. Grinberg, J. L. Plana, R. D. Freue, J. A. Manni, and L. Paz, "Primary central nervous system lymphoma in a patient with systemic lupus erythematosus," *Medicina*, vol. 63, no. 3, pp. 221–223, 2003.

[35] B. Svobodova, Z. Hruskova, R. Rysava, and V. Tesar, "Brain diffuse large B-cell lymphoma in a systemic lupus erythematosus patient treated with immunosuppressive agents including mycophenolate mofetil," *Lupus*, vol. 20, no. 13, pp. 1452–1454, 2011.

[36] H. H. L. Tsang, N. J. Trendell-Smith, A. K. P. Wu, and M. Y. Mok, "Diffuse large B-cell lymphoma of the central nervous system in mycophenolate mofetil-treated patients with systemic lupus erythematosus," *Lupus*, vol. 19, no. 3, pp. 330–333, 2010.

[37] P. F. Finelli, K. Naik, J. A. DiGiuseppe, and A. Prasad, "Primary lymphoma of CNS, mycophenolate mofetil and lupus," *Lupus*, vol. 15, no. 12, pp. 886–888, 2006.

[38] N. Dasgupta, A. C. Gelber, F. Racke, and D. M. Fine, "Central nervous system lymphoma associated with mycophenolate mofetil in lupus nephritis," *Lupus*, vol. 14, no. 11, pp. 910–913, 2005.

[39] M.-G. Kim, S. Y. Park, E. J. Kim et al., "Hepatitis B virus reactivation in a primary central nervous system lymphoma patient following intrathecal rituximab treatment," *Acta Haematologica*, vol. 125, no. 3, pp. 121–124, 2011.

[40] Y. Meng, S. He, Q. Liu, D. Xu, T. Zhang, and Z. Chen, "High prevalence of hepatitis B virus infection in primary central nervous system lymphoma," *International Journal of Clinical and Experimental Medicine*, vol. 8, no. 6, pp. 9937–9942, 2015.

[41] P. M. Bracci, "Obesity and hepatitis B infection and risk of primary CNS lymphoma," *Blood*, vol. 122, no. 21, 2013.

[42] G. Ruiz-Irastorza, A. Ugarte, M. V. Egurbide et al., "Antimalarials may influence the risk of malignancy in systemic lupus erythematosus," *Annals of the Rheumatic Diseases*, vol. 66, no. 6, pp. 815–817, 2007.

[43] R. F. Ambinder, "Gammaherpesviruses and "hit-and-run" oncogenesis," *American Journal of Pathology*, vol. 156, no. 1, pp. 1–3, 2000.

[44] P. L. Zinzani, A. Broccoli, V. Stefoni et al., "Immunophenotype and intermediate-high international prognostic index score are prognostic factors for therapy in diffuse large B-cell lymphoma patients," *Cancer*, vol. 116, no. 24, pp. 5667–5675, 2010.

[45] T. Y. Lin, H. Y. Zhang, Y. Huang et al., "Comparison between R-CHOP regimen and CHOP regimen in treating naive diffuse large B-cell lymphoma in China—a multi-center randomized trial," *Ai Zheng*, vol. 24, no. 12, pp. 1421–1426, 2005.

[46] M. Holdhoff, P. Ambady, A. Abdelaziz et al., "High-dose methotrexate with or without rituximab in newly diagnosed primary CNS lymphoma," *Neurology*, vol. 83, no. 3, pp. 235–239, 2014.

[47] B. Alchi, D. Jayne, M. Labopin et al., "Autologous haematopoietic stem cell transplantation for systemic lupus erythematosus: data from the European Group for Blood and Marrow Transplantation registry," *Lupus*, vol. 22, no. 3, pp. 245–253, 2013.

[48] E. Klyuchnikov, U. Bacher, T. Kroll et al., "Allogeneic hematopoietic cell transplantation for diffuse large B cell lymphoma: who, when and how?" *Bone Marrow Transplantation*, vol. 49, no. 1, pp. 1–7, 2014.

26

A Case of Amyopathic Dermatomyositis with Pneumomediastinum and Subcutaneous Emphysema

Aslıhan Gürün Kaya,[1] **Aydın Çiledağ,**[1] **Orhan Küçükşahin,**[2] **Özlem Özdemir Kumbasar,**[1] **and Çetin Atasoy**[3]

[1]*Department of Chest Diseases, Ankara University School of Medicine, Ankara, Turkey*
[2]*Department of Rheumatology, Ankara University School of Medicine, Ankara, Turkey*
[3]*Department of Radiology, Ankara University School of Medicine, Ankara, Turkey*

Correspondence should be addressed to Aslıhan Gürün Kaya; aslihangurun@hotmail.com

Academic Editor: Shigeko Inokuma

A 34-year-old man was admitted with dyspnea, cough, and fever. Thorax computed tomography revealed ground glass opacities and pneumomediastinum. The patient was diagnosed as amyopathic dermatomyositis due to skin lesions and radiological findings. Despite immunosuppressive treatment clinical deterioration and radiological progression were observed and the patient died because of severe hypoxemic respiratory failure. The patient presented with extremely rare occurrence of pneumomediastinum and subcutaneous emphysema in amyopathic dermatomyositis with a poor prognosis.

1. Introduction

Dermatomyositis (DM) is an inflammatory disease characterized by skin lesions with muscle weakness. Amyopathic dermatomyositis (ADM) is a subtype of DM with characteristic cutaneous manifestations but without muscle involvement. Respiratory diseases, especially interstitial lung diseases (ILD), present more than half of the patients. Several reports have documented cases of interstitial lung diseases and the most common histological findings are nonspecific interstitial pneumonia, organising pneumonia, diffuse alveolar damage, and usual interstitial pneumonia. Pneumomediastinum, pneumothorax, and subcutaneous emphysema are rare, but characteristic complications with poor prognosis [1, 2].

2. Case Report

A 34-year-old male patient was admitted with dyspnea, cough, and fever for two weeks. There was no history of any occupational exposure and he had a 10-pack-year smoking history. The patient had a diagnosis of undifferentiated arthritis four months ago. He received 21 days of salazopyrin treatment but the drug had been discontinued because of hepatotoxicity. The symptoms were developed after 3 months of the cessation of the drug. On physical examination, cyanosis, macular erythema at neck and extensor surfaces of the arms, and also Gottron papules in joints and dorsum of the hand were detected and bilateral fine crackles were heard. The erythrocyte sedimentation rate was 70 mm/h and CRP level was 32.3 mg/dL. Serum biochemistry and complete blood count were normal. ANA, ANCA, RF, and other immune markers were negative, while anti-SS-A(Ro) was positive. The smear and culture of sputum were negative for any microorganism and acid-fast bacilli. Chest X-ray revealed bilateral opacities and computed tomography (CT) showed bilateral ground glass opacity in subpleural areas, consolidation, and pneumomediastinum (Figure 1).

The patient was transferred to intensive care unit (ICU) due to severe hypoxemic respiratory failure. There was no clinical and radiological improvement despite broad-spectrum antibiotics. Corticosteroid treatment was started because of severe hypoxemic respiratory failure. He did not complain of dry eye and/or mouth. Schirmer's test was negative and biopsy of salivary gland revealed minimal chronic inflammation. Serum creatine kinase (CK) and aldolase levels

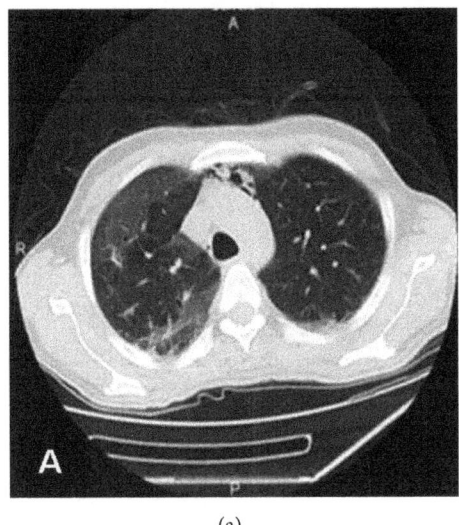
(a)

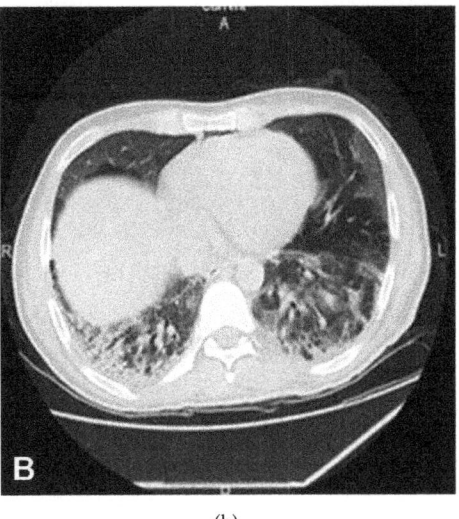
(b)

FIGURE 1: Thorax CT revealing bilateral ground glass opacity in subpleural areas, consolidation, and pneumomediastinum.

were normal. The patient was accepted as ADM due to skin lesions without myositis and radiological findings.

Cyclophosphamide 600 mg/m^2 per 21 days, methylprednisolone 60 mg/day, and hydroxychloroquine 400 mg/day were initiated. A biopsy of skin lesion was performed. Although pathologic examination revealed no specific pathology, we suggested that this might be secondary to the corticosteroid treatment. After second course of cyclophosphamide, although a clinical improvement was observed, chest radiograph and CT showed a progression with pneumomediastinum, interstitial and subcutaneous emphysema, thickening of interlobular septa, and reticular pattern (Figures 2 and 3). Cyclophosphamide treatment was discontinued, the dose of corticosteroids was increased, and mycophenolate mofetil (MMF) treatment was started. The patient was discharged with MMF and corticosteroid therapy. One month later, he was admitted with severe dyspnea on second admission. A radiological progression was observed. He was hospitalized in the ICU; however, the patient died because of severe hypoxemic respiratory failure despite immunosuppressive treatment and mechanical ventilation.

3. Discussion

Dermatomyositis is an inflammatory disease with characteristic cutaneous and musculoskeletal findings. Amyopathic dermatomyositis is a clinical subtype of DM and represents an estimated 20% of all DM cases [3]. It was first described by Pearson in 1979 as a rare skin disease that has the same cutaneous symptoms as classic DM without myopathy [4].

Onset usually occurs in early adulthood, although juvenile forms have been reported. The disease is more common in female. In a report including 291 adult-onset ADM cases, 73% of patients were female [5].

The diagnostic criteria for diagnosis of ADM vary. In 1993, Euwer and Sontheimer published four diagnostic criteria for ADM; (1) cutaneous changes pathognomonic of DM,

(2) skin biopsy specimen findings compatible with DM, (3) absence of clinical evidence of proximal motor weakness within 2 years of skin disease, and (4) normal skeletal enzyme levels for 2 years following the appearance of skin lesions [6]. However, Stonecipher et al. described different criteria and they divided patients with ADM into 3 main groups: (1) patients with cutaneous changes only, (2) patients with cutaneous changes at baseline and subsequent evolution to myositis, and (3) patients with cutaneous changes and normal muscle enzyme levels but in whom diagnostic evaluations showed subclinical myositis [7]. Also, Sontheimer et al. reported several major and minor criteria for the diagnosis of ADM and in our case the diagnosis was made according to presence of these two minor criteria and one major criterion [8]. Although the skin biopsy revealed no specific pathology in presented case, the biopsy had been performed under corticosteroid treatment.

The cutaneous findings in ADM are not different from those in classic D. Heliotrope rash and Gottron's papules are the most common skin changes. El-Azhary and Pakzad retrospectively reviewed 37 ADM cases and reported that Gottron's papules on the dorsa of the hands appear to be the most consistent presentation [9].

While the patients with DM-associated ILD are more likely to have the antiaminoacyl transfer RNA synthetase antibody (anti-Jo-1), this antibody is typically absent in patients with ADM even when ILD is present as in our case. In the study performed by El-Azhary and Pakzad, antinuclear antibodies (ANA) were positive in 20 of 28 patients [9]. In another report, ANA was positive in 2 of 8 ADM cases [10]. In 2005, Sato et al. reported a newly specific autoantibody in ADM patients which was named as anti-CADM-140 antibody [11]. This antibody may be detected in 50–73% of ADM patients. Gerami et al. reported that, in 72 of 115 ADM patients, ANA was positive (63%), while anti-Jo-1 antibodies were positive in 3 of 85 cases (4%) [5]. They also reported that assays for specific ANAs such as double-stranded DNA,

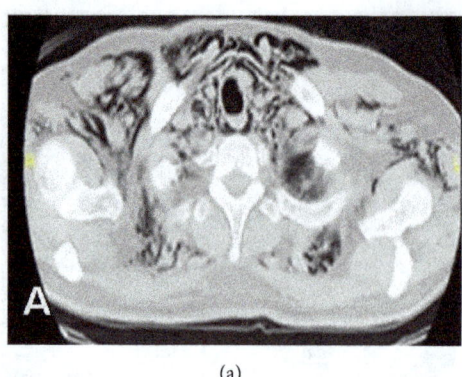 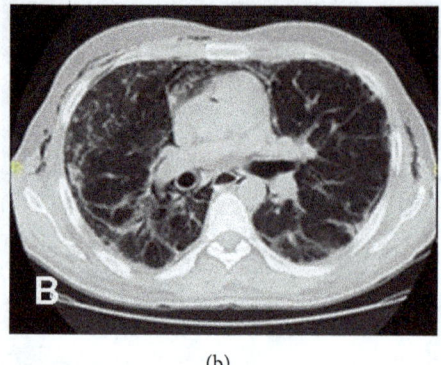

(a)   (b)

FIGURE 2: Thorax CT revealing pneumomediastinum, interstitial and subcutaneous emphysema, thickening of interlobular septa, and reticular pattern.

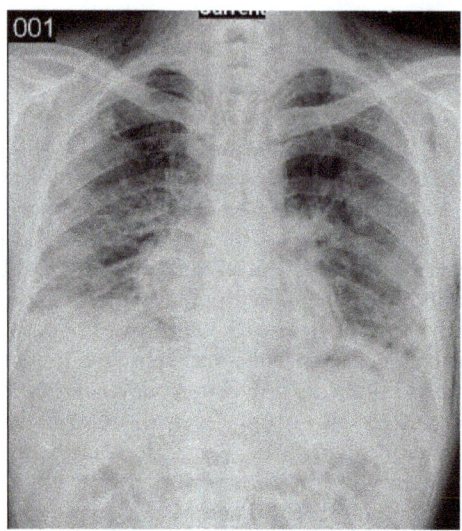

FIGURE 3: Chest radiograph showing bilateral opacities, pneumomediastinum, and subcutaneous emphysema.

Sm, Ro, and La were negative when reported. In contrast, in our case, only anti-SS-A(Ro) was positive, and, to our knowledge, this is the first case which is compatible with ADM with a positive anti-SS-A(Ro). We could not analyze the anti-CADM-140 antibody because of absence of this test in our laboratory.

Pulmonary involvement is seen in up to 50% of ADM patients and the most common radiographic abnormality is a diffuse reticulonodular pattern with patchy bilateral ground glass opacities. Spontaneous pneumomediastinum and subcutaneous emphysema are very rare and only several cases have been reported previously. Pulmonary involvement is the main cause of death in ADM and severe ILD and pneumomediastinum are the most potentially life-threatening complications. The presence of spontaneous pneumomediastinum is important, because it often leads to a rapid and aggressive course with fatal prognosis [1]. The rupture of subpleural blebs and cysts that developed from interstitial fibrosis and

a raised intra-alveolar pressure have been speculated as potential risk factors for development of pneumomediastinum. It has also been reported that corticosteroid treatment may lead to pneumomediastinum by weakening alveolar walls [12, 13].

There is no standard treatment strategy for ADM pulmonary complication. Cozzani et al. reviewed 55 ADM cases with pulmonary involvement and reported that high dose systemic corticosteroids were the first line therapy in all cases. Immunosuppressive or immunomodulant agents, like azathioprine, methotrexate, cyclosporine A, cycles of cyclophosphamide, high dose intravenous immunoglobulin, tacrolimus, or mycophenolate mofetil, were associated in 46 patients as first line therapy and in five cases as second line therapy [1]. The authors also reported a case of ADM with lung involvement in whom a successful outcome was achieved by mycophenolate mofetil without concomitant high dose corticosteroids. The efficacy of mycophenolate mofetil in ILD complicating ADM has also been shown in a few reports [14, 15]. Also, the potential effectiveness of an intensive therapy protocol with the addition of calcineurin inhibitor to glucocorticoid or more drug combination has been reported. (x) MMF suppresses lymphocyte proliferation via the inhibition of inosine monophosphate dehydrogenase, a rate-limiting enzyme for the de novo synthesis of guanosine nucleotides, and inhibits fibrosis via direct suppression of fibroblast function. In our case, initially we started with methylprednisolone, hydroxychloroquine, and cyclophosphamide. Due to absence of an improvement, the therapy was switched to corticosteroid and mycophenolate mofetil. Unfortunately, no improvement was observed and, after a rapid progression, the patient died.

In conclusion, since a rapidly progressive and fatal ILD with pneumomediastinum may develop, ADM cases must be followed closely. An effective and optimal treatment strategy is still needed.

References

[1] E. Cozzani, E. Cinotti, R. Felletti, D. Pelucco, A. Rebora, and A. Parodi, "Amyopathic dermatomyositis with lung involvement responsive to mycophenolate mofetil," *Immunopharmacology and Immunotoxicology*, vol. 35, no. 6, pp. 687–692, 2013.

[2] C. Powell, B. Kendall, R. Wernick, and J. E. Heffner, "A 34-year-old man with amyopathic dermatomyositis and rapidly progressive dyspnea with facial swelling," *Chest*, vol. 132, no. 5, pp. 1710–1713, 2007.

[3] M. J. Bendewald, D. A. Wetter, X. Li, and M. D. P. Davis, "Incidence of dermatomyositis and clinically amyopathic dermatomyositis: a population-based study in Olmsted County, Minnesota," *Archives of Dermatology*, vol. 146, no. 1, pp. 26–30, 2010.

[4] C. Pearson, "Polymyositis and dermatomyositis," in *Arthritis and Allied Conditions: a Textbook of Rheumatology*, D. J. McCarty, Ed., p. 742, Lea & Febiger, Philadelphia, Pa, USA, 9th edition, 1979.

[5] P. Gerami, J. M. Schope, L. McDonald, H. W. Walling, and R. D. Sontheimer, "A systematic review of adult-onset clinically amyopathic dermatomyositis (dermatomyositis siné myositis): a missing link within the spectrum of the idiopathic inflammatory myopathies," *Journal of the American Academy of Dermatology*, vol. 54, no. 4, pp. 597–613, 2006.

[6] R. L. Euwer and R. D. Sontheimer, "Amyopathic dermatomyositis: a review," *Journal of Investigative Dermatology*, vol. 100, no. 1, pp. 124–127, 1993.

[7] M. R. Stonecipher, J. L. Jorizzo, W. L. White, F. O. Walker, and E. Prichard, "Cutaneous changes of dermatomyositis in patients with normal muscle enzymes: dermatomyositis sine myositis?" *Journal of the American Academy of Dermatology*, vol. 28, no. 6, pp. 951–956, 1993.

[8] R. D. Sontheimer, P. Gerami, and H. W. Walling, "Clinically amyopathic dermatomyositis," in *Diagnostic Criteria in Autoimmune Diseases*, Y. Shoenfeld, R. Cervera, and M. E. Gershwin, Eds., pp. 159–163, Humana Press, Totowa, NJ, USA, 2008.

[9] R. A. El-Azhary and S. Y. Pakzad, "Amyopathic dermatomyositis: retrospective review of 37 cases," *Journal of the American Academy of Dermatology*, vol. 46, no. 4, pp. 560–565, 2002.

[10] R. Neri, S. Barsotti, V. Iacopetti et al., "Clinically amyopathic dermatomyositis: analysis of a monocentric cohort," *Journal of Clinical Neuromuscular Disease*, vol. 15, no. 4, pp. 157–160, 2014.

[11] S. Sato, M. Hirakata, M. Kuwana et al., "Autoantibodies to a 140-kd polypeptide, CADM-140, in Japanese patients with clinically amyopathic dermatomyositis," *Arthritis and Rheumatism*, vol. 52, no. 5, pp. 1571–1576, 2005.

[12] F. de Souza Neves, S. K. Shinjo, J. F. Carvalho, M. Levy-Neto, and C. T. L. Borges, "Spontaneous pneumomediastinum and dermatomyositis may be a not so rare association: report of a case and review of the literature," *Clinical Rheumatology*, vol. 26, no. 1, pp. 105–107, 2007.

[13] Y. Yamanishi, H. Maeda, F. Konishi et al., "Dermatomyositis associated with rapidly progressive fatal interstitial pneumonitis and pneumomediastinum," *Scandinavian Journal of Rheumatology*, vol. 28, no. 1, pp. 58–61, 1999.

[14] P. A. Morganroth, M. E. Kreider, and V. P. Werth, "Mycophenolate mofetil for interstitial lung disease in dermatomyositis," *Arthritis Care and Research*, vol. 62, no. 10, pp. 1496–1501, 2010.

[15] H. Tsuchiya, H. Tsuno, M. Inoue et al., "Mycophenolate mofetil therapy for rapidly progressive interstitial lung disease in a patient with clinically amyopathic dermatomyositis," *Modern Rheumatology*, vol. 24, no. 4, pp. 694–696, 2014.

27

Role of ^{18}F-FDG PET Scan in Rheumatoid Lung Nodule

Christine L. Chhakchhuak,[1] Mehdi Khosravi,[2] and Kristine M. Lohr[1]

[1] Division of Rheumatology, Department of Internal Medicine, University of Kentucky, 740 South Limestone Street, Room J-515, Lexington, KY 40536, USA
[2] Division of Pulmonary and Critical Care Medicine, Department of Internal Medicine, University of Kentucky, 740 South Limestone Street, Kentucky Clinic L 543, Lexington KY 40536, USA

Correspondence should be addressed to Christine L. Chhakchhuak; chrischkchk@gmail.com

Academic Editors: G. S. Alarcon, D. R. Alpert, and J. Mikdashi

Flourine-18 fluoro-2-deoxy-glucose (^{18}F-FDG) positron emission tomography combined with computed tomography (PET/CT) is a useful test for the management of malignant conditions. Inflammatory and infectious processes, however, can cause increased uptake on PET scanning, often causing diagnostic dilemmas. This knowledge is important to the rheumatologist not only because of the inflammatory conditions we treat but also because certain rheumatic diseases impose an increased risk of malignancy either due to the disease itself or as a consequence of medications used to treat the rheumatic diseases. There is an increasing body of evidence investigating the role of PET scans in inflammatory conditions. This paper describes a patient with rheumatoid arthritis who developed pulmonary nodules that showed increased uptake on PET/CT scan and reviews the use of PET scanning in the diagnosis and management of rheumatoid arthritis.

1. Introduction

Fluorine-18 fluoro-2-deoxyglucose (^{18}F-FDG) positron emission tomography combined with computed tomography (PET/CT) is a useful test to evaluate malignancies [1]. However, inflammatory diseases may also show increased uptake of ^{18}F-FDG and cause false-positive PET scan results, necessitating further investigations to rule out malignant conditions [2]. Positron emission tomography (PET) is an analytical imaging technology developed to use compounds labeled with positron-emitting radioisotopes as molecular probes to image and measure biochemical processes in vivo [3]. Numerous tracers have been used in conjunction with PET scanning to aid in the diagnosis of various disorders. ^{18}F-FDG has now become the most commonly used radiotracer for PET scanning. Because of the increased metabolic activity of the tumor cells, there is an increased uptake of glucose in tumor cells, thus forming the basis for widespread use of ^{18}F-FDG PET scan in the diagnosis, staging, and management of malignancies. However, the increased uptake of ^{18}F-FDG tracer is not limited to malignant states and has been seen in benign as well as inflammatory conditions such as sarcoidosis, large vessel vasculitis, inflammatory bowel disease, and rheumatoid arthritis (RA) [2, 4–8].

We describe a patient with RA who developed pulmonary nodules, showing increased uptake on ^{18}F-FDG PET/CT scan. We also review the current literature on the use of PET scanning in articular and extra-articular RA.

2. Case Report

A 50-year-old Caucasian woman with a history of RA presented with dyspnea on exertion. RA was diagnosed 4 years earlier and has been treated with methotrexate since the time of diagnosis. RA is currently in remission on oral methotrexate 15 mg weekly and folic acid 1 mg daily. Both rheumatoid factor and anticitrullinated peptide antibody are highly positive. Past medical history is significant for coronary artery disease with stent placement, chronic obstructive pulmonary disease (COPD), hypothyroidism, hypertension, and gastroesophageal reflux disease. She has a 60-pack-year smoking history and continues to smoke. Family history is positive for a mother and sister with lung cancer who were both heavy smokers and 2 sisters with COPD. She has lost 15–20 pounds of weight intentionally over a period of 3 months. There is history of loss of appetite. Physical examination including joint examination is normal except for decreased breath sounds in both upper lobes. Laboratory data revealed normal blood count, erythrocyte sedimentation rate (ESR), C-reactive protein (CRP), and renal and liver functions. A chest X-ray done for evaluation of dyspnea on exertion revealed a new right upper lobe (RUL) lung nodule. Her previous chest X-ray four years earlier showed multiple calcified nodules bilaterally and a small noncalcified RUL nodule less than a centimeter. CT chest revealed a 1.5 cm × 2.5 cm noncalcified pleural-based RUL nodule, a 1.1 cm calcified nodule in the left upper lobe, and an 8 mm noncalcified nodule in the right lower lobe (Figure 1). ^{18}F-FDG PET/CT scan showed moderately increased uptake in all nodules with a maximum standardized uptake value (SUV) of 3.7 in the RUL nodule (Figure 2). Given the patient's high risk based on tobacco use and family history of lung cancer, she underwent a CT-guided biopsy of the RUL nodule that was nondiagnostic. Subsequent video-assisted thoracic surgery (VATS) biopsy of the right upper and lower lobe nodules was performed. Pathology of both nodules revealed chronic inflammation with necrotizing granulomatous formation consistent with rheumatoid nodules and no evidence of malignancy (Figures 3 and 4). Fungal and acid-fast bacilli stains and cultures were negative.

3. Discussion

It has been noted that around 50 percent of solitary pulmonary nodules and a greater percentage of multiple pulmonary nodules turn out to be benign processes [9]. This, in the face of 200,000 cases of lung cancer diagnosed per year with mortality of 150,000 per year, creates a difficult conundrum in the management of pulmonary nodules in diseases known to cause lung nodules such as RA [10]. ^{18}F-FDG PET/CT scan has a sensitivity of 96-97% and a specificity of 83–85% in differentiating malignant pulmonary nodules [11–13]. However, the presence of inflammation and fibrosis significantly hinders PET scan accuracy. This is compromised even more so in the era of RA treatment with biologics that confers increased risk of mycobacterial and fungal infections which can potentially present as PET-positive lesions.

Reports of the use of PET and PET/CT in extra-articular RA are limited to subcutaneous nodules, lymph nodes, and the lung. Rodríguez et al. described two patients with RA in whom pulmonary nodules showed increased SUV on ^{18}F-FDG PET scan [14]. Biopsy of the nodules demonstrated bronchogenic carcinoma developing within preexisting rheumatoid nodules. Based on their experience they concluded that PET scan is a diagnostic test of high accuracy and can be used before surgical biopsy in patients with RA and pulmonary nodules who are suspected to have bronchogenic carcinoma. However, not all cases of increased uptake on PET scan are related to malignancy as is evidenced by the

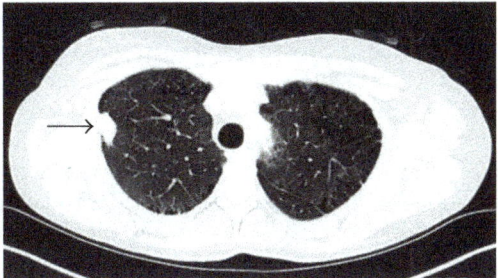

FIGURE 1: CT chest showing 1.5 cm × 2.5 cm RUL pleural-based nodule (arrow).

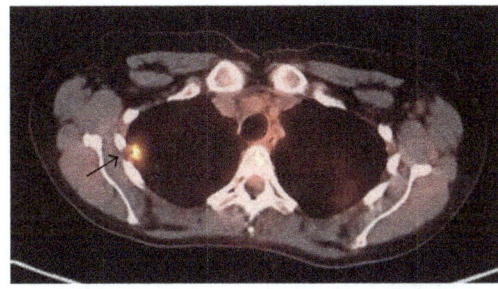

FIGURE 2: PET scan showing increased uptake in RUL nodule (arrow).

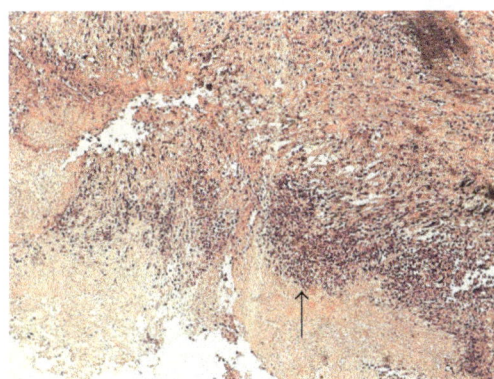

FIGURE 3: Mixed inflammatory infiltrate seen within the nodule.

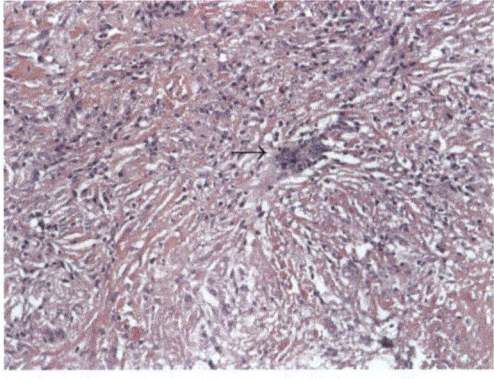

FIGURE 4: Multinucleated giant cells with lymphocytes, fibroblasts, and collagen in the granuloma wall.

following reports. Gupta et al. described a patient with RA found to have mild increased uptake in pulmonary nodules on PET scan [15]. Histological examination of these nodules revealed the presence of rheumatoid nodules. Bagga reported a case of a 63-year-old female with severe RA and long-standing smoking history [16]. The patient had multiple pulmonary nodules and a left pleural effusion. PET scan showed no uptake in the lung nodules but intense pleural uptake. A CT-guided biopsy of both the nodules and the pleura was performed, which confirmed the diagnosis of rheumatoid lung disease. dos Anjos et al. reported a patient with RA in whom increased ^{18}F-FDG uptake was found in subcutaneous nodules and lymph nodes including cervical, supraclavicular, axillary, and pelvic areas [17]. Similarly, Seldin et al. have published a series of nine patients with RA having increased FDG tracer uptake in the axillary lymph nodes [18]. Strobel et al. described a patient with RA with a soft tissue nodule on the left elbow [19]. Based on moderately increased activity on PET scan, the patient underwent excision of the nodule. It turned out to be a rheumatoid nodule.

4. Conclusion

The role of PET scan in diagnosis, staging, and management of malignancies is well known. There is an increasing body of evidence supporting the role of PET scans in nonmalignant conditions including vasculitis and granulomatous diseases such as sarcoidosis [20, 21]. The major factors limiting widespread use of PET/CT scanning appear to be cost, availability, and radiation exposure. The role of PET scan in cases of extra-articular involvement of RA has not been studied and is limited to a very small number of case reports and case series.

As evidenced by our case as well as other case reports, increased activity on PET scan does not necessarily translate into the diagnosis of malignancy. One would generally assume that the degree of maximum FDG uptake is lower in inflammatory lung nodules compared to malignancies. However, this is not always the case, as RA nodules have been reported with SUVs ranging from low to very high [15, 16, 19, 22, 23]. Thus, SUV cannot be used to differentiate between benign inflammatory and malignant lesions. Serial monitoring with PET/CT scans may show a more stable SUV uptake in benign inflammatory lesions compared to malignancies. Recently, the use of 11C-methionine PET scan has been shown to be more sensitive in differentiating between malignant and inflammatory lung lesions [24, 25]. ^{18}F-FDG PET scan provides valuable information on joint involvement as well as extra-articular disease in patients with RA. As promising as PET scanning is for inflammatory joint conditions, larger studies are necessary, especially pertaining to the cost effectiveness of routine PET scanning before its use in clinical practice. Clinicians need to be aware of the fact that rheumatoid nodules can have increased activity on PET scan. With the increasing use of PET scan for evaluation of lung nodules, rheumatologists will likely be confronted with more such cases of increased PET uptake in RA patients. Considering the lack of an established range of rheumatoid nodule metabolic activity, close monitoring, with or without

the use of invasive diagnostic methods such as needle biopsy or VATS, is prudent in the management of lung nodules in rheumatoid arthritis.

Disclosure

The paper has not been presented in any form in any meeting or forum. The contents of this paper have not been published in any journal and are not under consideration in any other journal. All authors have read the paper and agreed on the content.

Acknowledgment

The authors acknowledge Drs. William N. O'Connor and Jill A. Eickhoff from the Department of Pathology, University of Kentucky, for contributing histopathology slides.

References

[1] L. Kostakoglu, H. Agress Jr., and S. J. Goldsmith, "Clinical role of FDG PET in evaluation of cancer patients," *Radiographics*, vol. 23, no. 2, pp. 315–340, 2003.

[2] U. Metser and E. Even-Sapir, "Increased (18)F-fluorodeoxyglu-cose uptake in benign, nonphysiologic lesions found on whole-body positron emission tomography/computed tomography (PET/CT): accumulated data from four years of experience with PET/CT," *Seminars in Nuclear Medicine*, vol. 37, no. 3, pp. 206–222, 2007.

[3] S. Basu, T. C. Kwee, S. Surti, E. A. Akin, D. Yoo, and A. Alavi, "Fundamentals of PET and PET/CT imaging," *Annals of the New York Academy of Sciences*, vol. 1228, no. 1, pp. 1–18, 2011.

[4] S. Basu, H. Zhuang, D. A. Torigian, J. Rosenbaum, W. Chen, and A. Alavi, "Functional imaging of inflammatory diseases using nuclear medicine techniques," *Seminars in Nuclear Medicine*, vol. 39, no. 2, pp. 124–145, 2009.

[5] H. Engel, H. Steinert, A. Buck, T. Berthold, R. A. H. Böni, and G. K. von Schulthess, "Whole-body PET: physiological and arti-factual fluorodeoxyglucose accumulations," *Journal of Nuclear Medicine*, vol. 37, no. 3, pp. 441–446, 1996.

[6] U. Metser, E. Miller, H. Lerman, and E. Even-Sapir, "Benign nonphysiologic lesions with increased 18F-FDG uptake on PET/CT: characterization and incidence," *American Journal of Roent-genology*, vol. 189, no. 5, pp. 1203–1210, 2007.

[7] G. Treglia, M. V. Mattoli, L. Leccisotti, G. Ferraccioli, and A. Giordano, "Usefulness of whole-body fluorine-18-fluorodeoxy-glucose positron emission tomography in patients with large-vessel vasculitis: a systematic review," *Clinical Rheumatology*, vol. 30, no. 10, pp. 1265–1275, 2011.

[8] A. S. Teirstein, J. Machac, O. Almeida, P. Lu, M. L. Padilla, and M. C. Iannuzzi, "Results of 188 whole-body fluorodeoxyglucose positron emission tomography scans in 137 patients with sar-coidosis," *Chest*, vol. 132, no. 6, pp. 1949–1953, 2007.

[9] G. A. Higgins, T. W. Shields, and R. J. Keehn, "The solitary pulmonary nodule. Ten year follow up of Veterans Administra-tion—Armed Forces cooperative study," *Archives of Surgery*, vol. 110, no. 5, pp. 570–575, 1975.

[10] A. Jemal, R. Siegel, E. Ward et al., "Cancer statistics, 2008," *CA Cancer Journal for Clinicians*, vol. 58, no. 2, pp. 71–96, 2008.

[11] S. K. Kim, M. Allen-Auerbach, J. Goldin et al., "Accuracy of PET/CT in characterization of solitary pulmonary lesions," *Journal of Nuclear Medicine*, vol. 48, no. 2, pp. 214–220, 2007.

[12] C. A. Yi, S. L. Kyung, B.-T. Kim et al., "Tissue characterization of solitary pulmonary nodule: comparative study between helical dynamic CT and integrated PET/CT," *Journal of Nuclear Medicine*, vol. 47, no. 3, pp. 443–450, 2006.

[13] C.-Y. Chang, C. Tzao, S.-C. Lee et al., "Incremental value of integrated FDG-PET/CT in evaluating indeterminate solitary pulmonary nodule for malignancy," *Molecular Imaging and Biology*, vol. 12, no. 2, pp. 204–209, 2010.

[14] P. Rodríguez, T. Romero, F. Rodríguez de Castro, M. Hussein, and J. Freixinet, "Bronchogenic carcinoma associated with rheumatoid arthritis: role of FDG-PET scans," *Rheumatology*, vol. 45, no. 3, pp. 359–360, 2006.

[15] P. Gupta, F. Ponzo, and E. L. Kramer, "Fluorodeoxyglucose (FDG) uptake in pulmonary rheumatoid nodules," *Clinical Rheumatology*, vol. 24, no. 4, pp. 402–405, 2005.

[16] S. Bagga, "Rheumatoid lung disease as seen on PET/CT scan," *Clinical Nuclear Medicine*, vol. 32, no. 9, pp. 753–754, 2007.

[17] D. A. dos Anjos, G. F. do Vale, C. de Mello Campos et al., "Extra-articular inflammatory sites detected by F-18 FDG PET/CT in a patient with rheumatoid arthritis," *Clinical Nuclear Medicine*, vol. 35, no. 7, pp. 540–541, 2010.

[18] D. W. Seldin, I. Habib, and G. Soudry, "Axillary lymph node visualization on F-18 FDG PET body scans in patients with rheumatoid arthritis," *Clinical Nuclear Medicine*, vol. 32, no. 7, pp. 524–526, 2007.

[19] K. Strobel, A. R. von Hochstetter, and U. G. Exner, "FDG uptake in a rheumatoid nodule with imaging appearance similar to a malignant soft tissue tumor," *Clinical Nuclear Medicine*, vol. 34, no. 10, pp. 691–692, 2009.

[20] I. Zerizer, K. Tan, S. Khan et al., "Role of FDG-PET and PET/CT in the diagnosis and management of vasculitis," *European Journal of Radiology*, vol. 73, no. 3, pp. 504–509, 2010.

[21] G. Treglia, S. Taralli, and A. Giordano, "Emerging role of whole-body18F-fluorodeoxyglucose positron emission tomography as a marker of disease activity in patients with sarcoidosis: a systematic review," *Sarcoidosis Vasculitis and Diffuse Lung Diseases*, vol. 28, no. 2, pp. 87–94, 2011.

[22] S. M. B. Bakheet and J. Powe, "Fluorine-18-fluorodeoxyglucose uptake in rheumatoid arthritis-associated lung disease in a patient with thyroid cancer," *Journal of Nuclear Medicine*, vol. 39, no. 2, pp. 234–236, 1998.

[23] T. Saraya, R. Tanaka, M. Fujiwara, H. Koji, M. Oda, Y. Ogawa et al., "Fluorodeoxyglucose (FDG) uptake in pulmonary rheumatoid nodules diagnosed by video-assisted thoracic surgery lung biopsy: two case reports and a review of the literature," *Modern Rheumatology*, vol. 23, no. 2, pp. 393–396, 2013.

[24] H.-J. Hsieh, S.-H. Lin, K.-H. Lin, C.-Y. Lee, C.-P. Chang, and S.-J. Wang, "The feasibility of 11C-methionine-PET in diagnosis of solitary lung nodules/masses when compared with 18F-FDG-PET," *Annals of Nuclear Medicine*, vol. 22, no. 6, pp. 533–538, 2008.

[25] K. Kanegae, I. Nakano, K. Kimura et al., "Comparison of MET-PET and FDG-PET for differentiation between benign lesions and lung cancer in pneumoconiosis," *Annals of Nuclear Medicine*, vol. 21, no. 6, pp. 331–337, 2007.

28

Olecranon Bursitis Caused by *Candida parapsilosis* in a Patient with Rheumatoid Arthritis

Carla F. Gamarra-Hilburn, Grissel Rios, and Luis M. Vilá

Division of Rheumatology, Department of Medicine, University of Puerto Rico, Medical Sciences Campus, San Juan, PR 00936-5067, USA

Correspondence should be addressed to Luis M. Vilá; luis.vila2@upr.edu

Academic Editor: George S. Habib

Septic bursitis is usually caused by bacterial organisms. However, infectious bursitis caused by fungi is very rare. Herein, we present a 68-year-old woman with long-standing rheumatoid arthritis who developed pain, erythema, and swelling of the right olecranon bursa. Aspiration of the olecranon bursa showed a white blood cell count of $3.1 \times 10^3/\mu L$ (41% neutrophils, 30% lymphocytes, and 29% monocytes). Fluid culture was positive for *Candida parapsilosis*. She was treated with caspofungin 50 mg intravenously daily for 13 days followed by fluconazole 200 mg orally daily for one week. She responded well to this treatment but had recurrent swelling of the bursa. Bursectomy was recommended but she declined this option. This case, together with other reports, suggests that the awareness of uncommon pathogens, their presentation, and predisposing risk factors are important to establish an early diagnosis and prevent long-term complications.

1. Introduction

Septic bursitis occurs in the olecranon bursa very commonly [1]; this is due to its superficial location and vulnerability to trauma [1]. Among predisposing factors for septic bursitis are immunosuppression, surgical intervention, chronic diseases, and any occupation that can produce trauma to the area [1, 2]. Bacteria are the most frequent culprit, with *Staphylococcus aureus* producing the majority of the cases [1, 2]. Fungal infection is rare and there are only few cases published in the medical literature. Septic bursitis due to *Candida* (*parapsilosis*, *albicans*, *tropicalis*, and *glabrata*) species, *Penicillium* species, *Anthopsis deltoidea*, *Aspergillus terreus*, and *Phialophora richardsiae* has been reported [1–13]. Herein, we report a case of an elderly woman with long-standing rheumatoid arthritis (RA) who presented with septic olecranon bursitis secondary to *Candida parapsilosis*. We also present a literature review of bursitis caused by *Candida* species.

2. Case Presentation

A 68-year-old female was referred to our service for evaluation of erythema and swelling of the right elbow. She was admitted to the hospital 12 days before because of an infected left foot ulcer that required debridement and intravenous antibiotic therapy. Six weeks prior to admission she was seen by a pain management specialist for swelling of the right elbow and she was diagnosed with olecranon bursitis. She was treated with bursa aspiration and corticosteroid injection. Cultures were reportedly negative. One to two weeks after the procedure, she had worsening of swelling, as well as pain and erythema of the olecranon bursa. She did not report fever, weight loss, fatigue, or weakness.

Her past medical history was remarkable for RA diagnosed at 30 years of age, arterial hypertension, peripheral vascular disease, and asthma. Her surgical history included amputations of the first and second toes of the left foot and two tendon repairs (left hand and left shoulder). She received multiple therapies for RA including auranofin, methotrexate, leflunomide, and etanercept. Her last treatment was golimumab, which she used for 4 years. She did not have further follow-up with her rheumatologist and stopped this treatment about 2 years before onset of olecranon bursitis.

On initial evaluation, she had normal vital signs. Scleromalacia was noted bilaterally. Examination of the upper extremities showed ulnar deviation of the metacarpopha-langeal joints and swan neck deformities bilaterally. The left wrist had marked limitation of flexion and extension. The right olecranon bursa was tender and swollen, and the overlying skin was erythematous (Figure 1). Range of motion of the right elbow was not limited. She had multiple subcutaneous nodules in the right leg and a stage IV ulcer on the medial aspect of the left foot. Generalized muscle atrophy was observed. The rest of the examination was unremarkable.

Laboratory tests showed a white blood cell count of 6.8 × $10^3/\mu L$, lymphocytic count of $1.2 \times 10^3/\mu L$, hemoglobin of 9.6 g/dL, and platelet count of $344 \times 10^3/\mu L$. Serum creatinine was 0.5 mg/dL and blood urea nitrogen was 17 mg/dL. Wound cultures were negative. Chest X-ray showed mild prominence of the pulmonary markings in the right infrahilar region.

The olecranon bursa was aspirated and 9 mL of hemor-rhagic fluid was obtained. No crystals were observed under polarized microscopy. Fluid analysis showed a white blood cell count of $3.1 \times 10^3/\mu L$ (41% neutrophils, 30% lympho-cytes, and 29% monocytes). Bacterial cultures were negative. Fungal culture was positive for *Candida parapsilosis*; this was sensitive to anidulafungin, micafungin, caspofungin, 5-flucytosine, voriconazole, itraconazole, and fluconazole. The VITEK 2 system (bioMérieux, Inc., Hazelwood, Missouri, USA) was used for fungus identification. The Sensititre YeastOne system (Trek Diagnostic Systems, Cleveland, Ohio, USA) was utilized to determine antifungal susceptibility.

She was treated with caspofungin 50 mg intravenously daily for 13 days. Four aspiration procedures were required (every 3–5 days) due to fluid reaccumulation. All samples were cultured but only the first two were positive for *Candida parapsilosis*. After intravenous therapy, fluconazole 200 mg orally daily was prescribed for one week. She responded well to this therapy but had recurrent swelling of the bursa. Bursectomy was recommended but she did not wish to proceed with the intervention or receive further treatment. After 3 months of follow-up, she continued to have fluid in the olecranon bursa and had some discomfort in the area.

3. Discussion

Symptoms and signs of septic bursitis, either bacterial or fungal, are similar. However, fungal bursitis seems to have a more indolent course which may cause a delay in diagnosis and treatment [2, 4–7]. Among all bursae, the olecranon and the prepatellar bursae are the most commonly involved; this is because they are superficial, and pathogens can migrate transcutaneously through minor trauma [2]. Although septic bursitis is almost always secondary to direct inoculation, hematogenous spread can also occur [8, 9].

Fungal septic bursitis is rare. *Candida* (*parapsilosis, albi-cans, tropicalis,* and *glabrata*), *Penicillium* species, *Anthopsis deltoidea, Aspergillus terreus,* and *Phialophora richardsiae* have been isolated [1–13]. Specifically, very few cases of olecranon bursitis secondary to *Candida parapsilosis* have been reported in the medical literature [3, 7, 10, 11]. Unlike *Candida albicans* and *Candida tropicalis, Candida parapsilosis* is not an obligate human pathogen [14]. The clinical spectrum

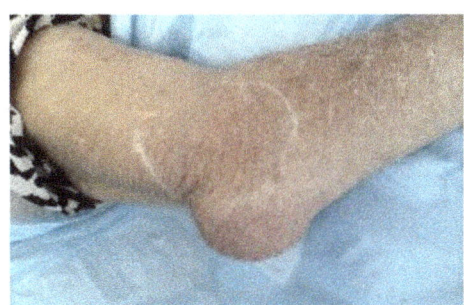

FIGURE 1: Erythema and swelling of the right olecranon bursa.

of *Candida parapsilosis* infection is variable, ranging from vulvovaginitis to fungemia and endocarditis. It is also known to cause arthritis which can be secondary to fungemia, intra-articular injections, or catheterizations or related to prosthetic joints [8, 9, 11, 15].

To the best of our knowledge, 11 cases of septic bursitis due to *Candida* species, including ours, have been reported in the medical literature (Table 1) [1, 3, 4, 7–13]. Five cases, including our case, were secondary to *Candida parapsilosis* [3, 7, 10, 11]. Two cases were secondary to *Candida tropicalis* [8, 9], and the other three were due to *Candida albicans* [1], Candida *lusitaniae* [13], and *Candida glabrata* [12] (one each). The subclass identification of *Candida* species was not done in one patient with subacromial bursitis and the diagnosis was achieved histopathologically after bursectomy was performed [4]. Regarding the site involved, the olecranon bursa was affected in 7 of the 11 cases including our patient [3, 7, 8, 11–13]; the subacromial bursa was affected in 3 patients [1, 4, 10]; and the popliteal bursa was affected in 1 case [9]. Six patients were immunosuppressed and 1 patient was receiving prednisone at low dose (10 mg daily) [1, 7–9, 11–13]. Our patient had severe joint damage from RA, but she was not receiving immunosuppressive therapy at the time of septic bursitis.

In the 11 cases reported with *Candida* bursitis, the probable source of infection was thought to be fungemia in 3 cases [1, 8, 9], one case was thought to be secondary to superficial trauma [13], and in 3 cases the source of infection was undetermined [7, 10, 11]. Four cases were likely related to corticosteroid injection, including our case [3, 4, 12]. In our patient, although her musculoskeletal deformities and her duties as an administrative assistant predisposed to continuous trauma to the area, her symptoms worsened after the intrabursal injection. This event suggests that the pathogen could have been inoculated during the aspiration and corticosteroid injection. She could have also acquired the infection through transient fungemia from the wound in her foot. However, wound cultures were negative.

The course of septic bursitis due to fungi can be chronic and this delays diagnosis and treatment. Six of the 10 reported cases had a chronic course ranging from 4 to 18 months [3, 4, 8, 10, 13]; the remaining cases had an acute onset [1, 7, 9, 12]. In one case, the duration of the disease was not described but it presented 7 months after infliximab therapy was started [11]. Regarding the age at presentation, more than 70% of

TABLE 1: Demographic features, clinical manifestations, treatment, and outcome of septic bursitis caused by *Candida* species.

Case number	*Candida* strain/culture site	Author/year of publication	Age/sex	Infected bursa	Clinical presentation of bursitis	Comorbidities	Other risk factors	Probable source of infection	Treatment	Outcome
1	*C. albicans* Bursal fluid	Rosochmann and Bell/1987 [1]	73/M	Subacromial	Acute, 5 days	SLE	Corticosteroids	Fungemia	Amphotericin B	Complete resolution
2	*C. glabrata* Phlegmon-like material form olecranon bursae	Skedros et al./2013 [12]	63/F	Olecranon	Acute, 2 weeks after corticosteroid injection	COPD Arterial hypertension Hypothyroidism Recurrent oropharyngeal candidiasis	Prednisone 10 mg daily	Corticosteroid injection	Caspofungin Debridement, irrigation, and bursectomy	Complete resolution
3	*C. lusitaniae* Bursal fluid	Behar and Chertow/1998 [13]	59/F	Olecranon	Chronic, 6 months	SLE Diabetes Asthma	Methotrexate 15 mg weekly Prednisone 30 mg daily	Superficial trauma	Fluconazole 100 mg a day; 5-fluorocytosine	Recurrence after several months
4	*C. parapsilosis* Bursal fluid	Schlesinger and Hoffman/1995 [7]	62/F	Olecranon	Acute	Breast cancer COPD	Prednisone 40 mg daily	Undetermined	Amphotericin B IV over 9 days Ketoconazole (400 mg/d for 2 months)	Complete resolution
5	*C. parapsilosis* Bursal fluid	Jiménez-Palop et al./2002 [3]	32/M	Olecranon	Chronic, around 3 months	None	None	Corticosteroid injection	Fluconazole 400 mg for 7 days, followed by 200 mg a day Bursectomy	Complete resolution
6	*C. parapsilosis* Bursa tissue culture	Miyamoto et al./2012 [11]	60/F	Olecranon	Duration of the disease not mentioned. It presented 7 months after infliximab therapy was started	RA	Infliximab Methotrexate Prednisolone	Undetermined	Bursectomy	Complete resolution of bursitis. Later developed wrist arthritis
7	*C. parapsilosis* Shoulder synovial fluid Tissue culture	Jeong et al./2013 [10]	74/M	Subacromial, subdeltoid, and subcoracoid	Chronic, >18 months	None	None	Undetermined	Fluconazole (neither dose nor length of therapy specified) Surgical exploration with drainage, debridement, and bursectomy	Complete resolution
8	*C. parapsilosis* Bursal fluid	Current case	68/F	Olecranon	Acute, 1-2 weeks after bursa aspiration and corticosteroid injection	RA Infected ulcer	None	Corticosteroid injection	Caspofungin 50 mg IV daily for 2 weeks, followed by fluconazole 200 mg a day for 1 week	Persistence
9	*C. tropicalis* Bursal fluid Urine Blood	Murray et al./1976 [8]	77/M	Olecranon	Chronic	Bladder cancer Syphilis Sepsis	Neutropenia Urethral and venous catheters	Fungemia	Amphotericin B IV for 9 weeks Bursectomy	Complete resolution

TABLE 1: Continued.

Case number	Candida strain/culture site	Author/year of publication	Age/sex	Infected bursa	Clinical presentation of bursitis	Comorbidities	Other risk factors	Probable source of infection	Treatment	Outcome
10	C. tropicalis Blood Fluid from ruptured bursae	Wall et al./1982 [9]	48/M	First, knee septic arthritis; later, popliteal bursitis	Acute, 2 weeks after chemotherapy	Lymphocytic lymphoma	Chemotherapy Methotrexate Corticosteroids Neutropenia	Fungemia	Amphotericin B IV for 5 months Bursectomy and calf dissection	Complete resolution
11	Candida species No cultures, diagnosis done by histopathology	Khazzam et al./2005 [4]	65/M	Subacromial	Chronic, >4 months	Myocardial infarction	None	Corticosteroid injection	Voriconazole 200 mg twice daily for 6 weeks Bursectomy	Complete resolution

C: Candida; M: male; F: female; SLE: systemic lupus erythematosus; COPD: chronic obstructive pulmonary disease; IV: intravenous; RA: rheumatoid arthritis.

the patients were older than sixty years of age, this including our patient.

Fungal bursitis is treated with oral or parenteral antifungals as well as drainage of infected bursal fluid; this is frequently done by needle aspiration. Bursectomy is indicated when there is no response to this treatment, when the bursal fluid cannot be drained with a needle, or when there is infection of the surrounding soft tissue [2]. All of the patients that we describe in Table 1 received antifungal therapy at some point, but 7 required bursectomy to achieve cure [3, 4, 8–12]. Two patients were cured with antifungal therapy alone [1, 7]. One of the patients, who had olecranon bursitis due to *Candida lusitaniae*, was severely immunosuppressed, had recurrent bursitis, and ultimately died of *Pneumocystis jirovecii* infection [13]. Our patient had reaccumulation of fluid and bursectomy was indicated but she declined this option.

In summary, fungal infection due to *C. parapsilosis* is rare and follows an indolent course. Immunosuppression and advanced age appear to be predisposing factors for bursitis caused by *Candida* species. Septic bursitis caused by bacterial organisms usually responds well to antimicrobial therapy and fluid aspiration. In contrast, this therapeutic approach is not entirely effective for fungal bursitis caused by *Candida* species as recurrent bursitis is quite common. Definite cure is attained with bursectomy for which this procedure should be highly considered early in the management of these cases.

Competing Interests

The authors have no competing interests to disclose.

References

[1] R. A. Rosochmann and C. L. Bell, "Septic bursitis in immunocompromised patients," *The American Journal of Medicine*, vol. 83, no. 4, pp. 661–665, 1987.

[2] B. Zimmermann III, D. J. Mikolich, and G. Ho Jr., "Septic bursitis," *Seminars in Arthritis and Rheumatism*, vol. 24, no. 6, pp. 391–410, 1995.

[3] M. Jiménez-Palop, M. Corteguera, R. Ibáñez, and R. Serrano-Heranz, "Olecranon bursitis due to *Candida parapsilosis* in an immunocompetent adult," *Annals of the Rheumatic Diseases*, vol. 61, no. 3, pp. 279–281, 2002.

[4] M. Khazzam, M. Bansal, and S. Fealy, "Candida infection of the subacromial bursa. A case report," *The Journal of Bone & Joint Surgery—American Volume*, vol. 87, no. 1, pp. 168–171, 2005.

[5] K. J. Kwon-Chung and D. D. Droller, "Infection of the olecranon bursa by *Anthopsis deltoidea*," *Journal of Clinical Microbiology*, vol. 20, no. 2, pp. 271–273, 1984.

[6] P. B. Cornia, G. J. Raugi, and R. A. Miller, "*Phialophora richardsiae* bursitis treated medically," *The American Journal of Medicine*, vol. 115, no. 1, pp. 77–79, 2003.

[7] N. Schlesinger and B. I. Hoffman, "Fungal bursitis: olecranon bursitis caused by candida parapsilosis with review of the literature," *Journal of Clinical Rheumatology*, vol. 1, no. 4, pp. 232–235, 1995.

[8] H. W. Murray, M. A. Fialk, and R. B. Roberts, "Candida arthritis. A manifestation of disseminated candidiasis," *The American Journal of Medicine*, vol. 60, no. 4, pp. 587–595, 1976.

[9] B. A. Wall, M. E. Weinblatt, J. T. Darnall, and H. Muss, "Candida tropicalis arthritis and bursitis," *Journal of the American Medical Association*, vol. 248, no. 9, pp. 1098–1099, 1982.

[10] Y. M. Jeong, H. Y. Cho, S.-W. Lee, Y. M. Hwang, and Y.-K. Kim, "*Candida* septic arthritis with rice body formation: a case report and review of literature," *Korean Journal of Radiology*, vol. 14, no. 3, pp. 465–469, 2013.

[11] H. Miyamoto, T. Miura, E. Morita et al., "Fungal arthritis of the wrist caused by *Candida parapsilosis* during infliximab therapy for rheumatoid arthritis," *Modern Rheumatology*, vol. 22, no. 6, pp. 903–906, 2012.

[12] J. G. Skedros, K. E. Keenan, and J. D. Trachtenberg, "Candida glabrata olecranon bursitis treated with bursectomy and intravenous caspofungin," *Journal of surgical orthopaedic advances*, vol. 22, no. 2, pp. 179–182, 2013.

[13] S. M. Behar and G. M. Chertow, "Olecranon bursitis caused by infection with *Candida lusitaniae*," *Journal of Rheumatology*, vol. 25, no. 3, pp. 598–600, 1998.

[14] J. J. Weems Jr., M. E. Chamberland, J. Ward, M. Willy, A. A. Padhye, and S. L. Solomon, "Candida parapsilosis fungemia associated with parenteral nutrition and contaminated blood pressure transducers," *Journal of Clinical Microbiology*, vol. 25, no. 6, pp. 1029–1032, 1987.

[15] E. C. Van Asbeck, K. V. Clemons, and D. A. Stevens, "Candida parapsilosis: a review of its epidemiology, pathogenesis, clinical aspects, typing and antimicrobial susceptibility," *Critical Reviews in Microbiology*, vol. 35, no. 4, pp. 283–309, 2009.

29

Pachymeningitis in Granulomatosis with Polyangiitis

Grigorios T. Sakellariou[1] and Nicoleta Kefala[2]

[1] Department of Rheumatology, 424 General Military Hospital, 564 03 Thessaloniki, Greece
[2] Department of Internal Medicine, 424 General Military Hospital, 564 03 Thessaloniki, Greece

Correspondence should be addressed to Grigorios T. Sakellariou; sakelgr@gmail.com

Academic Editors: J. V. Dunne and P. E. Prete

Central nervous involvement, mainly with symptoms of cranial neuropathies, occurs in 2–8% of patients with granulomatosis with polyangiitis (GPA). Meningeal involvement, with persistent and severe headache as main manifestation and abnormal thickening and enhancement of the dural mater on postcontrast magnetic resonance imaging, is extremely rare. We present a case of pachymeningitis due to limited GPA, providing simultaneously a literature review.

1. Introduction

Granulomatosis with polyangiitis (GPA, formerly known as Wegener) is a rare, systemic disease of unknown etiology, characterized by necrotizing granulomatous inflammation and vasculitis, which in its classic form chiefly affects the upper and lower respiratory tracts and kidney [1]. Involvement of the nervous system is seen in about 23–54% of cases. The most common neurological manifestations are mononeuritis multiplex or, less frequently, distal symmetric sensorimotor polyneuropathies [2, 3]. Involvement of the central nervous system occurs in 2–8% of the patients with GPA and is commonly associated with dysfunction of one or several cranial nerves, most commonly the second, third, sixth, and seventh nerves. Meningeal inflammation, also known as hypertrophic pachymeningitis due to the typical presentation of thickening and contrast enhancement seen on magnetic resonance imaging (MRI), is extremely rare. We describe a patient with limited GPA with nasal lesions, otitis media, mastoiditis, sensorineural hearing loss, pachymeningitis, and positive cytoplasmic and proteinase-3 (PR-3) anti neutrophil cytoplasmic antibodies (ANCA). A literature review of pachymeningitis due to GPA is also provided.

2. Case Presentation

In January 2012, a 50-year-old man presented with nasal obstruction, a "clogged" sensation in his left ear, tinnitus, vertigo, and severe headache on the left parietofrontal area of the face.

The patient reported that the nasal congestion with fluid-thickened secretion started one year ago. After 3 months, he presented with a "clogged" sensation in his left ear with headache, which led to a diagnosis of serous otitis media. Myringotomy was performed, without resolution of symptoms. In August 2011, arthralgias, especially of the large joints (knees, elbows), was initiated, which resolved with low-dose prednisone for one month. In October 2011, the "clogged" sensation in his left ear and headache were deteriorated, and brain computed tomography (CT) was performed, which showed left mastoiditis. The patient was treated with antibiotics and nonsteroidal anti-inflammatory drugs, and after one month mastoidectomy was performed, without relief of symptoms. Ten days ago, he reported tinnitus, vertigo, further deterioration of headache, joint pain of his hands and foot, morning stiffness, fatigue, and low-level fever.

Physical examination revealed synovitis of bilateral wrists. There were no findings for cutaneous, ocular, neurological and pulmonary involvement. Otolaryngologic

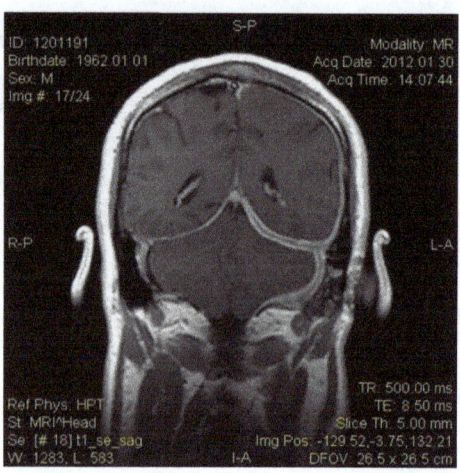

FIGURE 1: Gadolinium-enhanced coronal T1-weighted MRI scan showing pachymeningeal enhancement over the left temporal cerebral convexity, the left cerebellar convexity, and the left side of tentorium cerebelli. Also, there is left mastoiditis.

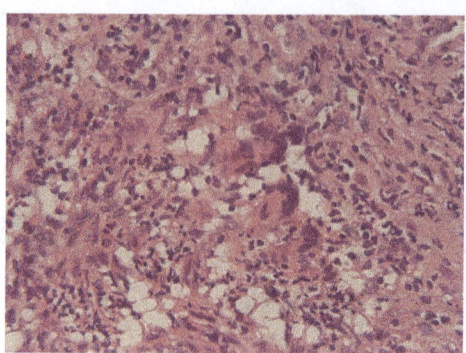

FIGURE 2: Nasal biopsy showing numerous multinucleated giant cells (haematoxylin-eosin staining).

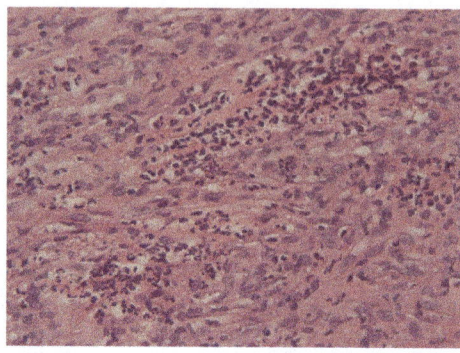

FIGURE 3: Nasal biopsy showing aggregate mainly consisting of neutrophils within and around blood vessel walls (haematoxylin-eosin staining).

examination found perforation of the nasal septum with crusting and left otitis media. The audiogram revealed sensor-ineural hearing loss of the left ear. A nasal biopsy was per-formed.

Laboratory tests showed increased inflammatory markers [erythrocyte sedimentation rate (ESR): 72 mm, C-reactive protein (CRP): 28.9 mg/L], leukocytosis (WBC: 16.500 K/μL), thrombocytosis (PLT: 533.000 K/μL), positive rheumatoid factor (RF) [RF: 39.4 IU/mL (>20 IU/mL, positive)], IgG: 3.980 mg/dL, positive cytoplasmic ANCA (c-ANCA), at a titer 1/320, and PR-3 ANCA antibodies [PR-3 ANCA: 24.08 U/mL (>8 U/mL, positive)], and normal renal function tests (serum creatinine: 1.0 mg/dL, serum urea nitrogen: 35 mg/dL). Urine test was normal, and perinuclear ANCA (p-ANCA) and MPO ANCA antibodies were negative.

Brain MRI on postgadolinium T1 sequence revealed thickness and pathological enhancement of dural mater along the left hemisphere of brain and cerebellum, with expansion to tentorium (Figure 1). Also, the mastoid air cells on the patient's left side were opacified. Chest X-ray was normal.

Histological examination of nasal mucosa showed inflammation with presence of confluent polykaryocyte giant cells type Langhans (Figure 2) and vessels with lesions of type leukocytoclastic vasculitis (Figure 3), findings suggesting GPA.

A diagnosis of limited GPA with involvement of the upper respiratory tract (nose, ear, and sinus) and central nervous system (meninges and auditory nerve) was made. The patient initiated prednisolone 32 mg daily with tapering and monthly pulses, totally seven, of cyclophosphamide (CYC) 1.5 gr in combination with hydrocortisone 1 gr. There was prompt resolution of all symptoms, with remaining mild sensorineural hearing loss of the left ear, improvement of abnormal laboratory tests (reduction of inflammatory markers to normal level and resolution of thrombocytosis in the 1st month, and negativity of positive c-ANCA and PR-3 ANCA antibodies in the 6th month), and moderate resolution of pachymeningitis on repeated brain MRI. At present, the patient takes methotrexate (MTX) 20 mg weekly and prednisolone 8 mg daily. Because any effort for reduction of prednisolone at a dose lower than 10 mg/day has led to headache regression, we consider to treat the patient with rituximab.

3. Discussion

Meningeal inflammation is a rare manifestation of GPA. In two large series, meningitis was observed in none of 158 (0%) and 2 of 324 (0.6%) patients with GPA, respectively [2, 3]. Review of the English literature including case reports uncovered 54 patients with GPA and meningitis. Meningeal involvement more frequently occurs early in the course (within 6 months of onset) of clinically active, limited GPA [4, 5], as in our patient. However, in only 2 patients with GPA and meningitis, mastoiditis has been reported [4].

Persistent and severe headache is the predominant and almost always the first symptom of meningeal involvement of GPA [5]. Because headache is a common symptom in patients with GPA, due to chronic sinusitis or orbital disease, meningeal involvement may remain unrecognized for a long time. In most of the patients with meningeal disease neurological manifestations of cranial nerves have been reported, most commonly the second, third, sixth, and seventh nerves.

Dysfunction of the eighth nerve rarely occurs [6, 7]. Seizures and encephalopathy have been described. In the majority of cases there were elevated inflammatory markers such as ESR and CRP. A positive serum ANCA, either cytoplasmic or perinuclear, is found in about two-thirds of patients. In accordance with these mentioned above, our patient had persistent headache as main symptom, dysfunction of cranial nerve, elevated inflammatory markers, and positive c-ANCA and PR-3 ANCA. Considering that there was improvement of hearing loss concomitant with imaging improvement of the meningeal inflammation, we suspect most likely a retrocochlear lesion such as fibrous entrapment of auditory nerve due to thickened and inflammatory dural mater than a cochlear lesion due to autoimmune process to be involved in the eighth cranial neuropathy.

The sensitivity of CT to detect meningeal disease is low, and in most cases the examination of cerebrospinal fluid (CSF) shows nonspecific abnormalities such as mild pleocytosis, consisting mainly of lymphocytes [8]. However, the widespread application of MRI has greatly facilitated early recognition and followup of patients with pachymeningitis. The typical finding on MRI is thickening and contrast enhancement of dural mater. Leptomeninges involvement is found less commonly [4, 5]. Two distinct MRI patterns have been described: (a) diffusely abnormal meninges unrelated to sinus or orbital disease; (b) focal enhancing thickening adjacent to sinus or orbital disease [9]. Meningeal biopsy has been reported in 26 cases and was performed because of either absence of involvement of other organs or tissues or nonspecific findings on extracranial biopsy [4]. The most common finding was necrotizing granulomatous inflammation, with limited or no signs of vasculitis. It is thought that the pathogenic mechanism of pachymeningitis in GPA is a remote granulomatous inflammation affecting only the meninges (diffuse dural thickening and enhancement on MRI), or, most frequently, the spreading of granulomatous tissue from the nasal or paranasal cavities and contiguously invasion to the adjacent structures including meninges (focal dural thickening and enhancement on MRI) [4, 10], as in our patient.

Early treatment of pachymeningitis in GPA is associated with improved outcome in terms of neurological recovery. A gratifying response to immunosuppressive therapy with resolution of headache, improvement or stabilization of cranial neuropathies and other neurological symptoms, reduction of ESR and CRP, and sometimes reversal of MRI abnormalities was observed in the majority of those with GPA-related pachymeningitis [5]. However, repeat brain MRI may show no [11, 12] or minimal [8] radiological improvement despite clinical recovery. This finding could represent residual postinflammatory fibrosis of dural mater [11, 12]. Therefore, to minimize treatment-related toxicity, the individual symptomatic response should be used to guide the rate of tapering the immunosuppressive drugs. Most cases, including our patient, initially received standard therapy with corticosteroids and CYC, either per os or intravenously on monthly courses, in doses similar to those used in generalized GPA, switching, after induction of remission, to oral MTX or azathioprine (AZA) for remission maintenance [5]. However,

rituximab [12–14] or infliximab [15] has been successfully used in refractory cases.

In conclusion, pachymeningitis is undoubtedly a rare manifestation of active limited GPA. Heightened awareness, early diagnosis, and timely therapy are important to prevent permanent neurological dysfunction. If the clinical findings, ANCA results, MRI abnormalities, and extracranial biopsies are inconclusive or nondiagnostic of GPA, a dural biopsy may be necessary to confirm the diagnosis. Although there are no controlled studies, most patients with GPA-associated pachymeningitis respond favorably to treatment with corticosteroids and cytotoxic drugs (CYC, MTX, or AZA), particularly when such therapy is initiated early, before irreversible neurological damage.

References

[1] J. C. Jennette, R. J. Falk, P. A. Bacon et al., "2012 revised International Chapel Hill consensus conference nomenclature of vasculitides," *Arthritis & Rheumatism*, vol. 65, pp. 1–11, 2013.

[2] G. S. Hoffman, G. S. Kerr, R. Y. Leavitt et al., "Wegener granulomatosis: an analysis of 158 patients," *Annals of Internal Medicine*, vol. 116, no. 6, pp. 488–498, 1992.

[3] H. Nishino, F. A. Rubino, R. A. DeRemee, J. W. Swanson, and J. E. Parisi, "Neurological involvement in Wegener's granulomatosis: an analysis of 324 consecutive patients at the Mayo Clinic," *Annals of Neurology*, vol. 33, no. 1, pp. 4–9, 1993.

[4] G. Di Comite, E. P. Bozzolo, L. Praderio, M. Tresoldi, and M. G. Sabbadini, "Meningeal involvement in Wegener's granulomatosis is associated with localized disease," *Clinical and Experimental Rheumatology*, vol. 24, supplement 41, pp. S60–S64, 2006.

[5] A. G. Fam, E. Lavine, L. Lee, B. Perez-Ordonez, and M. Goyal, "Cranial pachymeningitis: an unusual manifestation of Wegener's granulomatosis," *Journal of Rheumatology*, vol. 30, no. 9, pp. 2070–2074, 2003.

[6] Case Records of the Massachusetts General Hospital Weekly Clinicopathological Exercises, "Case 12-1988. A 72-year-old man with headache and multiple cranial-nerve palsies," *The New England Journal of Medicine*, vol. 318, pp. 760–768, 1988.

[7] N. J. Newman, T. L. Slamovits, S. Friedland, and W. B. Wilson, "Neuro-ophthalmic manifestations of meningocerebral inflammation from the limited form of Wegener's granulomatosis," *American Journal of Ophthalmology*, vol. 120, no. 5, pp. 613–621, 1995.

[8] U. Specks, K. G. Moder, and T. J. McDonald, "Meningeal involvement in Wegener granulomatosis," *Mayo Clinic Proceedings*, vol. 75, no. 8, pp. 856–859, 2000.

[9] J. M. Murphy, B. Gomez-Anson, J. H. Gillard et al., "Wegener granulomatosis: MR imaging findings in brain and meninges," *Radiology*, vol. 213, no. 3, pp. 794–799, 1999.

[10] R. Seror, A. Mahr, J. Ramanoelina, C. Pagnoux, P. Cohen, and L. Guillevin, "Central nervous system involvement in wegener granulomatosis," *Medicine*, vol. 85, no. 1, pp. 54–65, 2006.

[11] M. Spranger, S. Schwab, H.-M. Meinck et al., "Meningeal involvement in Wegener's granulomatosis confirmed and monitored by positive circulating antineutrophil cytoplasm in cerebrospinal fluid," *Neurology*, vol. 48, no. 1, pp. 263–265, 1997.

[12] S. Bawa, C. Mukhtyar, S. Edmonds, and M. Webley, "Refractory Wegener's meningitis treated with rituximab," *Journal of Rheumatology*, vol. 34, no. 4, pp. 900–902, 2007.

[13] A. Sharma, S. Kumar, A. Wanchu et al., "Successful treatment of hypertrophic pachymeningitis in refractory Wegener's granulomatosis with rituximab," *Clinical Rheumatology*, vol. 29, no. 1, pp. 107–110, 2010.

[14] N. Tamura, R. Matsudaira, M. Hirashima et al., "Two cases of refractory Wegener's granulomatosis successfully treated with rituximab," *Internal Medicine*, vol. 46, no. 7, pp. 409–414, 2007.

[15] J. Hermann, P. Reittner, M. Scarpatetti, and W. Graninger, "Successful treatment of meningeal involvement in Wegener's granulomatosis with infliximab," *Annals of the Rheumatic Diseases*, vol. 65, no. 5, pp. 691–692, 2006.

30

Elevated Tropon in Serum Levels in Adult Onset Still's Disease

Carlo Umberto Manzini,[1] Lucio Brugioni,[2] Michele Colaci,[1] Maurizio Tognetti,[2] Amelia Spinella,[1] Marco Sebastiani,[1] Dilia Giuggioli,[1] and Clodoveo Ferri[1]

[1]*Chair and Rheumatology Unit, Medical School, Azienda Ospedaliero-Universitaria, University of Modena and Reggio Emilia, Policlinico di Modena, Via del Pozzo 71, 41100 Modena, Italy*
[2]*Critical Care Unit, Azienda Ospedaliero-Universitaria Policlinico di Modena, Modena, Italy*

Correspondence should be addressed to Clodoveo Ferri; clferri@unimore.it

Academic Editor: Mehmet Soy

Adult onset Still's disease (AOSD) is a rare inflammatory systemic disease that occasionally may affect myocardium. Diagnosis is based on typical AOSD symptoms after the exclusion of well-known infectious, neoplastic, or autoimmune/autoinflammatory disorders. In the case of abrupt, recent onset AOSD, it could be particularly difficult to make the differential diagnosis and in particular to early detect the possible heart involvement. This latter event is suggested by the clinical history of the four patients described here, incidentally observed at our emergency room. All cases were referred because of acute illness (high fever, malaise, polyarthralgias, skin rash, and sore throat), successively classified as AOSD, and they presented abnormally high levels of serum troponin without overt symptoms of cardiac involvement. The timely treatment with steroids (3 cases) or ibuprofen (1 case) leads to the remission of clinicoserological manifestations within few weeks. These observations suggest that early myocardial injury might be underestimated or entirely overlooked in patients with AOSD; routine cardiac assessment including troponin evaluation should be mandatory in all patients with suspected AOSD.

1. Introduction

Adult onset Still's disease (AOSD) is a rare inflammatory disease characterized by spiking fevers >39°C, arthritis/arthralgias, typical salmon-colored bumpy rash, and possible involvement of visceral organs [1]. The etiology of AOSD remains obscure, but an autoimmune pathogenesis has been suggested [2]. The age peak of disease onset is between 16 and 35 years, with an incidence below 1/100,000 inhabitants, without gender differences. The diagnosis is exclusively based on clinical symptoms, according to the criteria proposed by Yamaguchi et al. [3] or Cush et al. [4], after the exclusion of well-known infectious, neoplastic, or other autoimmune/autoinflammatory disorders [5]. Corticosteroids and nonsteroidal anti-inflammatory drugs represent the first line therapy in the acute phase, while disease-modifying antirheumatic drugs (sulphasalazine, hydroxychloroquine, or methotrexate) or anti-TNFα blockers can be considered in the chronic subsets.

Among AOSD clinical manifestations, serositises, including pericardial effusion, are also described (approximately 30–40% of cases), as well as myocardium/endocardium involvement [6–13]. Pericardial complication can be one of the presenting symptoms [8, 14, 15] or manifestation of relapsing disease [16–18]. In this context, increased troponin levels have also been reported in anecdotal observations, probably related to heart involvement [14]. Troponin is a protein found only in cardiac myocytes; it exerts an important role in regulating the interaction of actin and myosin filaments during cardiac contraction. Because of its cardiac origin, troponin is commonly used as a very sensitive and specific marker of myocardial damage, not only in the case of myocardial ischemia, but also in inflammatory diseases inducing cardiac injury, such as AOSD [19].

We describe four consecutive patients, referred to the emergency room of our university-based hospital, who presented abnormally increased levels of serum troponin in the

TABLE 1: Clinicoserological features of the 4 patients affected by adult onset Still's disease (AOSD) with serum troponin levels elevation.

Patient number	Sex/age (years)	Clinical features	Troponin cTnI peak normal <0.06 ng/mL	EKG	ECHO-cg	Therapy	Troponin normaliza-tion time	AOSD outcome
1	M/19	High fever, rash, sore throat, arthralgias, and neutrophilia	0.5	Normal	Slight LV thickness	Steroids	3 days	Remission
2	M/27	High fever, cough, dyspnea, arthralgias, rash, and neutrophilia	3.04	Normal	Mild pericardial effusion	Steroids	4 days	Remission
3	M/49	High fever, rash, sore throat, arthralgias, and neutrophilia	0.33	Normal	Negative	Steroids	2 days	Remission
4	M/70	High fever, sore throat, arthralgias, and neutrophilia	2.0	Normal	Negative	Ibuprofen	15 days	Remission

absence of significant electrocardiographic and echocardiographic abnormalities, successively diagnosed as AOSD.

2. Case Reports

2.1. Case Number 1. A 19-year-old man was referred to the emergency room for sore throat and high fever up to 39°C, skin rash of the trunk and limbs, and polyarthralgias, poorly responsive to acetaminophen (Table 1). Blood exams revealed an increase of C-reactive protein (CRP 21.8 mg/dL; n.v. 0–0.7 mg/dL), erythrocyte sedimentation rate (ESR 74 mm/h, normal values 0–15 mm/h), ferritin (1,503 ng/mL, normal values 13–150 ng/mL), and WBC ($19 \times 10^3/\mu L$ with neutrophil count 92%). Liver cytolysis and cholestasis indexes were also increased: AST 84 U/L (normal < 31 U/L), ALT 155 U/L (normal < 31 U/L), gamma-GT 242 U/L (normal < 35 U/L), and alkaline phosphatase 483 U/L (reference range 35–129 U/L). Creatine kinase was in normal range. Blood culture, urine culture, and throat swab were negative, as well as virological serology for EBV, CMV, Parvovirus B19, HBV, HCV, and HIV. No abnormalities were observed at chest radiograph and EKG. An increase of troponin cTnI up to 0.5 ng/mL (normal < 0.06 ng/mL) was also noticed. Therefore, transthoracic echocardiography was performed to exclude the presence of possible myocarditis, showing a slight increase of thickness of left ventricular wall with normal systolic function (EF 60%).

According to the Yamaguchi criteria [3], AOSD was diagnosed by a rheumatologist. Intravenous steroid therapy (methylprednisolone) was started, from 60 mg/day (approximately 1 mg/kg body-weight), slowly tapered until the suspension after 40 days. The clinical and laboratory features dramatically improved; in particular, troponin levels were normalized since the third day of therapy. A complete disease remission was observed at subsequent clinical controls.

2.2. Case Number 2. A 27-year-old man presented to the emergency room with high fever, polyarthralgias, faint skin rash on the trunk, cough, and dyspnea; previous oral

antibiotic therapy prescribed by his family doctor was ineffective (Table 1). Laboratory examinations revealed abnormally increased serum levels of troponin (cTnI up to 3.04 ng/mL), in the absence of chest pain or other signs and/or symptoms suggestive of ischemic heart disease. The EKG was normal, while chest radiograph documented a bilateral parenchymal densification and mild pleural effusion. The echocardiogram and cardiac MRI did not show significant morphofunctional changes, but only a slight pericardial effusion; on the basis of these investigations, ischemic heart disease was excluded.

The patient was hospitalized in the critical care unit; blood pressure was 110/60 mmHg, heart rate 130 bpm (rhythmic), oxygen saturation 96%, and fever 38.8°C. Laboratory examinations showed CRP 14.15 mg/dL 8 (n.v. 0–0.7 mg/dL), WBC $12 \times 10^3/\mu L$ (neutrophils 88%), AST 80 U/L and ALT 127 U/L (normal < 31 U/L), and CK 123 (normal < 170 U/L); moreover, antinuclear antibody and rheumatoid factor were negative.

Even if microbiology and virology investigations were negative, broad-spectrum antibiotic intravenous therapy was administered. However, the clinical picture gradually improved only with the use of steroid therapy (methylprednisolone 80 mg/day iv, slowly tapered and discontinued within 38 days); therefore the diagnosis of AOSD was formulated. This treatment leads to stable symptom remission, resolution of lung radiological alteration, and normalization of inflammatory indexes. In particular, serum troponin normalized within the first 4 days of steroid treatment. No flares were observed in the follow-up, up to date.

2.3. Case Number 3. A 49-year-old man presented to the emergency room with persistent fever > 40°C for 10 days; he also showed sore throat, polyarthralgias, and faint skin rash on the trunk and neck, not responsive to antibiotic therapy. The physical examination was normal, except for the presence of some painful submandibular lymph nodes (Table 1).

Laboratory examinations revealed leukocytosis (WBC $24 \times 10^3/\mu L$, neutrophils 84.9%), increase of inflammatory indexes (CRP 14.68 mg/dL, ESR 64 mm/h), ferritin

(3147 ng/mL), and transaminases (AST/ALT 83/99 U/L); CK was normal. Seriate controls showed slight elevation of troponin cTnI levels up to 0.33 ng/mL (normal < 0.06 ng/mL), in absence of EKG abnormalities. During hospitalization, blood and urine cultures, throat swab, and feces samples, as well as microbiology and virology analysis (Treponema Pallidum, HHV-6, HHV-8, HIV-1, HIV-2, HBV, HCV, Monotest, Parvovirus B19, *B. burgdorferi*, *T. gondii*, *L. pneumophila*, and Quantiferon-TB test) were negative.

The echocardiographic examination permitted excluding endocardial vegetations, while ejection fraction was normal. A total-body computed tomography showed only reactive cervical and abdominal lymph node enlargement.

AOSD diagnosis was performed and steroid therapy at low doses was started (prednisone 25 mg/day, tapered until suspension within the following 3 months); the treatment produced the gradual normalization of inflammatory markers and troponin levels (0.02 after 2 days), with consistent clinical remission.

2.4. Case Number 4. A 70-year-old man, with a past clinical history of myocardial infarction in 2008, presented to the emergency room of cardiology unit because of the presence of malaise, fatigue, relapsing high fever, slightly sore throat, and severe arthralgias, during the last 3 months. At the admission, elevated troponin cTnI level (2 ng/mL; Table 1) was found, without new cardiac symptoms or signs suggestive for heart attack. Blood examinations showed leukocytosis (WBC 23 × $10^3/\mu L$, neutrophils 78.6%) and CRP 18.47 mg/dL. Moreover, antinuclear autoantibodies, rheumatoid factor, and microbiological investigations were negative, as well as EKG, transthoracic echocardiography, and coronary angiography.

The diagnosis of AOSD was formulated. Since the patient refused steroid treatment, ibuprofen 600 mg bid for 6 weeks was prescribed. The symptoms gradually disappeared in 6 weeks, as well as laboratory alterations; in particular, leukocytes, CRP, and troponin levels normalized during the following 7–15 days. No flares were observed in the follow-up, up to date.

3. Discussion

The present report described 4 patients with AOSD who presented abnormally increased troponin serum levels at the disease onset; all cases were characterized by monocyclic course of AOSD successfully treated with first line therapy.

AOSD is an inflammatory disorder of unknown etiology, characterized by typical but nonpathognomonic clinical and laboratory features, commonly used to correctly classify the disease after the exclusion of infectious, neoplastic, or autoimmune disorders [20]. To date, even if classification criteria for AOSD have been proposed [1, 2], no specific clinical, serological, and/or instrumental diagnostic markers for AOSD have been identified.

Pericarditis is the most common cardiac manifestation detectable in up to 50% of patients; it is usually subclinical, whereas myocarditis is quite rare [1]. The latter may lead to congestive heart failure and arrhythmias in childhood Still's disease, but these manifestations have rarely been reported in adult patients [12]. In the literature, several cases of AOSD with cardiac manifestation were anecdotally reported. In some patients chest X-ray and cardiac ultrasound showed heart enlargement or pleural effusion; left ventricular hypokinesis and a decreased ejection fraction are also described. Moreover, electrocardiogram could show nonspecific ST-segment and T-wave abnormalities such as T-wave inversion in some leads [14]. More interestingly, Sachs et al. found fibrinoid necrosis at histological examination of myocardial vessels in an AOSD patient [21]. Again, Yamazoe et al. [22] described the case of a 36-year-old female with AOSD complicated by diffuse myocardial hypokinesis at echocardiography and massive pericardial effusion; diagnostic endomyocardial biopsy was performed, revealing fibrosis and infiltration of neutrophils. Acute myocarditis was diagnosed by means of histology for the first time [22]; after pulse intravenous steroids the patient showed marked clinical improvement with complete resolution within one month. Choi et al. [23] reported the case of 37-year-old male with AOSD patient showing T-wave inversions at EKG and increase of troponin serum level, in the absence of significant echocardiographic alterations. Magnetic resonance imaging confirmed the presence of myocarditis, usefully treated with anakinra. Another young man described by Gonzalez et al. [24], who was referred to emergency room for a typical AOSD clinical picture, presented increase of troponin level, ST elevation in leads V1–V5, and diffuse hypokinesia of the left ventricle at echocardiography; remission was achieved by means of high-dosage prednisolone.

The four AOSD patients described here were hospitalized after the initial referring to emergency room, where troponin serum level is routinely measured. This fortuitous chance permitted evidencing the abnormal troponin elevation in all cases; this specific marker alteration prompts us to detect the presence of possible concurrent myocardial damage. The EKG and echocardiography were substantially normal, excluding coronary thrombotic events, while a number of clinical and laboratory features permitted classifying the patients as having AOSD complicated by myocardial inflammatory injury.

Interestingly, early anti-inflammatory treatment induced a rapid remission of the clinical features in all patients, suggesting the presence of possible mild AOSD variants.

Our clinical observations confirmed, at least in part, previous data in the literature, suggesting that myocardial involvement might represent a relatively frequent complication in patients with AOSD. Besides, it is possible to hypothesize that this harmful complication might be underestimated or entirely overlooked in a number of patients, mainly in those with troponin alteration appearing early in the course of AOSD. Therefore, routine cardiac assessment, including troponin evaluation, should be mandatory in all patients with high fever and other inflammatory clinicoserological features evocative of AOSD.

Ethical Approval

The present work was approved by the local ethical committee.

Authors' Contribution

All authors contributed to the writing, review, and editing of this report.

References

[1] M. Gerfaud-Valentin, Y. Jamilloux, J. Iwaz, and P. Sève, "Adult-onset Still's disease," *Autoimmunity Reviews*, vol. 13, no. 7, pp. 708–722, 2014.

[2] Y. Jamilloux, M. Gerfaud-Valentin, F. Martinon, A. Belot, T. Henry, and P. Sève, "Pathogenesis of adult-onset Still's disease: new insights from the juvenile counterpart," *Immunologic Research*, vol. 61, no. 1-2, pp. 53–62, 2015.

[3] M. Yamaguchi, A. Ohta, T. Tsunematsu et al., "Preliminary criteria for classification of adult Still's disease," *Journal of Rheumatology*, vol. 19, no. 3, pp. 424–430, 1992.

[4] J. J. Cush, T. A. Medsger Jr., W. C. Christy, D. C. Herbert, and L. A. Cooperstein, "Adult-onset Still's disease. Clinical course and outcome," *Arthritis and Rheumatism*, vol. 30, no. 2, pp. 186–194, 1987.

[5] V. Bagnari, M. Colina, G. Ciancio, M. Govoni, and F. Trotta, "Adult-onset Still's disease," *Rheumatology International*, vol. 30, no. 7, pp. 855–862, 2010.

[6] A. Falkenbach, B. Lembcke, M. Schneider, R. Wigand, R. Mulert-Ernst, and W. Caspary, "Polyserositis with adult Still's disease onset during pregnancy," *Clinical Rheumatology*, vol. 13, no. 3, pp. 513–517, 1994.

[7] D. Zenagui and J. P. de Coninck, "Atypical presentation of adult Still's disease mimicking acute bacterial endocarditis," *European Heart Journal*, vol. 16, no. 10, pp. 1448–1450, 1995.

[8] F. Vandergheynst, J. Gosset, P. Van de Borne, and G. Decaux, "Myopericarditis revealing adult-onset Still's disease," *Acta Clinica Belgica*, vol. 60, no. 4, pp. 205–208, 2005.

[9] T. Ikeue, A. Fukuhara, S. Watanabe, and T. Sugita, "A case of severe adult-onset Still's disease presenting with pleuropericarditis," *Nihon Kokyuki Gakkai Zasshi*, vol. 44, pp. 389–393, 2006.

[10] I. Ben Ghorbel, M. Lamloum, M. Miled, N. Aoun, M.-H. Houman, and J. Pouchot, "Adult-onset Still's disease revealed by a pericardial tamponade: report of two cases," *Revue de Medecine Interne*, vol. 27, no. 7, pp. 546–549, 2006.

[11] S. J. Buss, D. Wolf, D. Mereles, N. Blank, H. A. Katus, and S. E. Hardt, "A rare case of reversible constrictive pericarditis with severe pericardial thickening in a patient with adult onset Still's disease," *International Journal of Cardiology*, vol. 144, no. 2, pp. e23–e25, 2010.

[12] G. García-García, V. Fernández-Auzmendi, F. Olgado-Ferrero, D. Magro-Ledesma, and S. Sánchez Giralt, "Acute mioperi-carditis as the presenting feature of adult-onset Still's disease," *Reumatología Clínica*, vol. 8, no. 1, pp. 31–33, 2012.

[13] A. Bilska, E. Wilińska, M. Szturmowicz et al., "Recurrent effusive pericarditis in the course of adult-onset Still's disease—case reports of two patients," *Pneumonologia i Alergologia Polska*, vol. 79, no. 3, pp. 215–221, 2011.

[14] A. Miczke, M. Waśniewski, E. Straburzyńska-Migaj, P. Leszczyński, R. Ochotny, and S. Grajek, "Myocarditis—the first symptom of adult Still's disease," *Kardiologia Polska*, vol. 67, no. 8, pp. 884–886, 2009.

[15] S. Hosaka, N. Takashina, A. Ishikawa, H. Kondo, and S. Kashiwazaki, "Adult Still's disease with myocarditis and peritonitis," *Internal Medicine*, vol. 31, no. 6, pp. 812–815, 1992.

[16] W. H. Yoo, "Adult onset Still's disease flared with pericardial effusion," *Rheumatology International*, vol. 28, no. 3, pp. 285–287, 2008.

[17] J. A. Cavallasca, C. A. Vigliano, C. E. Perandones, and G. A. Tate, "Myocarditis as a form of relapse in two patients with adult Still's disease," *Rheumatology International*, vol. 30, no. 8, pp. 1095–1097, 2010.

[18] A. Acosta, J. Thierer, D. Conde et al., "Acute heart failure as a form of relapse in a patient with adult-onset Still disease," *The American Journal of Emergency Medicine*, vol. 32, no. 9, pp. 1151.e5–1151.e6, 2014.

[19] A. S. Jaffe, "Troponin—past, present, and future," *Current Problems in Cardiology*, vol. 37, no. 6, pp. 209–228, 2012.

[20] Q. Hu, Z. Yan, and J. Zhong, "Adult-onset Still's disease: how to make a diagnosis in an atypical case," *Rheumatology International*, vol. 32, no. 10, pp. 3299–3302, 2012.

[21] R. N. Sachs, O. Talvard, and J. Lanfranchi, "Myocarditis in adult Still's disease," *International Journal of Cardiology*, vol. 27, no. 3, pp. 377–380, 1990.

[22] M. Yamazoe, A. Mizuno, Y. Suyama et al., "Endomyocardial biopsy and magnetic resonance imaging of acute myocarditis with adult-onset still's disease," *Korean Circulation Journal*, vol. 44, no. 6, pp. 437–440, 2014.

[23] A. D. Choi, V. Moles, A. Fuisz, and G. Weissman, "Cardiac magnetic resonance in myocarditis from adult onset Still's disease successfully treated with anakinra," *International Journal of Cardiology*, vol. 172, no. 1, pp. e225–e227, 2014.

[24] F. A. Gonzalez, P. Beirão, J. Adrião, and M. L. Coelho, "Adult-onset Still's disease presenting as myopericarditis," *BMJ Case Reports*, Article ID bcr2013202754, 2014.

31

Pyogenic Sacroiliitis and Pyomyositis in a Patient with Systemic Lupus Erythematous

Wafa Chebbi,[1] **Saida Jerbi,**[2] **Wassia Kessomtini,**[3] **Asma Fradi,**[1] **Baha Zantour,**[1] **and Mohamed Habib Sfar**[1]

[1] *Department of Internal Medicine, University Hospital Taher Sfar, 5100 Mahdia, Tunisia*
[2] *Department of Radiology, University Hospital Taher Sfar, 5100 Mahdia, Tunisia*
[3] *Department of Physical Medicine, University Hospital Taher Sfar, 5100 Mahdia, Tunisia*

Correspondence should be addressed to Wafa Chebbi; chebbiwafamedimegh@yahoo.fr

Academic Editor: Mario Salazar-Paramo

Pyogenic sacroiliitis and pyomyositis are uncommon infectious diseases and their diagnoses are often delayed. They are typically seen in children and young adults and are rare in middle-aged people especially in those affected by rheumatic diseases. We present the first case of a Staphylococcus aureus related pyogenic sacroiliitis associated with iliacus and gluteal pyomyositis occurring in a patient with systemic lupus erythematosus. Antibiotic treatment was administered for a total of 6 weeks with a total recovery. Pyogenic sacroiliitis and pyomyositis, although remaining rare events, should be remembered as severe complications in immunosuppressed patients with inflammatory diseases. Early clinical suspicion, imaging diagnosis, and adequate therapy are decisive for the satisfactory outcome.

1. Introduction

Pyogenic sacroiliitis and pyomyositis are very rare infectious diseases. Diagnoses are often delayed because of their variable clinical presentations, low suspicion by the examining physician, and rare findings on radiographs. They are typically seen in children and young adults and are rare in middle-aged people especially in those affected by rheumatic diseases [1].

Systemic lupus erythematosus (SLE) is a chronic inflammatory condition associated with systemic features and multiple organ involvement. It is an immunodepression condition due to both the disease itself and its medicamentous treatment. Thus, SLE patients are at risk for developing infections [2].

We report a case of a *Staphylococcus aureus* related pyogenic sacroiliitis associated with iliacus and gluteal pyomyositis occurring in a patient with SLE.

2. Case Report

A 52-year-old woman was diagnosed to have SLE according to the American College of Rheumatology 1997 criteria (photosensitivity, malar rash, polyarthritis, leucolymphopenia, and positive antinuclear and anti-DNA native antibodies) and Sjögren's syndrome in April 1999. She was treated with hydroxychloroquine and corticosteroids 10 mg/day. In August 2012, she developed lower-extremity edema, and her urinalysis showed an active urine sediment and proteinuria of 1.4 g/24 h. The serum creatinine was normal (0.82 mg/dL). Both C3 and C4 titers were low. SLE disease activity index (SLEDAI) was 13. A renal biopsy showed a focal proliferative lupus nephritis, World Health Organization (WHO) class III, and International Society of Nephrology/Renal Pathology Society (ISN/RPS) class III(A), with mild activity and essentially no chronicity. Treatment with intravenous methylprednisolone (1 g/day for three days) followed by oral prednisolone with a daily dose of 60 mg and monthly pulses of intravenous cyclophosphamide for six months was started. After 8-month follow-up, her lupus nephritis was in remission on prednisone 10 mg/day, hydroxychloroquine, and mycophenolate mofetil (1.5 g/day).

In October 2013, she was admitted with a 7-day history of acute pain, in the right hip area and buttock, and fever. The pain was progressively worsened to the point that she was unable to walk. The patient had no history of prior trauma, genitourinary problems, illicit drug use, or recent infection but she reported intramuscular injections of nonsteroidal anti-inflammatory drugs two days preceding the onset of symptoms. She was on combination of prednisolone (7.5 mg/day), hydroxychloroquine (400 mg/day), and mycophenolate mofetil (1.5 g/day). Physical examination disclosed tenderness over the right hip, and limitation of movement and pelvic compression elicited severe pain in the right sacroiliac joint. The patient had a temperature of 38.6°C, a blood pressure of 120/70 mm Hg, and a pulse rate of 100 beats per minute. There was no cutaneous lesion, adenopathy, erythema, or induration. Chest, abdominal, neurological, and gynecological examinations were normal. SLEDAI at this time was 2. Laboratory investigations showed a C-reactive protein level of 86.4 mg/L (normal range, <6 mg/L), an elevated erythrocyte sedimentation rate (108 mm/h), a white blood cell count of 8100 μL, haemoglobin of 10.7 g/dL, and platelet count of 320000 × μL. The liver and renal function tests were within normal ranges. Radiographs of the chest and right hip were unrevealing. Intravenous antibiotherapy (cefotaxime with fosfomycin) was initiated for suspected septic arthritis of the right hip or right pyogenic sacroiliitis. Technetium-99 methylene diphosphonate (Tc-99m MDP) bone scintigraphy performed two days after admission revealed increased uptake in the right sacroiliac joint (Figure 1). Magnetic resonance imaging (MRI) of the pelvis performed ten days after admission revealed an increased signal intensity of the right sacroiliac joint and diffuse hyper intensity of the adjacent iliacus and gluteal muscles on coronal T2-weighted fat-suppressed image (Figure 2). Post-contrast coronal T1-weighted MRI of the pelvis shows areas of diffuse enhancement of the right sacroiliac joint and the adjacent iliacus and gluteal muscles (Figure 3). Blood cultures disclosed *Staphylococcus aureus* sensitive to cefotaxime and fosfomycin. Tuberculin skin test and serological tests for *Salmonella* and *Brucella* were negative. A transesophageal echocardiography was normal. Treatment was continued with the same antibiotics, with disappearance of fever and improvement of pain. Rehabilitation programme was initiated so that the patient might recover her strength and mobility. The patient responded promptly to 30 days of intravenous antibiotherapy followed by an additional two weeks of oral antibiotherapy (ofloxacin). A significant improvement in her blood parameters (CRP: 2 mg/L, erythrocyte sedimentation: 18 mm/h) was obtained. Followed up six months later, the patient improved well without sequelae.

3. Discussion

This case deals with pyogenic sacroiliitis and iliacus and gluteal pyomyositis in a patient with SLE. The patient experienced acute pain in the right hip area and fever 2 days after intramuscular injections of nonsteroidal anti-inflammatory drugs. Infection was suspected and the patient was treated with cefotaxime and fosfomycin. The MRI confirmed the diagnosis of sacroiliitis and showed an iliacus and gluteal myositis. Additionally, *Staphylococcus aureus* was discovered

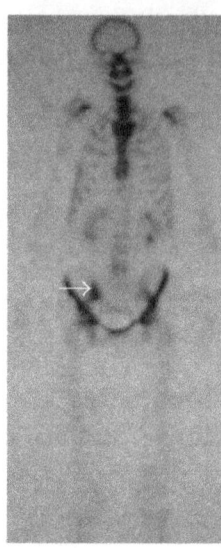

FIGURE 1: Technetium-99m MDP bone scintigraphy of the anterior pelvis shows increased uptake in the right sacroiliac joint (arrow).

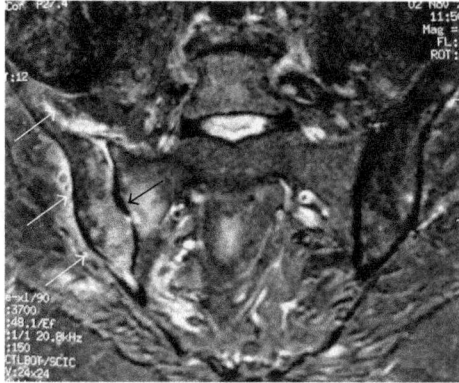

FIGURE 2: Coronal T2-weighted fat-suppressed MR image of the pelvis shows an increased signal intensity of the right sacroiliac joint (black arrow) and diffuse hyper intensity of the adjacent iliacus and gluteal muscles (white arrows).

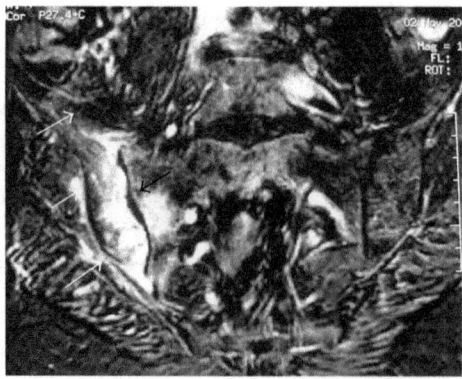

FIGURE 3: Post-contrast coronal T1-weighted MR image of the pelvis shows areas of diffuse enhancement of the right sacroiliac joint and the adjacent iliacus and gluteal muscles.

TABLE 1: Clinical features of pyomyositis in patients with systemic lupus erythematous.

Reference	Age/sex	Country	Therapy	Muscles	Organism	Antibiotics	Outcome
Dede et al. [3]	23/F	Turkey	HCQ	Gastrocnemius	*S. aureus*	yes	Recovery
Claudepierre et al. [4]	32/F	France	Pred + Cyclo	Quadriceps	*S. aureus*	4 weeks	Recovery
Ravindran and Duke [5]	34/F	UK	Pred + HCQ	Pronator teres	*S. aureus*	4 weeks	Recovery
Souza et al. [6]	25/F	Brazil	—	Iliacus muscle	*S. aureus*	6 weeks	Recovery
Baaj et al. [7]	47/F	Morocco	Pred	Quadriceps	*E. coli*	3 weeks	Recovery
Present case	52/F	Tunisia	HCQ + Pred + MMF	Iliacus, gluteal	*S. aureus*	6 weeks	Recovery

F: female; HCQ: hydroxychloroquine; Pred: prednisolone; Cyclo: cyclophosphamide; MMF: mofetil mycophenolate; S: staphylococcus; E: *Escherichia*.

in the blood culture. Antibiotic treatment was administered for a total of 6 weeks with a total recovery.

Pyogenic sacroiliitis and pyomyositis are very rare infections especially among rheumatic diseases and no case in SLE patients has been described up to now. To the best of our knowledge, our case is the first one reported in course of SLE and again it stresses the likely predisposing role played by glucocorticoids and immunosupressive treatment in a patient whose underlying disease state may have contributed to the development of infectious complication.

Pyogenic sacroiliitis is a rare disorder, affecting between 1% and 2% of all patients with septic arthritis, which is probably due to the poor vascularisation of this joint, resulting in a low risk of infection via the haematogenous route [1, 8]. The diagnosis is difficult and often delayed owing to its clinical heterogeneity and the lack of symptom specificity [9]. The mean age of presentation is twenty years but approximately one third of the cases occur in children. The sacroiliac joint is a complex joint and an integral component of the spinal axial support system. It is a true synovial (diarthrodial) joint with a capsule and synovial fluid and, thus, subject to various forms of arthritis. Hyalin cartilage is found on the sacral side of the joint and fibrocartilage on the iliac contribution of the joint [10]. The pathophysiology of pyogenic sacroiliitis is presumed to be the hematogenous spread of bacteria from a distant source of infection to the sacroiliac joint [11]. The joint space is invaded by bacteria by either direct penetration, hematogenous, or by nearby structures such as the gut. The subchondral circulation on the iliac side of the sacroiliac joint is an end-arterial site and so may act as an entry point for inoculation of organisms with subsequent extension into the joint. Other mechanisms include direct invasion of the joint capsule or iatrogenic infection following surgical intervention or invasive procedures [12]. In adults, the most common predisposing risk factors are intravenous drugs use, pelvic trauma, infectious endocarditis, haemoglobinopathy, immunosuppressive treatment, and infections of the skin, respiratory, gastrointestinal, gynecological, and genitourinary tracts [8, 11].

Pyomyositis is a bacterial infection of the skeletal muscle. The etiology of pyomyositis is frequently classified as primary or secondary to a contiguous infection of the skin, bone, or soft tissue. Pyomyositis is most common in tropical areas, and there is a high rate of incidence in children, especially ages 2–5 [13, 14]. The pyomyositis is believed to be a complication of transient bacteremia, which is sometimes associated with a concomitant muscle tissue structure abnormality after trauma or exercise creating a locus minoris resistentiae for implantation of bacteria [13]. The most prevalent organism is *Staphylococcus aureus* with the bacteria accounting for 50–90% of cases [13, 15, 16]. Individuals with a history of diabetes, alcoholism, drug abuse, HIV infection, cancer, and systemic sclerosis are at higher risk for pyomyositis [15]. Association of pyomyositis and SLE is very rare and is limited to only a few case reports (Table 1) [3–7]. All the patients were females and made full recovery. *Staphylococcus aureus* is the most causative agent [3–6]. At the time of the event, three patients received prednisolone associated with cyclophosphamide in one case [4, 5, 7].

Pyomyositis is characterized by a three-stage clinical course beginning with a subacute stage. The second stage is formation of a muscle abscess with associated local and systemic findings. The diagnosis is most often confirmed at this stage as the involved muscle becomes increasingly swollen and tender. If not adequately treated, the third stage is reached, which includes toxicity and septic shock [13, 14, 17]. Our case presented in the second stage of iliacus pyomyositis associated with septic sacroiliitis and responded well to antibiotics. MRI is the most sensitive investigation to confirm the diagnosis. It shows increased signal intensity on T2 weighted images within the affected muscle in addition to a rim of fluid intra/perimuscular. It will also show if the infection has spread from any nearby joints [13, 17]. The hip and the muscles of the lower part of the body are most prone to pyomyositis. The muscles most commonly affected are quadriceps, gluteus, and psoas muscles [15]. Pyomyositis rarely affects the iliacus muscle and very few cases have been reported in the literature [14–16, 18–22]. Most cases occurred in children, and the diagnosis of septic arthritis of the hip was initially suspected in the majority of cases. Moreover, in two patients, both conditions, pyomyositis of the iliacus muscle and septic arthritis of the hip, presented simultaneously [17, 18]. Pyogenic sacroiliitis has been reported to be a complication of primary pyomyositis after 2 weeks of adequate treatment only in one case [15].

In our case, it is difficult to determine which occurred first, pyogenic sacroiliitis or pyomyositis. It seems more likely that pyomyositis of the iliacus and gluteal muscle first occurred, followed by infection of the sacroiliac joint. Intramuscular injections may have been the trauma and facilitated the *Staphylococcus aureus* colonisation. Therefore, we cannot exclude the possibility that pyomyositis and pyogenic sacroiliitis occurred due to hematogenous origin. The use of glucocorticoids and immunosuppressive treatment increases the possibility of infection.

In conclusion, pyogenic sacroiliitis and pyomyositis, although remaining rare events, should be remembered as severe complications in immunosuppressed patients with inflammatory diseases. Their insidious onset can delay diagnosis, limiting prognosis. MRI is the most valuable diagnostic tool and should be utilised in the early stage of the process. Early clinical suspicion, imaging diagnosis, and adequate therapy are decisive for the satisfactory outcome of such cases.

References

[1] L. Mancarella, M. de Santis, N. Magarelli, A. M. Ierardi, L. Bonomo, and G. Ferraccioli, "Septic sacroiliitis: an uncommon septic arthritis," *Clinical and Experimental Rheumatology*, vol. 27, no. 6, pp. 1004–1008, 2009.

[2] A. G. Iliopoulos and G. C. Tsokos, "Immunopathogenesis and spectrum of infections in systemic lupus erythematosus," *Seminars in Arthritis and Rheumatism*, vol. 25, no. 5, pp. 318–336, 1996.

[3] H. Dede, H. Ozdogan, A. Dumankar, Y. Aktuglu, F. Tabak, and H. Yazic, "Tropical pyomyositis in a temperate climate," *The British Journal of Rheumatology*, vol. 32, no. 5, pp. 435–436, 1993.

[4] P. Claudepierre, B. Saint-Marcoux, J. Allain, J. L. Montazel, B. Larget-Piet, and X. Chevalier, "Value of magnetic resonance imaging in extensive pyomyositis," *Arthritis and Rheumatism*, vol. 39, no. 10, p. 1760, 1996.

[5] V. Ravindran and O. Duke, "Non-tropical pyomyositis in a patient with systemic lupus erythematosus," *Lupus*, vol. 18, no. 4, pp. 379–380, 2009.

[6] H. C. B. de Souza, B. N. de Carvalho, M. G. V. de Morais, G. Z. Monteiro, F. T. Emori, and L. C. Latorre, "Tropical pyomyositis in a patient with systemic lupus erythematosus and HTLV 1/2 infection," *Revista Brasileira de Reumatologia*, vol. 51, no. 1, pp. 97–103, 2011.

[7] M. El Baaj, F. Tabache, K. Modden et al., "Pyomyositis: an infectious complication in systemic lupus erythematous," *Revue de Medecine Interne*, vol. 31, no. 3, pp. e4–e6, 2010.

[8] M. Doita, S. Yoshiya, Y. Nabeshima et al., "Acute pyogenic sacroiliitis without predisposing conditions," *Spine*, vol. 28, no. 18, pp. E384–E389, 2003.

[9] G. T. Abbott and H. Carty, "Pyogenic sacroiliitis, the missed diagnosis?" *The British Journal of Radiology*, vol. 66, no. 782, pp. 120–122, 1993.

[10] H. C. Hansen and H. Standiford, "Sacroiliac joint pain and dysfunction," *Pain Physician*, vol. 6, no. 2, pp. 179–189, 2003.

[11] M. Bindal and B. Krabak, "Acute bacterial sacroiliitis in an adult: a case report and review of the literature," *Archives of Physical Medicine and Rehabilitation*, vol. 88, no. 10, pp. 1357–1359, 2007.

[12] R. Raman, H. Dinopoulos, and P. V. Giannoudis, "Management of pyogenic sacroiliitis: an update," *Current Orthopaedics*, vol. 18, no. 4, pp. 321–325, 2004.

[13] G. G. Moran, C. G. Duran, and J. Albiñana, "Imaging on pelvic pyomyositis in children related to pathogenesis," *Journal of Children's Orthopaedics*, vol. 3, no. 6, pp. 479–484, 2009.

[14] D. Zlotkin, "Pyomyositis of the iliacus muscle in an adolescent," *Southern Medical Journal*, vol. 98, no. 12, pp. 1224–1225, 2005.

[15] B. Roca and V. Torres, "Pyomyositis of the iliacus muscle complicated with septic sacroiliitis," *QJM*, vol. 101, no. 12, pp. 983–984, 2008.

[16] W. R. C. Peckett, A. Butler-Manuel, and L. A. Apthorp, "Pyomyositis of the iliacus muscle in a child," *The Journal of Bone & Joint Surgery*, vol. 83, no. 1, pp. 103–105, 2001.

[17] S. J. Theodorou, D. J. Theodorou, and D. Resnick, "MR imaging findings of pyogenic bacterial myositis (pyomyositis) in patients with local muscle trauma: illustrative cases," *Emergency Radiology*, vol. 14, no. 2, pp. 89–96, 2007.

[18] I. Jou, N. Chiu, K. Lai, and Y. Chuang, "Synchronous pyomyositis and septic hip arthritis," *Clinical Rheumatology*, vol. 19, no. 5, pp. 385–388, 2000.

[19] S. Romeo and S. Sunshine, "Pyomyositis in a 5-year-old child," *Archives of Family Medicine*, vol. 9, no. 7, pp. 653–656, 2000.

[20] S. Thomas, G. Tytherleigh-Strong, and R. Dodds, "Pyomyositis of the iliacus muscle in a child," *The Journal of Bone and Joint Surgery B*, vol. 83, no. 4, pp. 619–620, 2001.

[21] J. F. Maillefert, C. Mischis-Troussard, A. A. Proy, C. Piroth, and C. Tavernier, "Pyomyositis of the psoas and the iliacus muscles mimicking infective sacroiliitis," *Journal of Clinical Rheumatology*, vol. 2, no. 4, p. 231, 1996.

[22] W.-S. Chen and Y.-L. Wan, "Iliacus pyomyositis mimicking septic arthritis of the hip joint," *Archives of Orthopaedic and Trauma Surgery*, vol. 115, no. 3-4, pp. 233–235, 1996.

32

Response to Rituximab in a Case of Lupus Associated Digital Ischemia

Orhan Küçükşahin,[1] **Nurşen Düzgün,**[1] **Alexis K. Okoh,**[2] **and Emre Kulahçioglu**[2]

[1] *Department of Rheumatology, Ankara University Medical Faculty, Sihhiye, 06410 Ankara, Turkey*
[2] *Department of Internal Medicine, Ankara University Medical Faculty, Sihhiye, 06410 Ankara, Turkey*

Correspondence should be addressed to Orhan Küçükşahin; orhankcs@hotmail.com

Academic Editor: Jamal Mikdashi

We report the case of a 38-year-old female patient with systemic lupus erythematosus (SLE) and Jaccoud arthritis (JA) that sequentially developed digital ischemic lesions of the hands. In spite of follow-up treatment with glucocorticoids, immunosuppressant, antiaggregant, and potent vasodilatator agents, a serious progression to digital gangrene over a one-month period was observed. Surprisingly, her nonhealing digital lesions improved after two cycles of rituximab (RTX) administration.

1. Introduction

Systemic lupus erythematosus (SLE) is a multisystemic autoimmune disease that is associated with considerable morbidity and mortality. Digital ischemia, digital ulcer, or gangrenous lesions have been described in SLE [1, 2]. Vascular damage in SLE most likely occurs due to vasculitis, premature atherosclerosis, and hypercoagulability related to antiphospholipid antibodies. Vasculitic ulcers tend to be chronic if not well treated and may lead to significant impact on the psychosocial as well as physical well-being of the individual. The gangrene could also contribute to other conditions such as anatomical changes [1].

Presented here is an SLE-JA patient with subluxation of MCPs swan neck deformities who sequentially developed digital ischemic lesions after stopping immunosuppressive treatment at her own discretion due to exorbitant side effects. Digital ischemia of hands showed a serious progression to digital gangrene over a month in spite of follow-up treatment with glucocorticoids, immunosuppressant, antiaggregant, and potent vasodilatator agents.

Surprisingly, her nonhealing ulcers improved dramatically after two cycles of rituximab RTX administration. To the best of our knowledge, this is the first SLE-JA case presenting with nonhealing digital ischemic lesions responding dramatically to RTX therapy in the medical literature.

2. Case Presentation

A 38-year-old Turkish woman with a history of SLE presented in 2003 with photosensitive rash on her face and chest, oral aphthous lesions, and arthritis with pain and motion restriction in hands, wrists, elbows, ankles, and knees. A diagnosis of SLE associated arthritis was made and treatment with 5 mg of prednisone once daily and 200 mg of hydroxychloroquine twice daily was started requiring the addition of methotrexate in escalation until 25 mg weekly was reached. Her joint manifestations were partially responsive; however, arthritis remained active in the small joints of her hands with pain and swelling. Six years later, the patient developed avascular necrosis during follow-up for which she was operated on at an outside setting and a hip prosthesis was implanted.

Two years following surgical treatment for avascular necrosis, the patient presented to our rheumatologic polyclinic with complaints of pain, swelling, warmth, and cyanosis over the fingers of both hand and toe tips. Physical

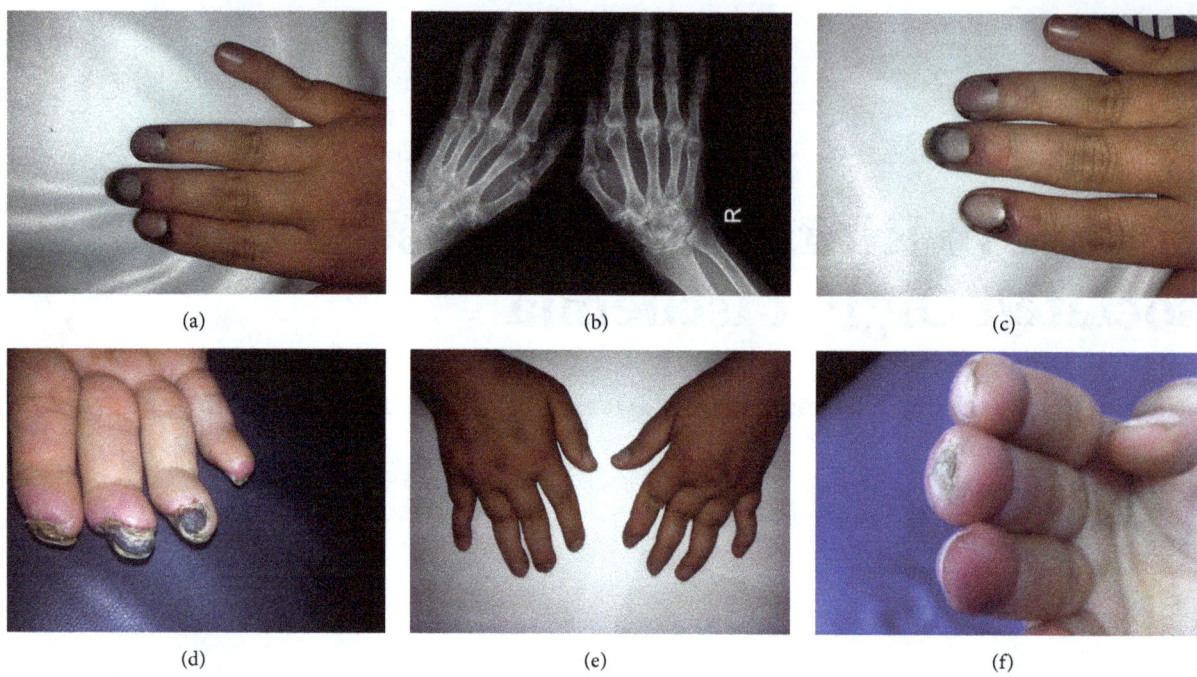

(a)   (b)   (c)

(d)   (e)   (f)

FIGURE 1: (a) Right hand with swan neck and Z deformity of the thumb (before treatment). (b) Radiograph; AP of bilateral hands suggesting Jaccoud radiological features. (c) Digital ulcers of the second to fourth digits of the right hand (2 weeks after initial treatment with cyclophosphamide). (d) Unresponsiveness to initial treatment demonstrated by a serious progression from ischemic lesions to digital gangrene lesions of the second to fourth digits of the right hand (one month after initial treatment regimen; cyclophosphamide, corticosteroids, and prostaglandins). (e) Response to treatment observed after first cycle of rituximab therapy (5 months following the start of RTX treatment). (f) Complete remission of digital gangrenous lesions after 2 cycles of rituximab therapy (10th month of the RTX treatment protocol (rituximab, glucocorticoid, aspirin, azathioprine, and hydroxychloroquine)).

examination revealed swelling, warmth, and tenderness in the proximal interphalangeal (PIP) joints of both hands, Ulnar deviation, and bilateral swan neck deformities. Right is greater than left. "Z" deformities of thumbs (Figure 1(a)) and cyanotic ulcers were seen on the third to fifth digits (Figure 1(c)) and on both digits of feet. All described deformities were reducible. Peripheral pulses were normal. In addition, she had a history of photosensitivity and two gestations with two uneventful births. On further interrogation, the patient was admitted to stopping medical treatment at her own discretion three years before presentation due to exorbitant side effects.

Laboratory findings were as follows: WBC: $5.6 \times 109/L$, Hb: 11.9 g/dL, platelet: $276 \times 109/L$, Hct: 35.4%, ESR: 120 mm/h, CRP: 80 mg/L, microscopic hematuria and trace proteinuria on urinalysis.

Immunologic studies revealed an ANA titer of 1 : 3200, (++++, speckled pattern), U1RNP (+++), p-ANCA (+), anti-beta 2 GP1-IgA isotype (43,5 U/mL; normal: <5 U/mL). There was hypocomplementemia (C3: 0,647 g/L, C4: 0,0758 g/L; normal: 0.9–2 g/L and 0.1–0.4 g/L, respectively.). ds-DNA and Sm antibodies and rheumatoid factor were negative.

Review of hand radiographs showed no erosive changes consistent with a diagnosis of JA (Figure 1(b)). Electrocardiographic, echocardiographic, and computed tomography (CT) imaging studies of the thorax did not show any pathological findings.

Results from laboratory studies showed high disease activity of lupus. Initial treatment was started with glucocorticoid (1 mg/kg/day), aspirin (300 mg/day), IV prostaglandin (2 mcg/kg/min), and IV cyclophosphamide (500 mg/m^2).

Unexpectedly, digital ischemia of hands showed a serious progression to digital gangrene (Figure 1(d)) over a one-month period in spite of treatment with glucocorticoids, immunosuppressant, antiaggregant, and potent vasodilatator agents.

Following the first month of unsuccessful treatment with the initial treatment regimen, a new treatment protocol including rituximab (RTX) with 2 infusions of 1 g at a 14-day interval in combination with hydroxychloroquine and aspirin was initiated during the second month. Clinical and laboratory response to treatment began to be observed during the third month of RTX therapy. Laboratory evaluation revealed the following: ESR: 22, CRP: 3 mg/dL, and normal levels of C3 and C4 complement levels. (Results from a complete blood count panel were unremarkable). A combining dosage of 100 mg/day azathioprine (AZA) was added to the treatment protocol after two infusions of RTX therapy. Also, corticosteroid dosage which was started at 1 mg/kg was tapered gradually by 10% per kilogram for every 10 days till it reached 5 mg/day over the three-month period. Eventually, digital gangrenous lesions started to regress after the first cycle (5 months) of RTX therapy (Figure 1(e)). A second cycle of RTX therapy was started during which a complete recovery of digital lesions (Figure 1(f)) and the regression of active disease signs and acute phase responses were seen. The patient has been in clinical remission with glucocorticoid (5 mg/day), aspirin (100 mg/day), azathioprine (2.5 mg/kg/day), and hydroxychloroquine (200 mg/day) for the last 2 years.

3. Discussion

Vasculitis and digital gangrene have been described in SLE. Thromboembolism, premature atherosclerosis, overlap syndrome, and especially antiphospholipid antibodies (aPLs) may contribute to the development of gangrene [3, 4]. In a study of 485 SLE patients, critical peripheral ischemia was observed in 7 patients (1.4%). 4 of the 7 patients had a positive aPl/LAC [5]. Liu et al. found that 18 of 2684 SLE patients had digital gangrene and Raynaud phenomenon, the long disease duration and elevated serum CRP may be predictive factors for SLE patients to develop the digital gangrene [3].

The prevalence of digital gangrene in APS patients has been reported to be between 3.3 and 7.5% and the presence of a positive anti-RNP has been described in some APS digital ulcer cases [6]. The relationship between a positive anti-RNP and Raynaud phenomenon has been shown [7, 8] and thought to play a role in the development of digital gangrene. To date, the exact etiology of SLE digital gangrene remains unclear and complex with the presence of APS, overlap syndrome, atherosclerosis, or vasculitis appearing as potential causes. A complication of APS is seen as the most probable cause. In our patient, active lupus disease, positive RNP, and antiphospholipid antibodies may play a role in the development of digital vascular lesions.

RTX has been shown to be effective in the reduction of B-cell production and used in the treatment of refractory SLE or vasculitis. In a prospective study conducted by Smith et al., rituximab was shown to play a role in B-cell depletion offering the prospect of sustained disease remission and improved disease control with low toxicity in patients with active refractory SLE or ANCA associated vasculitis (AAV) [9].

In the presence of Apl/LAC, patients were first anticoagulated with IV heparin or low molecular weight heparin (LMWH) before long-term treatment with warfarin [5]. Clinical response was not seen in one of the seven patients and a RTX dosage of 1gram/day was started. An IV dosage of 500 mg cyclophosphamide was added to his treatment regimen during follow-up. An improvement in lesions on day 20 after the first dose with RTX was not recorded [10]. In another case series a low dose of Epoprostenol (0.5 ng/kg/min) was used in the treatment of SLE patients presenting with peripheral ischemic findings and its efficacy was found to be the same as that of higher doses with lesser side effects [5, 11]. Epoprostenol has been shown to be useful in the treatment of necrotic digital ulcers secondary to APS [12]. In the treatment of patients with severe ischemia, a combination with LMWH is preferred. It is described to be effective against microvascular thrombotic occlusions due to its anticoagulant properties [10].

In our patient, digital ischemic lesions were seen two years after stopping treatment at her own will. We added a treatment regimen of Iloprost and acetyl salicylic acid to her traditional immunosuppressive agents which included steroids, hydroxychloroquine, and cyclophosphamides. Her nonhealing ulcers however prompted us to start an infusion dosage of 1000 mg rituximab (per 0–15 days) therapy considering its role in B-cell depletion and low toxicity in patients with ischemic lesions. Surprisingly, her digital ulcers responded dramatically to rituximab therapy after 2 cycles and a recession in acute phase markers was observed.

To the best of our knowledge, our case is the first case in the medical literature reporting an SLE-JA association developing digital ischemic lesions as a late clinical complication and responding dramatically to rituximab therapy.

As a conclusion in lupus patients with arthritis associated nonhealing digital ulcers under traditional immunosuppressive agents, RTX can be a treatment option.

References

[1] Y. Nagai, A. Shimizu, M. Suto et al., "Digital gangrene in systemic lupus erythematosus," *Acta Dermato-Venereologica*, vol. 89, no. 4, pp. 398–401, 2009.

[2] Y. Braun-Moscovici, Y. Butbul-Aviel, L. Guralnik et al., "Rituximab: rescue therapy in life-threatening complications or refractory autoimmune diseases: a single center experience," *Rheumatology International*, vol. 33, no. 6, pp. 1495–1504, 2013.

[3] A. Liu, W. Zhang, X. Tian, X. Zhang, F. Zhang, and X. Zeng, "Prevalence, risk factors and outcome of digital gangrene in 2684 lupus patients," *Lupus*, vol. 18, no. 12, pp. 1112–1118, 2009.

[4] R. A. Asherson, R. Cervera, and Y. Shoenfeld, "Peripheral vascular occlusions leading to gangrene and amputations in antiphospholipid antibody positive patients," *Annals of the New York Academy of Sciences*, vol. 1108, pp. 515–529, 2007.

[5] R. C. Jeffery, C. B. Narshi, and D. A. Isenberg, "Prevalence, serological features, response to treatment and outcome of critical peripheral ischaemia in a cohort of lupus patients," *Rheumatology*, vol. 47, no. 9, pp. 1379–1383, 2008.

[6] G. E. Gibson, W. P. D. Su, and M. R. Pittelkow, "Antiphospholipid syndrome and the skin," *Journal of the American Academy of Dermatology*, vol. 36, no. 6 I, pp. 970–982, 1997.

[7] R. A. Asherson, C. Francès, L. Iaccarino et al., "The antiphospholipid antibody syndrome: diagnosis, skin manifestations and current therapy," *Clinical and Experimental Rheumatology*, vol. 24, no. 40, pp. S46–S51, 2006.

[8] R. W. Hoffman, G. C. Sharp, and S. L. Deutscher, "Analysis of anti-U1 RNA antibodies in patients with connective tissue disease: association with HLA and clinical manifestations of disease," *Arthritis and Rheumatism*, vol. 38, no. 12, pp. 1837–1844, 1995.

[9] C. Montecucco, R. Caporali, A. Ravelli et al., "Frequency and clinical significance of anti-RNP antibodies in Italian SLE

patients," *Annali Italiani di Medicina Interna*, vol. 9, no. 1, pp. 12–15, 1994.

[10] K. G. C. Smith, R. B. Jones, S. M. Burns, and D. R. W. Jayne, "Long-term comparison of rituximab treatment for refractory systemic lupus erythematosus and vasculitis: remission, relapse, and re-treatment," *Arthritis & Rheumatism*, vol. 54, no. 9, pp. 2970–2982, 2006.

[11] S. Miyakis, M. D. Lockshin, T. Atsumi et al., "International consensus statement on an update of the classification criteria for definite antiphospholipid syndrome (APS)," *Journal of Thrombosis and Haemostasis*, vol. 4, no. 2, pp. 295–306, 2006.

[12] G. E. Gibson, S. W. P. Daniel, and M. R. Pittelkow, "Antiphospholipid syndrome and the skin," *Journal of the American Academy of Dermatology*, vol. 36, no. 6, pp. 970–982, 1997.

33

Henoch-Schönlein Purpura with Adalimumab Therapy for Ulcerative Colitis

Joseph J. LaConti,[1] Jean A. Donet,[2] Jeong Hee Cho-Vega,[3] Daniel A. Sussman,[2] Dana Ascherman,[1] and Amar R. Deshpande[2]

[1]Division of Rheumatology, University of Miami Leonard Miller School of Medicine, Miami, FL 33136, USA
[2]Division of Gastroenterology, University of Miami Leonard Miller School of Medicine, Miami, FL 33136, USA
[3]Department of Pathology, University of Miami Leonard Miller School of Medicine, Miami, FL 33136, USA

Correspondence should be addressed to Joseph J. LaConti; joseph.laconti@jhsmiami.org

Academic Editor: Gregory J. Tsay

Tumor necrosis factor-α (TNFα) inhibitor therapy has signified an important milestone in the fight against many rheumatological disorders and inflammatory bowel disease (IBD). Cutaneous adverse events caused by this class of medications are well known but relatively uncommon. Most reactions are mild and rarely warrant treatment withdrawal. Henoch-Schönlein purpura (HSP) is a disease with cutaneous vasculitis, arthritis, and gastrointestinal and renal involvement that is usually seen in children, though the worst complications are typically seen in adults. We present a case of HSP complicating adalimumab treatment in a patient with ulcerative colitis who had achieved endoscopic remission. We review similar cases reported in the literature and discuss the consequences of these autoimmune diseases.

1. Introduction

Tumor necrosis factor alpha (TNFα) inhibitors have widespread use in patients with rheumatological and gastrointestinal conditions, especially inflammatory bowel disease, where they have been shown to improve symptoms, lead to bowel mucosal healing, reduce hospitalizations and surgeries, and spare corticosteroid use [1]. A wide variety of adverse events including infections, malignancies, and cutaneous reactions have been reported with use of these medications. Cutaneous side effects are found in 29% of patients with IBD while receiving anti-TNFα treatment, but discontinuation of therapy is rarely required [2]. Small vessel vasculitis is a rare contributor to the cutaneous adverse effects seen during anti-TNFα treatment, and the majority of cases show resolution with drug discontinuation [3]. Henoch-Schönlein purpura (HSP) is an acute vasculitic syndrome presenting with cutaneous purpura, arthritis, and gastrointestinal and renal impairment generally seen in children; it has rarely been associated with anti-TNFα

treatment. Here we present a case of an adult male with ulcerative colitis who developed HSP while being treated with adalimumab.

2. Case Presentation

A 33-year-old Caucasian man with ulcerative colitis for three years in endoscopic and near histologic remission three months before, on adalimumab 40 mg every two weeks (Abbvie, North Chicago, IL), with therapeutic trough levels and no antidrug antibodies, was admitted to our hospital for workup of a recurrent erythematous, palpable, nonblanching rash on his bilateral lower extremities associated with joint pain and swelling of his ankles, knees, and elbows (Figure 1). He first noticed this rash two months before and was treated with empiric oral antibiotics, with incomplete resolution. The rash then recurred with more severity and ascended to his buttocks, lower back, and abdomen; biopsy at an outside facility was suggestive of a superficial perivascular dermatitis.

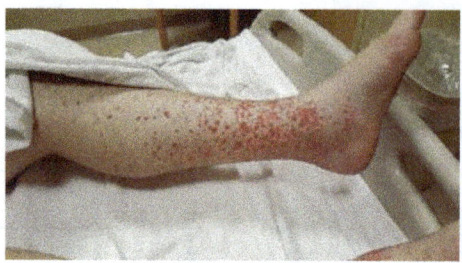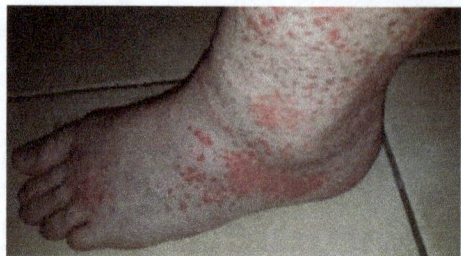

FIGURE 1: Palpable purpura on the lower extremities with ankle edema and arthritis.

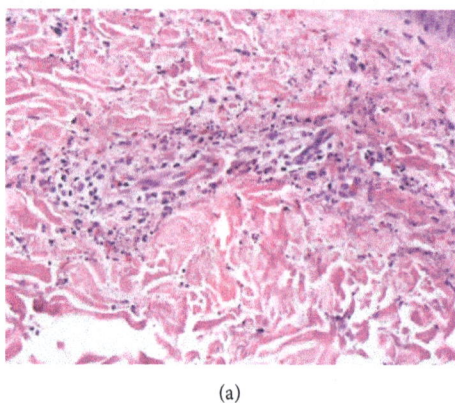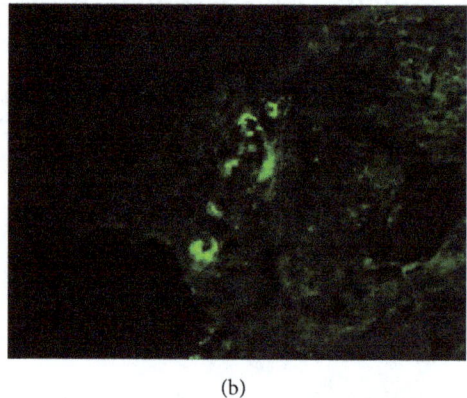

(a)   (b)

FIGURE 2: (a) High power hematoxylin and eosin stained slide showing leukocytoclastic vasculitis. (b) Direct immunofluorescence showing superficial dermal vascular depositions of IgA.

His adalimumab was stopped and he was treated with a week of oral steroids which resulted in resolution of the rash. However, when his oral steroids were completed, his rash reappeared in the same locations, and he was subsequently admitted to our hospital for lack of response of the rash thus far. He denied any fevers, chills, night sweats, weight loss, abdominal pain, change in bowel habits, gross hematuria, or blood in the stools since the onset of the rash. He denied recent respiratory, genitourinary, or gastrointestinal infections, recent travel, sick contacts, or exposure to new foods or medications. In his family history, he has two uncles with chronic kidney disease but the patient did not know the etiology. He had no allergies. The patient was a married male with no smoking or alcohol use history.

On physical exam, a palpable purpuric rash was present on his bilateral lower extremities from his toes up to his knees and then less prominently on his upper thighs along with several scattered lesions on his abdomen up to his umbilicus, buttocks, and lower back. Ankles were mildly tender and swollen without other signs of synovitis. Abdominal examination was otherwise normal. Laboratory data was significant for a mild leukocytosis of 11,600 (90% neutrophils), mild acute kidney injury with creatinine of 1.11 mg/dL, and slight proteinuria and hematuria; hemoglobin, platelet count, liver chemistries, and ESR were normal. HIV, viral hepatitis serologies, antinuclear antibody, antineutrophil cytoplasmic antibody (ANCA), cryoglobulins, and complement levels were all negative or within normal limits. Punch skin biopsies from the patient's right lower extremity revealed leukocytoclastic vasculitis with frequent eosinophils and direct immunofluorescence was positive for small vessel IgA deposition (Figure 2).

On the basis of these findings, the patient was diagnosed with HSP. Without a clear infectious trigger, we concluded that this episode was likely related to anti-TNFα treatment with adalimumab. The patient received treatment with methylprednisolone 20 mg intravenously every eight hours with almost complete resolution of the rash. His renal injury resolved as well. He was discharged on an oral prednisone taper. Several weeks later he had persistent resolution of the rash off steroids and adalimumab. The patient has been seen in follow-up every three months by either the gastroenterology or rheumatology team. The initial treatment of steroids and cessation of adalimumab resulted in resolution of his purpura and arthritis. He had no proteinuria on urinalysis. He continued to have up to 10 nonbloody bowel movements per day. A repeat colonoscopy showed mild, focal, active colitis. He is being treated with mesalamine with good control of his symptoms.

3. Discussion

We describe here an unusual case of HSP in an adult patient who had been treated with adalimumab for ulcerative colitis. Without any other clear trigger for the development of HSP, we attribute this to the use of anti-TNFα therapy.

The annual incidence of HSP ranges in different reports from 13 to 20/100,000 for children and infants. The incidence is much less for adults, closer to 1-2/100,000. The disease is often described as seasonal due to the fact that cases increase during the fall and winter months, when a preceding infection of the respiratory tract is more likely to act as the trigger. The classic findings comprise a tetrad of nonthrombocytopenic palpable purpura, arthritis, abdominal pain, and renal involvement such as proteinuria or hematuria. The arthritis is usually symmetric and has a predilection for the ankles and knees. Involvement of the gastrointestinal tract can range from symptoms of cramping and pain to the more feared complications of intussusception, hemorrhage, or perforation, which are more commonly seen in infants and children. Skin involvement is common and is a nearly universal sign of the disease. Crops of nonblanching purpura develop predominately in the dependent areas of the lower extremities and buttocks. The classic finding on skin biopsy is leukocytoclastic vasculitis with IgA deposits in the vasculature on direct immunofluorescence, similar to what was seen on the skin biopsy of our patient [4].

In adult patients with HSP, involvement of the kidney must be identified early, as an increased proportion of adults have persistent hematuria, proteinuria, or renal failure relative to children. While our patient initially had microhematuria and modest increase in creatinine, both of these parameters were corrected with administration of intravenous fluids and corticosteroids.

Our patient did not have clear evidence of a preceding infection to trigger the development of HSP. Group A beta-hemolytic *Streptococcus* (GAS) was seen in 20–50% of patients with acute HSP. Other pathogens such as parvovirus B19, *Bartonella henselae*, *Staphylococcus aureus*, *Helicobacter pylori*, *Haemophilus parainfluenzae*, Coxsackievirus, adenovirus, hepatitis A, and hepatitis B have also been implicated as infectious triggers of the disease [4]. However, the evidence linking these pathogens to the development of HSP consists of small reports of a descriptive nature and a true pathophysiological link has yet to be established.

Our patient was being treated with the TNFα blocker adalimumab for his ulcerative colitis. There are rare reports that have highlighted a case similar to ours, where a patient without a clear inciting event developed HSP while receiving an antagonist of TNFα. A 19-year-old male with Crohn's disease being treated with adalimumab developed purpura, joint pain, proteinuria, and hematuria. A skin biopsy showed leukocytoclastic vasculitis, consistent with HSP. Adalimumab was stopped as a precaution and then restarted with the rationale that this agent had no previous evidence to link it to HSP development. Upon reinitiation of the agent, the patient's symptoms returned [5]. In a similar case, a 36-year-old woman with Crohn's disease on adalimumab developed purpura, arthritis, proteinuria, and hematuria, with evidence of leukocytoclastic vasculitis on biopsy. Adalimumab was stopped and her symptoms resolved, but on rechallenge with the agent in order to better control her Crohn's disease the multisystem effects recurred [6].

This association with HSP is not unique to adalimumab, extending to other members of the TNFα inhibitor class.

In two separate reports, a twelve-year-old female and a 69-year-old female both developed HSP while being treated with infliximab for ulcerative colitis [7, 8]. Beyond these cases, a sixty-year-old female with rheumatoid arthritis developed purpura and hematuria while receiving etanercept; both skin and kidney biopsies showed IgA and C3 deposition diagnostic of HSP. This patient also saw resolution of her disease with cessation of etanercept, only to have the signs and symptoms reappear when etanercept was restarted [9]. Overall, this limited but seemingly growing body of literature suggests that many members of the TNFα inhibitor class may illicit an HSP reaction. Interestingly, however, there have been reports of patients with TNFα inhibitor-induced HSP being treated with a different TNFα without recurrence of HSP [6].

More generally, it has been long known that skin reactions can be seen during treatment with TNFα antagonists. In an analysis of a Spanish database of 5437 patients treated with etanercept, infliximab, or adalimumab representing 17,300 years of exposure, the most common reactions were psoriasiform changes, alopecia areata, cutaneous lupus, vitiligo, lichenoid eruption, morphea, granuloma annulare, and vasculitis [10]. Similarly, in a review of published reports of autoimmune diseases that developed while taking TNFα targeted therapy, 118 cases of vasculitis were found among 379 diagnoses of a new autoimmune disease. Of these 118 cases, 102 of the cases had cutaneous involvement, 44 were documented as leukocytoclastic vasculitis, and two were confirmed HSP cases [11]. Other reports include a 37-year-old female who developed leukocytoclastic vasculitis while being treated with golimumab for ankylosing spondylitis [12], a 20-year-old male who developed leukocytoclastic vasculitis while being treated with adalimumab for Crohn's and juvenile idiopathic arthritis [13], and a 30-year-old female who developed cutaneous vasculitis while being treated with infliximab for juvenile idiopathic arthritis [14]. Cumulatively these data underscore the fact that skin reactions are not limited to a specific TNFα inhibitor, gender, or diagnosis that required TNFα inhibition.

While autoimmune reactions such as HSP are rare among patients being treated with TNFα antagonists, these cases raise the question whether there is a pathophysiological link between the inhibition of TNFα and the cascade that leads to deposition of IgA complexes in skin and other organs. While genetic factors may predispose certain individuals to the development of HSP, large scale genome-wide association studies have not been performed in patients with this disease, and the evidence that has been reported thus far has not provided a link between specific genetic changes and risk of HSP. The current literature offers some interesting candidates that compromise pathways already linked to other autoimmune and inflammatory conditions (CTLA-4, HLA gene family, TLR-2, TLR-4, IL-1, IL-6, and IL-18) [15].

Beyond these genetic considerations, the observation that many patients who developed HSP while receiving TNFα antagonists were being treated for inflammatory bowel disease is provocative. IBD and HSP involve a breach of similar mucosal tissues (gut and respiratory mucosa, resp.), though IgA has not typically been considered a major player in the predominately T cell mediated pathogenesis of IBD.

However, recent work suggested that differential coating of bacteria by IgA can help identify those organisms most likely to cause colitis [16]. Studies such as this and the clinical reports featured above suggest that more scientific inquiry into the role of IgA in autoimmune diseases such as HSP and IBD is warranted.

Competing Interests

The authors declare that they have no competing interests.

Authors' Contributions

Joseph J. LaConti and Jean A. Donet performed the literature review and wrote the paper. Jeong Hee Cho-Vega provided pathology slides and expert opinion. Daniel A. Sussman, Dana Ascherman, and Amar R. Deshpande reviewed the paper and provided expert opinion.

References

[1] G. S. Seo and S.-C. Chae, "Biological therapy for ulcerative colitis: an update," *World Journal of Gastroenterology*, vol. 20, no. 37, pp. 13234–13238, 2014.

[2] I. Cleynen, W. Van Moerkercke, T. Billiet et al., "Characteristics of skin lesions associated with anti-tumor necrosis factor therapy in patients with inflammatory bowel disease: A Cohort Study," *Annals of Internal Medicine*, vol. 164, no. 1, pp. 10–22, 2016.

[3] E. B. Hawryluk, K. R. Linskey, L. M. Duncan, and R. M. Nazarian, "Broad range of adverse cutaneous eruptions in patients on TNF-alpha antagonists," *Journal of Cutaneous Pathology*, vol. 39, no. 5, pp. 481–492, 2012.

[4] F. T. Saulsbury, "Henoch-Schönlein purpura," *Current Opinion in Rheumatology*, vol. 13, no. 1, pp. 35–40, 2001.

[5] F. Z. Rahman, G. K. Takhar, O. Roy et al., "Henoch-Schönlein purpura complicating adalimumab therapy for Crohn's disease," *World Journal of Gastrointestinal Pharmacology and Therapeutics*, vol. 1, no. 5, pp. 119–122, 2010.

[6] I. Marques, A. Lagos, J. Reis, A. Pinto, and B. Neves, "Reversible Henoch-Schönlein purpura complicating adalimumab therapy," *Journal of Crohn's and Colitis*, vol. 6, no. 7, pp. 796–799, 2012.

[7] S. Nobile, C. Catassi, and L. Felici, "Herpes zoster infection followed by Henoch-Schönlein purpura in a girl receiving infliximab for ulcerative colitis," *Journal of Clinical Rheumatology*, vol. 15, no. 2, article 101, 2009.

[8] Y. Song, Y.-H. Shi, C. He et al., "Severe Henoch-Schönlein purpura with infliximab for ulcerative colitis," *World Journal of Gastroenterology*, vol. 21, no. 19, pp. 6082–6087, 2015.

[9] T. N. Duffy, M. Genta, S. Moll, P.-Y. Martin, and C. Gabay, "Henoch Schönlein purpura following etanercept treatment of rheumatoid arthritis," *Clinical and Experimental Rheumatology*, vol. 24, no. 2, p. S106, 2006.

[10] M. V. Hernández, R. Sanmartí, J. D. Cañete et al., "Cutaneous adverse events during treatment of chronic inflammatory rheumatic conditions with tumor necrosis factor antagonists: study using the Spanish registry of adverse events of biological therapies in rheumatic diseases," *Arthritis Care & Research*, vol. 65, no. 12, pp. 2024–2031, 2013.

[11] M. Ramos-Casals, P. Brito-Zerón, M.-J. Soto, M.-J. Cuadrado, and M. A. Khamashta, "Autoimmune diseases induced by TNF-targeted therapies," *Best Practice and Research: Clinical Rheumatology*, vol. 22, no. 5, pp. 847–861, 2008.

[12] A. Pàmies, S. Castro, M. J. Poveda, and R. Fontova, "Leucocytoclastic vasculitis associated with golimumab," *Rheumatology*, vol. 52, no. 10, pp. 1921–1923, 2013.

[13] U. N. Shivaji, A. K. Awasthi, and R. Aherne, "Cutaneous vasculitis caused by anti-tumor necrosis factor therapy: a case report," *Clinical Gastroenterology and Hepatology*, vol. 14, no. 1, pp. e1–e2, 2016.

[14] I. Pontikaki, E. Shahi, L. A. Frasin et al., "Skin manifestations induced by TNF-alpha inhibitors in juvenile idiopathic arthritis," *Clinical Reviews in Allergy and Immunology*, vol. 42, no. 2, pp. 131–134, 2012.

[15] X. He, C. Yu, P. Zhao et al., "The genetics of Henoch-Schönlein purpura: a systematic review and meta-analysis," *Rheumatology International*, vol. 33, no. 6, pp. 1387–1395, 2013.

[16] N. W. Palm, M. R. de Zoete, T. W. Cullen et al., "Immunoglobulin A coating identifies colitogenic bacteria in inflammatory bowel disease," *Cell*, vol. 158, no. 5, pp. 1000–1010, 2014.

34

Heparin-Related Thrombocytopenia Triggered by Severe Status of Systemic Lupus Erythematosus and Bacterial Infection

Satoshi Suzuki,[1,2] **Shihoko Nakajima,**[1] **Taiki Ando,**[3] **Keisuke Oda,**[1] **Manabu Sugita,**[4] **Kunimi Maeda,**[5] **Yutaka Nakiri,**[1] **and Yoshinari Takasaki**[3]

[1]*Department of Internal Medicine and Rheumatology, Juntendo University Nerima Hospital, Tokyo 177-8521, Japan*
[2]*Department of Internal Medicine Research, Sasaki Institute, Sasaki Foundation, Tokyo 101-0062, Japan*
[3]*Department of Internal Medicine and Rheumatology, Juntendo University School of Medicine, Tokyo 113-8431, Japan*
[4]*Department of Emergency and Critical Care Medicine, Juntendo University Nerima Hospital, Tokyo 177-8521, Japan*
[5]*Department of Internal Medicine and Nephrology, Juntendo University Nerima Hospital, Tokyo 177-8521, Japan*

Correspondence should be addressed to Satoshi Suzuki; satsuzu@juntendo.ac.jp

Academic Editor: Tsai-Ching Hsu

A patient with severe lupus nephritis developed thrombocytopenia during treatment with high-dose steroids. In addition to viral- or disease-induced cytopenia, the pathology was believed to arise from diverse contributing factors, such as thrombotic microangiopathy and heparin-related thrombocytopenia (HIT). By combining plasma exchange therapy and intravenous cyclophosphamide, we successfully controlled the SLE activity and improved the thrombocytopenia. An antecedent bacterial infection or SLE activity is believed to have contributed to the concurrent HIT.

1. Introduction

Systemic lupus erythematosus (SLE) is an autoimmune disease that can involve all bodily organs, including the lungs, kidneys, and skin. Diagnosis of SLE in Japan is primarily based on the diagnostic criteria of the American College of Rheumatology (ACR) as revised in 1997 [1]. However, there are cases that do not satisfy the diagnostic criteria yet involve symptoms or autoantibodies typical of SLE. Conversely, there are other autoimmune diseases, such as Sjögren's syndrome, that present with a pathology that would end up being misdiagnosed as SLE when judged purely on the diagnostic criteria [2]. Recently, the Systemic Lupus Collaborating Clinics (SLICC) have proposed new criteria for classifying SLE [3], but neither their sensitivity nor their specificity greatly exceeds those of the ACR diagnostic criteria. There are also individual differences in how symptoms manifest, varying from mild pathology limited to skin rashes and arthritis to severe pathology involving major organs. Accordingly, treatment needs to be tailored to suit individual symptoms. SLE is a refractory autoimmune disease that challenges a rheumatologist's competence in both diagnosis and treatment.

Representative forms of severe pathology with organ involvement include central nervous system lupus and glomerulonephritis (lupus nephritis), but patients so often exhibit severe thrombocytopenia that has also been included in the diagnostic criteria.

2. Case Report

A 52-year-old man with an unremarkable past medical history had anemia noted in a 2014 health check and, by the end of the year, lower limb edema was observed but was left untreated. In March 2015, he was admitted to a nearby clinic with a diagnosis of nephrotic syndrome. Renal dysfunction was observed when the nephrotic syndrome was diagnosed, and blood purification therapy was being considered, for which he was transferred to our hospital. Since progressive renal dysfunction had been observed, methylprednisolone (mPSL) pulse therapy (mPSL 1000 mg/day for 3 days) was initiated on the day of hospital transfer. This was followed by treatment with 100 mg/day (1 mg/kg) of prednisolone (PSL), beginning on hospital day 4. Testing conducted in parallel showed anti-nuclear antibody titers of ×320 (Homo

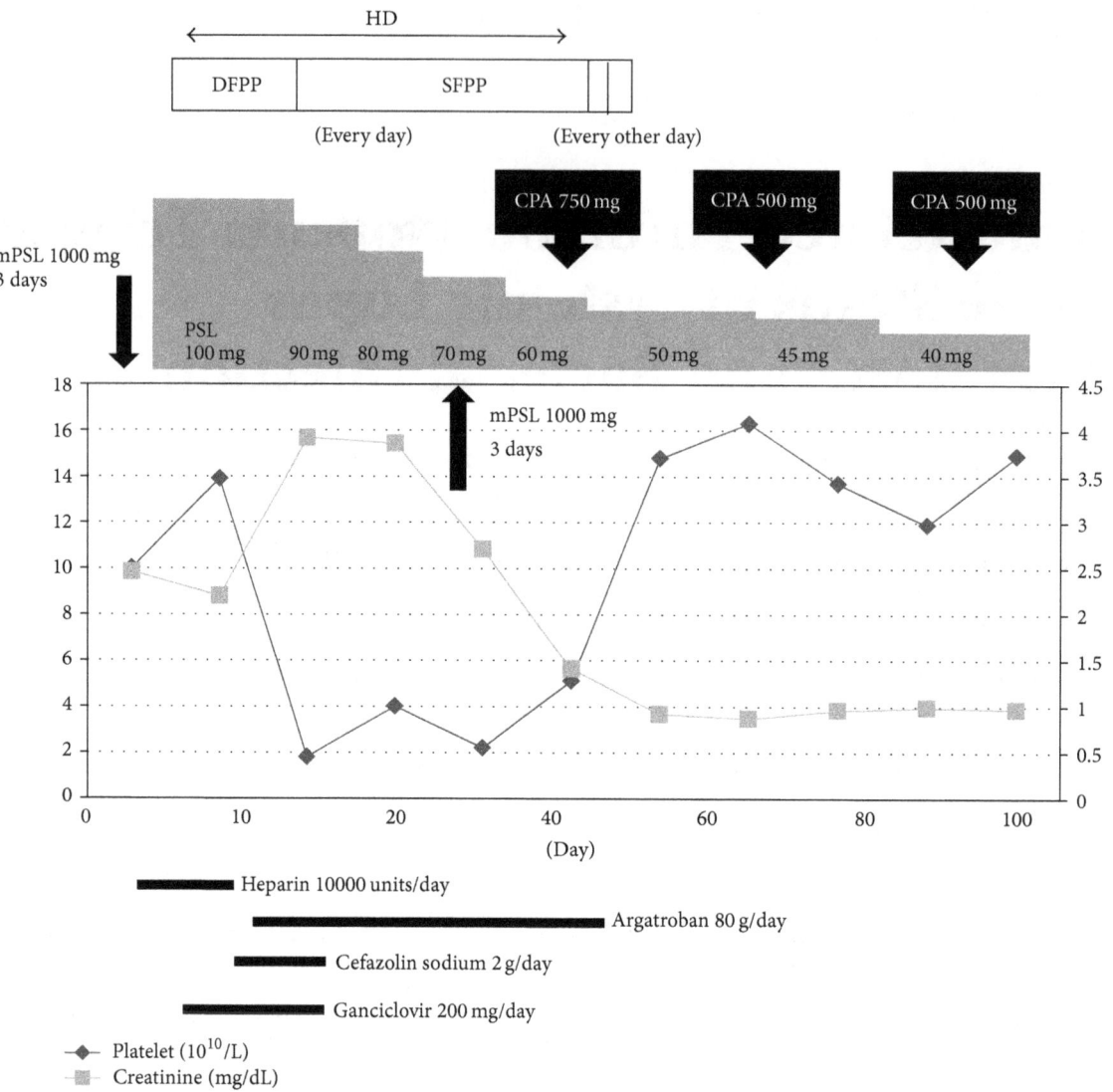

FIGURE 1: Clinical course.

×320, Spe ×320), anti-ds DNA antibody (ELISA) 300 IU/mL, anti-cardiolipin antibodies (IgG-aCL) at 16 U/mL, leukocytes at 1000/L, platelets at 100,000/L, and urine protein levels of 2.6 g/gCre, and he was diagnosed with SLE. With such significant systemic edema, difficulty with hemostasis was anticipated, and the patient was unable to lie prone, making it impossible to obtain a renal biopsy to differentiate the type of lupus nephritis. High disease activity persisted, and plasma exchange therapy (double filtration plasmapheresis) was initiated on hospital day 9. On hospital day 11, dialysis (hemodialysis, HD) was initiated. A fever was observed on hospital day 21, and *Staphylococcus aureus* (methicillin-sensitive *Staphylococcus aureus*, MSSA) was detected from a blood culture. At first, vancomycin was selected as an antibiotic, but after sensitivity was confirmed, the antibiotics were deescalated to cefazolin. On hospital day 23, decreases in oxygen saturation and blood pressure were observed, and the patient was admitted to the intensive care unit (ICU) with congestive heart failure. His circulation was

supported medically and the antibiotics were continued. The patient's testing did not support a diagnosis of acute coronary syndrome nor poor drainage during HD; myocardial damage from cytokine storm was believed to be the cause of his heart failure. High-level SLE activity persisted, and the patient was deemed to have a steroid-resistant pathology. We considered introducing cyclophosphamide (CPA) or mycophenolate mofetil (MMF). Laboratory test findings are shown in Table 1. Clinical course is shown in Figure 1.

Platelet count had been gradually decreasing since hospital day 10, and no improvement was observed despite changes in and discontinuation of the drugs used. A search for the cause of his thrombocytopenia identified CMV antigenemia (C7-HRP: 3/50,000 infected cells). He was also positive for CMV-DNA, and the possibility of thrombocytopenia associated with CMV viremia was considered. ADAMTS13 activity, which was submitted at the same time, also exhibited a mild decrease at 53%, and concurrent thrombotic microangiopathy (TMA) was considered, in light of the findings of fever,

TABLE 1: Laboratory test findings.

Test	Result
Blood cell count	WBC 1000/μL
	Neu 505/μL
	Lym 100/μL
	Eosi 0/μL
	RBC 280万/μL
	Hb 6.9 g/dL
	Hct 24.3%
	Plt 10000/μL
Coagulation	PT 114%
	(PT-INR 0.95)
	APTT 30.5 sec
	FDP 25.2 μg/mL
Biochemistry	T-Bil 0.3 mg/dL
	D-Bil 0.1 mg/dL
	AST 22 IU/L
	ALT 11 IU/L
	γ-GTP 21 IU/L
	BUN 62 mg/dL
	Cre 2.46 mg/dL
	eGFR 23.31
	UA 10.4 mg/dL
	Na 134 mEq/L
	K 5.0 mEq/L
	Cl 105 mEq/L
	TP 5.0 g/dL
	Alb 1.9 g/dL
Serology	CRP 1.87 mg/dL
	ANA ×320
	Homogeneous ×320
	Speckled ×320
	Anti-DNA antibody 300 IU/mL
	Anti-RNP antibody (−)
	Anti-SS-A antibody (−)
	Anti-cardiolipin antibody (IgG) 16 IU/mL
	CH50 12/mL
	C3 24 mg/dL
	C4 5 mg/dL
	IgG 1554 mg/dL
	IgA 148 mg/dL
	IgM 290 mg/dL
Urinalysis	pH 5.0
	Protein (4+)
	Ketone body (−)
	Occult blood (±)
Urinary sediment	RBC 10–19 HPF
	WBC 20–29 HPF
	Hyaline cast (2+)
	Epithelial cast (1+)
	Granular cast (1+)
	Waxy cast (1+)

WBC: white blood cell, RBC: red blood cell, Hb: hemoglobin, Hct: hematocrit, Plt: platelet, PT: prothrombin time, INR: international normalized ratio, APTT: activated partial thromboplastin time, FDP: fibrinogen and fibrin degradation products, Bil: bilirubin, AST: aspartate transaminase, ALT: alanine transaminase, BUN: blood urea nitrogen, eGFR: estimated glomerular filtration rate, TP: total protein, CRP: C-reactive protein, ANA: anti-nuclear antibody, LAC: lupus anticoagulant, CH50: total complement activity, Ig: immunoglobulin, and HPF: high power field.

peripheral blood schistocytes, hemolytic anemia, confusion, and progressive renal failure. In addition, he was found to be positive for heparin-related thrombocytopenia (HIT) antibodies, and we considered the possibility that he was experiencing HIT caused by the heparin used in thrombosis prophylaxis since hospital day 2. We found a deep vein thrombosis at left popliteal artery by ultrasonography, so 4T's score ran to 7 points. The viremia forced cyclophosphamide and MMF to be postponed, and simple plasma exchange therapy (single filtration plasmapheresis, SFPP) was initiated on hospital day 23 while the patient also was undergoing antiviral therapy with ganciclovir. Beginning on hospital day 24, a second course of mPSL pulse therapy (mPSL 1000 mg/day for 3 days) was begun to treat the cytokine storm, following which the steroid dosage would be reduced. Vital signs stabilized, and he was discharged from the ICU on hospital day 29, but hemoptysis occurred on hospital day 31 while he was undergoing HD. He was found to have decreased oxygen saturation and a decreased level of consciousness and started on ventilator management with endotracheal intubation. Chest computed tomography and bronchoscopy identified an alveolar hemorrhage, and again he was admitted to the ICU. Although this hemorrhage was believed to be the result of his low platelet count, he still had high SLE activity, and the possibility of alveolar hemorrhage secondary to SLE was considered. On hospital day 36, CMV C7-HRP was still positive; we made the decision to perform intermittent intravenous therapy (intravenous cyclophosphamide therapy, IVCY) with 750 mg of CPA to control SLE activity. Later, platelet count increased, in tandem with improved TMA pathology due to SFPP, reduced HIT due to heparin cessation, and an improvement in viremia due to a relatively fast decrease in steroid dosage.

The patient had a favorable therapeutic response to cyclophosphamide, and we were able to conclude mechanical ventilation and discharge him from the ICU on hospital day 39. We also discontinued HD and SFPP, and he underwent a second course of IVCY on hospital day 71 and a third course on hospital day 107, with a favorable course that allowed him to be discharged from the hospital on hospital day 127. Medical treatment has been continuing on an outpatient basis; SLE has maintained low disease activity, and there has been no decrease in his platelet count.

3. Discussion

Cytopenias frequently complicate SLE, including anemia (63.0%), lymphopenia (40.3%), leukopenia (30.0%), and thrombocytopenia (10.9%) [4]. In particular, thrombocytopenia has very diverse causes, including hemophagocytic syndrome (HPS), TMA, and antiphospholipid antibody syndrome, all involving the underlying disease, and viral infection, drug-induced cytopenia, and thrombosis caused by steroids, which involve the treatment. Depending on the cause, steroids and other such immunosuppressive therapies may be effective, but they have an inverse effect if the cause is infection or thrombosis [5]. The present case is believed to have had simultaneous onset of TMA and HIT, in addition to viral infection. TMA is a severe manifestation of SLE pathology, and, if left untreated, it is frequently fatal. TMA occurs frequently in highly active SLE with renal complications [6]. SFPP is an effective treatment for TMA and lowers the mortality rate, said to be 85–100% in the absence of treatment, down to 10–30% [7–9]. However, there are cases where SFPP is ineffective at treating or stopping recurrence, and in such cases, rituximab is reportedly effective [10, 11]. HIT is a pathology where, for some reason, pathogenic HIT antibodies are produced out of the autoantibodies (anti-heparin/PF4 antibodies) against platelet factor 4 (PF4) and the heparin complex [12]. HIT antibodies activate the vascular endothelium and induce thrombosis from excessive thrombin production [12]. To diagnose HIT, it is useful to measure HIT antibodies directly, a test which is covered by insurance even in Japan, but it is necessary to have a comprehensive approach by combining the 4T's score using the extent of thrombocytopenia, history of heparin use, and the presence or absence of thrombosis [13]. Anticoagulation therapy is required for thrombosis prophylaxis, but heparin exacerbates the thrombocytopenia, in which case argatroban, which is a thrombin inhibitor, is used. Approximately 19% of SLE patients have antibodies against PF4 (anti-PF4 antibodies) [14]. Anti-PF4 antibodies are believed to be synonymous with anti-heparin/PF4 antibodies in that they react to the heparin/PF4 complex (are heparin-dependent). However, heparin-independent anti-PF4 antibodies, which are believed to react only to PF4, have been discovered recently. The appearance of heparin-dependent anti-PF4 antibodies is associated with thrombocytopenia, while the appearance of heparin-independent anti-PF4 antibodies is related to SLE disease activity [14]. The patient presented tested positive for HIT antibodies, and therefore it was believed that autoantibodies against the heparin/PF4 complex (heparin-dependent anti-PF4 antibodies) were being produced, even though disease activity remained extremely high. Anti-heparin/PF4 antibodies are reportedly produced due to a cross-reaction between the complex of PF4 and bacteria (in particular, *Staphylococcus aureus* and *Escherichia coli*) [15]. This patient developed MSSA bacteremia, and it was possible that he experienced an abnormal immune response to the complex of bacteria and PF4 and produced anti-heparin/PF4 antibodies due to enhanced SLE activity. The pathology presented with the production of diverse autoantibodies, including anti-DNA, IgG-aCL, and HIT antibodies, and he was believed to have an abnormal enhancement of B-cell function. A malignant lymphoma test (7-amino-actinomycin-D, 7AAD) performed on peripheral blood ruled out B-cell lymphoproliferative disease. Finally, he responded to cyclophosphamide, which is a DNA synthesis inhibitor; in such cases, we feel that a treatment strategy targeting B-cells, such as rituximab or belimumab, may be effective and useful in terms of the risk of adverse reactions.

4. Conclusion

The causes of thrombocytopenia complicating SLE with high disease activity include those associated with the underlying disease, but numerous reports show that TMA, HPS, and similar conditions are also possible. In the present case, HIT antibodies appeared, and the patient is believed to have had concurrent heparin-related thrombocytopenia. In patients who are receiving high-dose steroids and have a high risk of thrombosis, there are some cases where heparin is used prophylactically, but we feel it is necessary to pay attention to the onset of heparin-related thrombocytopenia when the patient is being treated for autoimmune disease with high disease activity or when relatively severe bacterial infection is concurrent.

Competing Interests

The authors declare that they have no conflict of interests.

References

[1] E. M. Tan, A. S. Cohen, J. F. Fries et al., "The 1982 revised criteria for the classification of systemic lupus erythrematosus," *Arthritis and Rheumatism*, vol. 25, no. 11, pp. 1271–1277, 1982.

[2] S. Noah, "Sjögren syndrome and systemic lupus erythematosus are distinct conditions," *Dermatology Online Journal*, vol. 12, no. 1, article 4, 2006.

[3] M. Petri, A.-M. Orbai, G. S. Alarcón et al., "Derivation and validation of the systemic lupus international collaborating clinics classification criteria for systemic lupus erythematosus," *Arthritis and Rheumatism*, vol. 64, no. 8, pp. 2677–2686, 2012.

[4] A. Aamer, S. A. A. Abdurahman, K. Najma et al., "Haematological abnormalities in systemic lupus erythematosus," *Acta Rheumatologica Portuguesa*, vol. 39, pp. 236–241, 2014.

[5] K. Newman, M. B. Owlia, I. El-Hemaidi, and M. Akhtari, "Management of immune cytopenias in patients with systemic lupus erythematosus—old and new," *Autoimmunity Reviews*, vol. 12, no. 7, pp. 784–791, 2013.

[6] P. Letchumanan, H.-J. Ng, L.-H. Lee, and J. Thumboo, "A comparison of thrombotic thrombocytopenic purpura in an inception cohort of patients with and without systemic lupus erythematosus," *Rheumatology*, vol. 48, no. 4, pp. 399–403, 2009.

[7] F. Peyvandi, R. Palla, and L. A. Lotta, "Pathogenesis and treatment of acquired idiopathic thrombotic thrombocytopenic purpura," *Haematologica*, vol. 95, no. 9, pp. 1444–1447, 2010.

[8] J. N. George, "How I treat patients with thrombotic thrombocytopenic purpura: 2010," *Blood*, vol. 116, no. 20, pp. 4060–4069, 2010.

[9] G. B. Raimundo, M. S. Eva, M. S. Maria et al., "Systemic lupus erythematosus and thrombotic thrombocytopenia purpura: a refractory case without lupus activity," *Clinical Rheumatology*, vol. 9, no. 6, pp. 373–375, 2013.

[10] D. Caramazza, G. Quintini, I. Abbene et al., "Relapsing or refractory idiopathic thrombotic thrombocytopenic purpura-hemolytic uremic syndrome: the role of rituximab," *Transfusion*, vol. 50, no. 12, pp. 2753–2760, 2010.

[11] K. Kamiya, K. Kurasawa, S. Arai et al., "Rituximab was effective on refractory thrombotic thrombocytopenic purpura but induced a flare of hemophagocytic syndrome in a patient with systemic lupus erythematosus," *Modern Rheumatology*, vol. 20, no. 1, pp. 81–85, 2010.

[12] H. Yamamoto and S. Miyata, "Ischemic stroke and heparin-induced thrombocytopenia," *Clinical Neurology*, vol. 51, no. 5, pp. 316–320, 2011.

[13] G. K. Lo, D. Juhl, T. E. Warkentin, C. S. Sigouin, P. Eichler, and A. Greinacher, "Evaluation of pretest clinical score (4 T's) for the diagnosis of heparin-induced thrombocytopenia in two clinical

settings," *Journal of Thrombosis and Haemostasis*, vol. 4, no. 4, pp. 759–765, 2006.

[14] T. Satoh, Y. Tanaka, Y. Okazaki, J. Kaburaki, Y. Ikeda, and M. Kuwana, "Heparin-dependent and -independent anti-platelet factor 4 autoantibodies in patients with systemic lupus erythematosus," *Rheumatology*, vol. 51, no. 9, pp. 1721–1728, 2012.

[15] K. Krauel, C. Pötschke, C. Weber et al., "Platelet factor 4 binds to bacteria-inducing antibodies cross-reacting with the major antigen in heparin-induced thrombocytopenia," *Blood*, vol. 117, no. 4, pp. 1370–1378, 2011.

35

Catastrophic Antiphospholipid Syndrome

Rawhya R. El-Shereef,[1] Zein El-Abedin,[2] Rashad Abdel Aziz,[3] Ibrahim Talat,[4] Mohammed Saleh,[4] Hanna Abdel-Samia,[4] Amro Sameh,[5] and Mahmoud Sharha[5]

[1]Rheumatology Department, Faculty of Medicine, Minia, Egypt
[2]Neurology Department, Faculty of Medicine, Minia, Egypt
[3]Cardiology Department, Faculty of Medicine, Minia, Egypt
[4]ICU Department, Faculty of Medicine, Minia, Egypt
[5]Radiology Department, Faculty of Medicine, Minia, Egypt

Correspondence should be addressed to Rawhya R. El-Shereef; rawhyaelshereef@yahoo.com

Academic Editor: Gregory J. Tsay

This paper reports one case of successfully treated patients suffering from a rare entity, the catastrophic antiphospholipid syndrome (CAPS). Management of this patient is discussed in detail.

1. Introduction

The antiphospholipid syndrome (APS) is a systemic autoimmune disease characterized by the occurrence of arterial and venous thrombosis and/or obstetric complications (miscarriage, fetal death in utero) associated with the presence of antiphospholipid antibodies [1]. The catastrophic antiphospholipid syndrome (CAPS) is the most severe manifestation; CAPS is rare affecting less than 1% of patients with APS and is characterized by the occurrence of thrombosis in multiple organs over a short period of time [2]. It is acute in onset, with majority of cases developing thrombocytopenia, less frequently hemolytic anemia, and disseminated intravascular coagulation. Lupus anticoagulant and anticardiolipin antibodies have been reported as predominant antibodies associated with CAPS. The mortality rate is approaching 50%. It was first recognized in patients with systemic lupus erythematosus (SLE) and later found in association with other autoimmune disorders. This condition has also been recognized as a syndrome that can develop independent of any underlying disease, known as primary APS [3]. The high rate of mortality should warrant greater awareness among clinicians for timely diagnosis and treatment of this life-threatening condition. We report a case of a 32-year-old female admitted with clinical and laboratory findings consistent with CAPS which were successfully treated. Their management was discussed in detail later.

2. Clinical Case

A 32-year-old Egyptian physiotherapist female patient was admitted in the ICU of Al-Rashid Hospital, complaining from altered mental status, dyspnea, fever, and epileptic fit. The patient had no medical problems and had been in her usual state of health until 3 days before admission and then she developed frequent resistant headaches and blurring vision; CT of brain was done and was normal before admission in ICU by 3 days. This patient was admitted under neurology and received phenytoin and antibiotics vials. She was diagnosed as status epilepticus. After 2 days the patient experienced worsening of her neurological condition, presenting drowsiness, diplopia, squint, reduction of vision, severe headache, and developed quadriparesis. The patient was deteriorated into spastic quadriplegia within few hours. CT of brain showed slightly ill-defined hypodense lesions in both parietal lobes with faint blood density in left sided and white matter edema are noted. MRI of brain showed bilateral venous sinus thrombosis. The patient was subjected to the following laboratory: HIV antibody, HIBs antigen, which was negative. Blood culture showed no growth. D-dimer test was negative. INR was 0.88%. Platelet count was low, 100.000 mm^3. All liver, renal function, and electrolyte were normal. An initial diagnosis of bilateral stroke was retained. The treatment started by IV drip of heparin in maximum dose with no response clinically; also INR was not affected. The dose of oral anticoagulant (warfarin) was increased up to 11 mg with IV heparin with INR ranging from 1.2 to 1.3% in normal range.

After complete history taking from her husband, we found that there was past history of fetal miscarriage and history of abortion and intrauterine fetal death. There was history of preeclampsia in first baby with blood pressure of 200/110 during her delivery. In all her pregnancies, she received juspirin and low molecular weight heparin (clexane vial). There was also past history of receiving oral contraceptive pill for one year before this attack. There was family history of death of two of her relatives from preeclampsia during labor. Then the patient referred to consultant of rheumatology to complete the management.

Complete neurological and rheumatological examinations were done; there was spastic quadriplegia. There was severe abdominal tenderness with tenderness in right hip and right lower limb. The patient's vision was deteriorated rapidly, with developing diplopia and severe headache.

At that time, brain imaging demonstrated an increase in the feature discussed before. Echocardiography showed signs of cardiac failure with aortic, mitral, and tricuspid valve insufficiencies but no segmental hypokinesia. Laboratory tests showed moderate inflammation (CRP at 30 mg/L); D-dimer test was negative. Lupus anticoagulant (LA) and anticardiolipin IGG and IGM were done in higher centre, and positive PTT-LA was 162.3 seconds (reference value: 32–51 seconds in this laboratory), DRVV time (dilute Russell's viper venom time) was 99.5 seconds, and screen ratio was 2.51 (reference value not more than 1.5 in this laboratory). Thrombin time was more than 240 seconds (reference value: 14–22 seconds in this laboratory) and anti-beta 2GP1 IgG antibodies were positive and measured 33 AU/mL (Arbitrary Units/mL, reference < 20 AU/mL). Elevated LDH was 650 U/L (reference value: 225–400 U/L in our laboratory). Anticardiolipin IgG and IgM were negative. Antinuclear antibodies and the anti-dsDNA antibodies were negative, with normal complement and normal P and C ANCA.

The diagnosis of CAPS was suspected, and our therapeutic strategy combined curative anticoagulation with unfractionated heparin, and methylprednisolone (sulomedrol vial) was given as pulse dose at dose of 1 g/d for 5 days. Then prednisone was maintained at 1 mg/kg/day with daily intravenous immunoglobulin of 400 mg/kg/5 days with physiotherapy 2 times daily. With this treatment, evolution was rapidly favorable. Neurological symptoms regressed within few days, spasticity was absent, the movement of limbs started more in left side, and the muscle strength increased gradually, as well as dyspnea. Inflammatory parameters and thrombocytopenia were corrected within few days.

After 10 days from starting of medication of sulomedrol and gamma globulin the patient developed severe pain and swelling in right lower limb. Doppler for arteries and veins of right lower limb was done and showed totally thrombosed external iliac and common femoral, deep femoral, and popliteal vein with no colour flow inside, with mild subcutaneous oedema at the leg and calf region. Anterior and posterior tibial veins and peroneal vein were patent. Doppler ultrasound of all arteries was normal.

The patient received full anticoagulation again with the maximum time of 10 days and heparin IV drip 35000 IU daily with addition of dabigatran (pradaxa tablet 110 mg twice daily). Treatment with methylprednisolone was repeated by the same regimen, and this was relayed by a maintenance dose of 2 mg/kg/day. Cyclophosphamide 1 g was also added to the initial regimen. The administration of cyclophosphamide was repeated monthly for six months. With this treatment, the initial evolution was favorable. The right lower limb for first time started to move and strength of muscle reached grade 3 in few days.

After 15 days from beginning of second regimen of medication, Doppler of both lower limbs was done again and showed evidence of recanalization of the previously described deep venous thrombus of the right lower limb with sluggish blood flow inside. Left common femoral vein and deep femoral vein were patent with normal blood flow inside. But there was thrombosed left popliteal vein with no blood flow inside. Arterial supply was normal in both lower limbs.

Recurrence of thrombosis made us take the decision of doing filter to avoid pulmonary embolism. So, we stopped heparin infusion; the patient was maintained on pradaxa (thrombin inhibitor) and warfarin tablet 13 mg daily, and then the patient was shifted to do inferior venae cava filter in Al-Kaser El-Aini Hospital, Cairo university.

The first elevation in INR was after 10 weeks from starting steroid and cyclophosphamide. INR reached 2.8 then 3 then 3.5 percent. We started to decrease the dose of warfarin gradually after 3 months from initial treatment especially after autoantibody started to decrease in her blood.

So, during her stay in the ICU (45 days), the patient presented multiple thrombotic complications: bilateral venous sinus thrombosis, thrombosis of the right external iliac, common femoral, deep femoral, popliteal vein, and left popliteal vein. Also, there was avascular necrosis in right hip which was diagnosed by CT scan. There was diplopia with blurring of vision which was suggestive of retinal thrombosis.

Patient currently has improved significantly since her initial presentation. Her vision has improved allowing her to see shades of light and shapes and she has not had any further thrombotic episodes on clinical presentation and imaging. She is now able to ambulate while she was spastic and quadriplegic at presentation (after 3 months, she walked on crutches and then walked with cane and then walked without support after 6 months). Her LDH has normalized to 166 U/L. Of particular note is that improvement in patient's symptoms, visual acuity, and functional status as well as LDH has occurred after receiving medication. Lupus anticoagulant started to decrease after 2 months and the INR started for the first time to increase. The first symptom of this patient started on 11 April 2015; on October 2015, she went to her work as physiotherapist without any support. Now, on 1 May 2016, the patient stopped steroid and finished cyclophosphamide; she received warfarin sodium 8 mg only without any thrombosis in any organ.

3. Discussion

Antiphospholipid syndrome is a systemic autoimmune disorder characterized by arterial and/or venous thrombosis and recurrent fetal loss and can be associated with thrombocytopenia [3]. CAPS, a fatal variant of APS, was first described in 1992 and defined as thrombosis of at least three different organ systems over a very short period of time with histopathologic evidence of multiple small vessel occlusions and high titers of antiphospholipid antibodies (APL) [3–7].

The clinical manifestation of CAPS depends on the organ involvement affected by thrombosis. The major organs involved during the catastrophic episode were renal (71%), followed closely by lung (64%), brain (62%), heart (51%), and skin (50%) [8]. Our patient presented with epilepsy, cerebrovascular accident, spastic quadriplegia, blurring of vision with diplopia, acute avascular necrosis in right hip with acute DVT in both lower limbs, heart involvement, thrombocytopenia, and severe hypertension. All these organs were affected within few days. Interestingly, our patient's hypertension was initially worked up as a possible etiologic source for our patient's severe disease manifestation. However, it has been reported and also implemented in the preliminary criteria for classification of CAPS that hypertension tends to occur in conjunction with renal involvement [7].

Laboratory findings in CAPS patients may include thrombocytopenia, hemolytic anemia which is often accompanied by schistocytes, and disseminated intravascular coagulations (DIC) [8]. The autoantibodies of interest to diagnose APS are anti-B2-glycoprotein which was detected by enzyme-linked immunosorbent assay (ELISA), anticardiolipin (aCL), or lupus anticoagulant (LA) assay [3, 9]. The recent 2006 revised classification criteria for APS updated the timeframe for the presence of elevated titers of antiphospholipid antibodies from >6 weeks to its persistence for >12 weeks [1, 9]. In our study, lupus anticoagulant was highly positive during the admission and six weeks after being hospitalized and then transient decrease of antibody started. Review of the literature was unrevealing regarding length of time it may take to develop recurrent positive antibody testing after treatment, given that our patient has lost the antibody (LA delta 6.3–7.7 seconds) transiently after 12 weeks. It may also be worth researching this timeline further as repeating antibody testing prior to 12 weeks may be sufficient.

Laboratory studies have become important diagnostic criteria for detecting APS. LA activity is detected by coagulation assays that adhere to guidelines from the International Society of Thrombosis and Haemostasis (ISTH), updated in 2009 by Pengo et al., which include (a) prolonged phospholipid-dependent coagulation time found on a screening test (activated partial thromboplastin time and dilute Russell's viper venom time), (b) failure to correct prolonged coagulation time during mixing studies, (c) correction of prolonged coagulation time found on screening test by adding excess phospholipids, and finally (d) exclusion of other coagulopathies [3, 10]. The screening test criteria cutoff in the updated ISTH guidelines includes cutoff value above 99th percentile of the distribution [10].

Diagnosis and aggressive therapies are mandatory. Besides treating the trigger, including infection, specific treatment targets thrombosis and SIRS (systemic inflammatory response syndrome). Early anticoagulation is of utmost importance regardless of the severity of thrombocytopenia [11]. Intravenous unfractionated heparin is usually preferred to low molecular weight heparin in case of DVT. If the patient has a lupus anticoagulant, monitoring is based on heparin blood level instead of aPTT. Heparin is followed by VKA for an INR of approximately 3. Corticosteroids inhibit aPL-mediated thrombosis [12]. Some authors suggest very high doses (1 g/day of methylprednisolone) before a relay with usual doses of 1 mg/kg·day methylprednisolone equivalent. Duration depends on the clinical response. Intravenous immunoglobulin (IVIG) is proposed instead of plasma exchanges in case of hemodynamic instability [13, 14], usually at a dose of 2 g/kg in 4 to 5 days [6, 9]. The combination of anticoagulation with corticosteroids and IVIG provides 69% of success [15]. Some treatments have a specific indication. In our case cyclophosphamide was used successfully in treatment of CAPS monthly. Cyclophosphamide is indicated only in refractory CAPS, particularly in the presence of lupus flare [16].

4. Conclusion

Catastrophic antiphospholipid syndrome is a rare disease with high mortality. Its early identification is crucial in order to establish an effective treatment: anticoagulation, corticosteroids, and immunoglobulin. Cyclophosphamide could be a promising treatment in cases of refractory CAPS. We have used it successfully for our patient. Careful postpartum anticoagulation management is mandatory. Dabigatran, a new oral direct inhibitor of thrombin, has prevented thrombus development through direct, competitive inhibition of thrombin (thrombin enables fibrinogen conversion to fibrin during the coagulation cascade). It also inhibits free and clot bound thrombin and thrombin-induced platelet aggregation. Currently well-defined indications for treatment of DVT and pulmonary embolism in patients who have been treated with a parental anticoagulant for 5–10 days and to reduce the risk of recurrence of DVT and PE in patient who has been previously treated and its prescription outside these specific contexts should be argued. The dabigatran may be a new line of anticoagulation in treatment of DVT in catastrophic antiphospholipid syndrome. Also, cyclophosphamide gives successful result in treatment of CAPS. Contraceptive pill is serious risk factor for thrombosis in APS patient.

Competing Interests

The authors declare that there are no competing interests regarding the publication of this paper.

References

[1] S. Miyakis, M. D. Lockshin, T. Atsumi et al., "International consensus statement on an update of the classification criteria for definite antiphospholipid syndrome (APS)," *Journal of Thrombosis and Haemostasis*, vol. 4, no. 2, pp. 295–306, 2006.

[2] R. A. Asherson, R. Cervera, P. G. De Groot et al., "Catastrophic antiphospholipid syndrome: international consensus statement on classification criteria and treatment guidelines," *Lupus*, vol. 12, no. 7, pp. 530–534, 2003.

[3] R. Cervera, J.-C. Piette, J. Font et al., "Antiphospholipid syndrome: clinical and immunologic manifestations and patterns of disease expression in a cohort of 1,000 patients," *Arthritis and Rheumatism*, vol. 46, no. 4, pp. 1019–1027, 2002.

[4] R. A. Asherson, G. Espinosa, S. Menahem et al., "Relapsing catastrophic antiphospholipid syndrome: report of three cases," *Seminars in Arthritis and Rheumatism*, vol. 37, no. 6, pp. 366–372, 2008.

[5] S. Sciascia, C. Lopez-Pedrera, D. Roccatello, and M. J. Cuadrado, "Catastrophic antiphospholipid syndrome (CAPS)," *Best Practice and Research: Clinical Rheumatology*, vol. 26, no. 4, pp. 535–541, 2012.

[6] R. A. Asherson, R. Cervera, J.-C. Piette et al., "Catastrophic antiphospholipid syndrome: clinical and laboratory features of 50 patients," *Medicine*, vol. 77, no. 3, pp. 195–207, 1998.

[7] R. Cervera, J. Font, J. A. Gómez-Puerta et al., "Validation of the preliminary criteria for the classification of catastrophic antiphospholipid syndrome," *Annals of the Rheumatic Diseases*, vol. 64, no. 8, pp. 1205–1209, 2005.

[8] R. Cervera, S. Bucciarelli, M. A. Plasín et al., "Catastrophic antiphospholipid syndrome (CAPS): descriptive analysis of a series of 280 patients from the <CAPS Registry>," *Journal of Autoimmunity*, vol. 32, no. 3-4, pp. 240–245, 2009.

[9] B. Giannakopoulos and S. A. Krilis, "The pathogenesis of the antiphospholipid syndrome," *The New England Journal of Medicine*, vol. 368, no. 11, pp. 1033–1044, 2013.

[10] V. Pengo, A. Tripodi, G. Reber et al., "Update of the guidelines for lupus anticoagulant detection," *Journal of Thrombosis and Haemostasis*, vol. 7, no. 10, pp. 1737–1740, 2009.

[11] M. A. Khamashta, M. J. Cuadrado, F. Mujic, N. A. Taub, B. J. Hunt, and G. R. V. Hughes, "The management of thrombosis in the antiphospholipid-antibody syndrome," *The New England Journal of Medicine*, vol. 332, no. 15, pp. 993–997, 1995.

[12] R. Cervera and CAPS Registry Project Group, "Catastrophic antiphospholipid syndrome (CAPS): update from the 'CAPS Registry'," *Lupus*, vol. 19, no. 4, pp. 412–418, 2010.

[13] C. M. Neuwelt, D. I. Daikh, J. A. Linfoot et al., "Catastrophic antiphospholipid syndrome. Response to repeated plasmapheresis over three years," *Arthritis and Rheumatism*, vol. 40, no. 8, pp. 1534–1539, 1997.

[14] P. Boura, S. Papadopoulos, K. Tselios et al., "Intracerebral hemorrhage in a patient with SLE and catastrophic antiphospholipid syndrome (CAPS): report of a case," *Clinical Rheumatology*, vol. 24, no. 4, pp. 420–424, 2005.

[15] S. Bucciarelli, G. Espinosa, R. Cervera et al., "Mortality in the catastrophic antiphospholipid syndrome: causes of death and prognostic factors in a series of 250 patients," *Arthritis and Rheumatism*, vol. 54, no. 8, pp. 2568–2576, 2006.

[16] U. D. Bayraktar, D. Erkan, S. Bucciarelli, G. Espinosa, R. Asherson, and Catastrophic Antiphospholipid Syndrome Project Group, "The clinical spectrum of catastrophic antiphospholipid syndrome in the absence and presence of lupus," *Journal of Rheumatology*, vol. 34, no. 2, pp. 346–352, 2007.

36

Effective Administration of Rituximab in Anti-MDA5 Antibody–Positive Dermatomyositis with Rapidly Progressive Interstitial Lung Disease and Refractory Cutaneous Involvement

Yuka Ogawa,[1] Dai Kishida,[1] Yasuhiro Shimojima,[1] Koichi Hayashi,[2] and Yoshiki Sekijima[1]

[1]*Department of Medicine (Neurology and Rheumatology), Shinshu University School of Medicine, 3-1-1 Asahi, Matsumoto 390-8621, Japan*
[2]*Department of Dermatology, Shinshu University School of Medicine, 3-1-1 Asahi, Matsumoto 390-8621, Japan*

Correspondence should be addressed to Yasuhiro Shimojima; yshimoji@shinshu-u.ac.jp

Academic Editor: Gregory J. Tsay

We describe the case of a 48-year-old man with dermatomyositis (DM) who demonstrated rapidly progressive interstitial lung disease (RP-ILD) and refractory cutaneous involvement together with high levels of anti-melanoma differentiation-associated gene 5 antibody (anti-MDA5-Ab). Even after combination immunosuppressive therapy including a corticosteroid, cyclosporine A, and intravenous cyclophosphamide, his respiratory insufficiency and cutaneous involvement progressively worsened. However, the administration of rituximab (RTX) resulted in clinical remission as well as a visible reduction in anti-MDA5-Ab levels, suggesting that RTX could be a useful remedy in cases refractory to conventional immunosuppressive agents, especially those of RP-ILD related to anti-MDA5-Ab–positive DM.

1. Introduction

Dermatomyositis (DM) is an autoimmune inflammatory myopathy with characteristic cutaneous involvement such as Gottron's papules, a heliotrope rash, and/or an erythematous eruption around the neck and shoulders [1]. As a subtype of DM, clinically amyopathic DM (CADM), which is characterized by a typical skin lesion of DM with no or subclinical muscular manifestations, is substantially differentiated from classic DM [2]. In both CADM and classic DM, interstitial lung disease (ILD) has been recognized as the complication impacting on the prognosis; moreover, numerous studies have recently described that the development of rapidly progressive ILD (RP-ILD) is implicated in the positivity of anti-melanoma differentiation-associated gene 5 antibody (anti-MDA5-Ab), which is more frequently detected in patients with CADM than in those with classic DM [3–6].

Although combination immunosuppressive therapy consisting of a corticosteroid, calcineurin inhibitor, and intravenous cyclophosphamide (IVCY) is sometimes selected to prevent patients with DM-related RP-ILD from developing fatal disease, such an intensive therapeutic strategy is not entirely sufficient to ensure a favorable prognosis [7–9]. Rituximab (RTX), a chimeric monoclonal antibody for depleting B cells showing CD20 protein, was recently demonstrated to be effective for intractable muscular and/or cutaneous involvement in polymyositis or DM [10, 11]. It was also suggested that RTX could be useful for severe ILD in antisynthetase syndrome [12, 13]; meanwhile, there are only a few case reports in which RTX was used in anti-MDA5-Ab–positive DM with ILD [14–18].

Here we describe a case in which RTX ameliorated RP-ILD as well as refractory cutaneous involvement in a patient with anti-MDA5-Ab–positive DM despite the resistance to the conventional immunosuppressive therapy. We also review the literature for studies of RTX in anti-MDA5-Ab–positive DM with ILD.

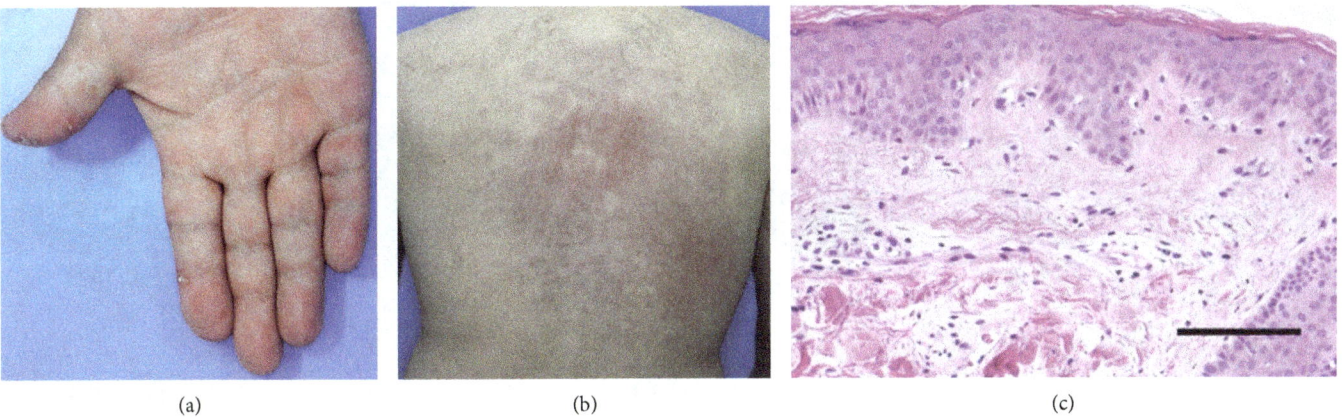

FIGURE 1: Skin lesions including palmar papules (a) and erythema on the back (b) before the initiation of treatment. A skin biopsy from the back indicates liquefactive degeneration with perivascular inflammation between the epidermis and dermis (c) (hematoxylin and eosin staining; scale bar = 100 μm).

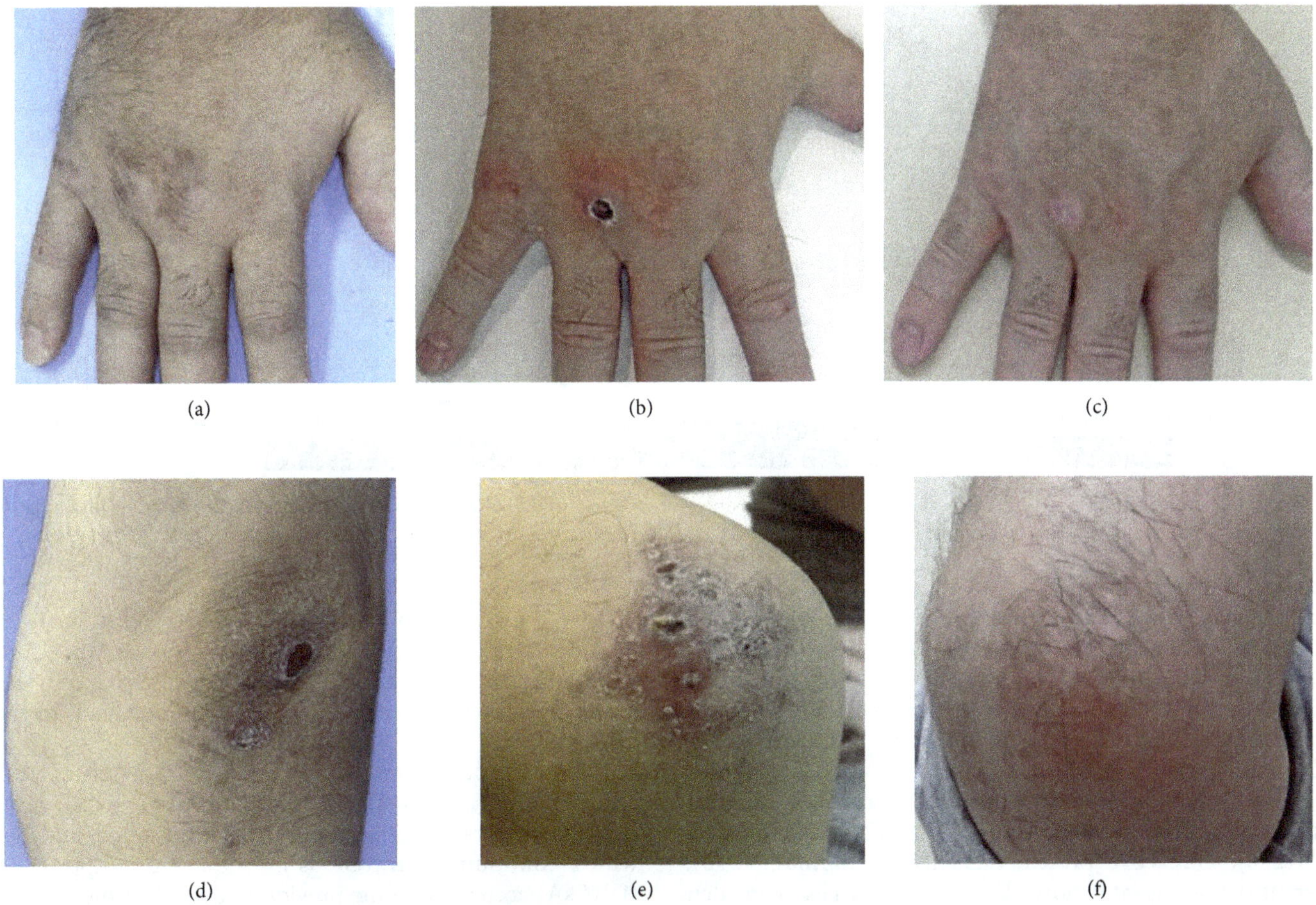

(a)

(b)

(c)

(d)

(e)

(f)

FIGURE 2: Sequential findings of cutaneous lesions on the dorsum of the hand and elbow before the initiation of treatment (a, d), before the addition of rituximab (RTX) (b, e), and after RTX administration (c, f).

2. Case Presentation

A 48-year-old man with a 1-month history of fatigue, appetite loss, and fever was admitted to our hospital. He reported experiencing arthralgia and a dry cough as well as mild exertional dyspnea prior to admission. A physical examination demonstrated a body temperature of 37.7°C, mild muscular weakness of the proximal lower limbs, edematous hands, and cutaneous manifestations including a heliotrope rash, Gottron's papules, mechanic's hands,

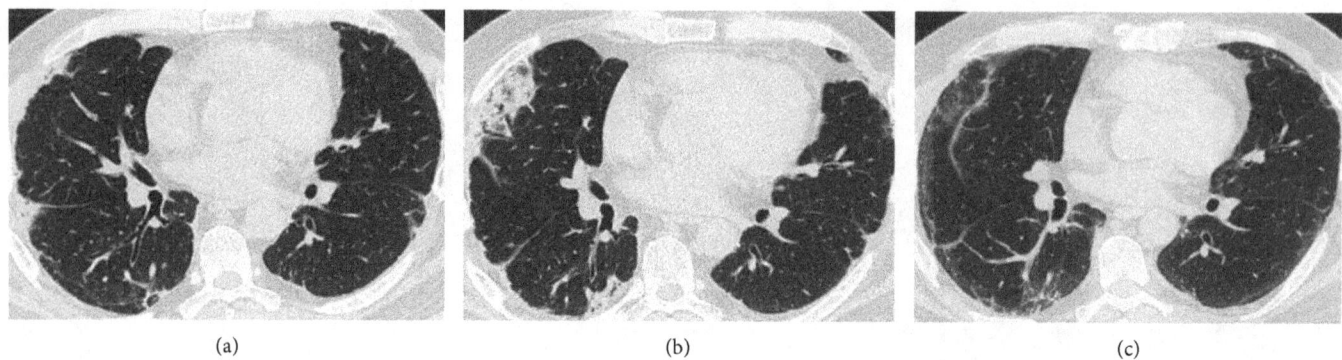

FIGURE 3: Chest computed tomography findings at admission (a), before the addition of rituximab (RTX) (b), and after RTX administration (c).

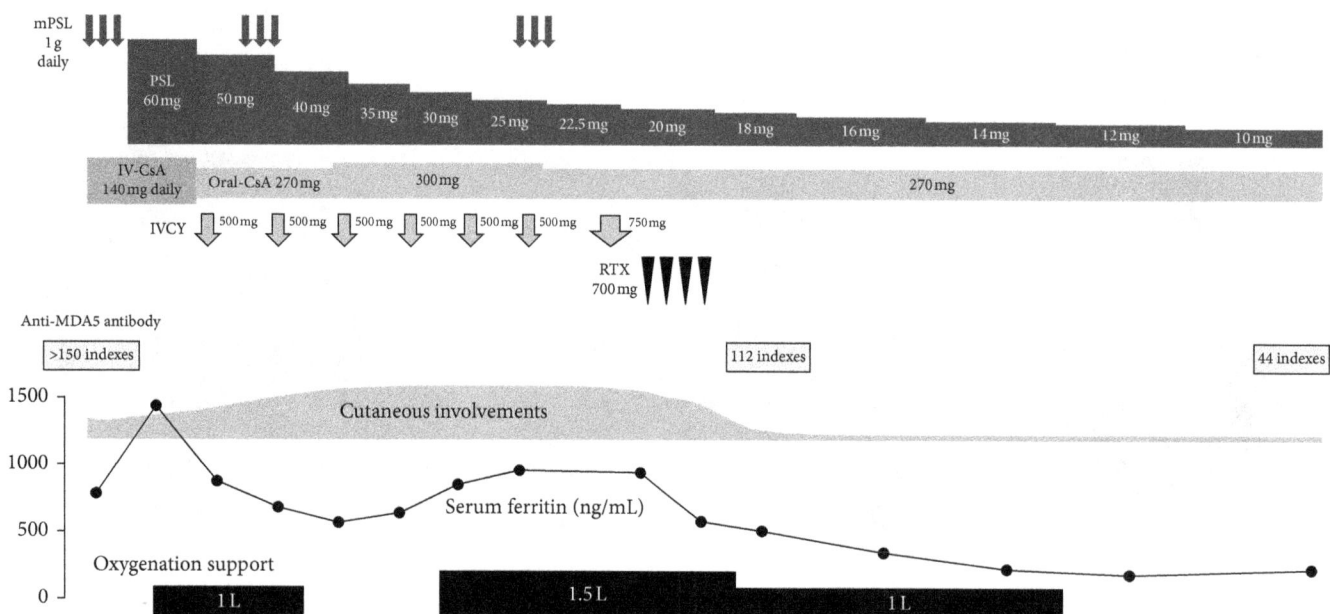

FIGURE 4: Clinical course of this patient. mPSL, methylprednisolone; PSL, prednisolone; IV-CsA, continuous intravenous infusion of cyclosporine A; oral-CsA, oral administration of cyclosporine A; IVCY, intravenous infusion of cyclophosphamide; RTX, rituximab.

palmar papules, and an erythematous rash on his face and back; in particular, ulcerative and erosive erythema was visible on his elbows (Figures 1 and 2). The pathological finding of the biopsied skin from his back demonstrated perivascular infiltration of inflammatory cells with lique-factive degeneration through the epidermis to the dermis (Figure 1(c)). Laboratory examinations revealed elevated serum levels of creatine kinase (CK) (278 U/L; normal, 43–230), C-reactive protein (0.59 mg/dL; normal, <0.10), ferritin (781 ng/mL; normal, 25–280), Krebs von den Lungen-6 (602 U/mL; normal, 105–435), and lactate de-hydrogenase (453 U/L; normal, 120–230). Anti-aminoacyl-tRNA synthetase (anti-ARS) antibodies were not detected; meanwhile, a high titer of anti-MDA5-Ab was seen (>150 indexes; normal, <32). The detection of anti-MDA5-Ab was performed by enzyme-linked immunosorbent assay. Tests for anti-nuclear antibody, rheumatoid factor, anti-citrullinated protein antibody, and anti-neutrophil cytoplasmic antibodies specific for either myeloperoxidase or proteinase-3 were negative. Arterial blood gas analysis revealed a PaO_2 of 66.4 mmHg and $PaCO_2$ of 32.9 mmHg on room air. Chest computed tomography (CT) revealed reticular shadows and ground-glass opacity on the middle to inferior fields of the bilateral lung (Figure 3(a)).

Since the patient was diagnosed with DM-related ILD and a low PaO_2, methylprednisolone (mPSL) (1 g daily for 3 consecutive days) was immediately administered together with a continuous intravenous infusion of cyclosporine A (IV-CsA) according to the previously described therapeutic protocol [9] (Figure 4). Subsequently, prednisolone (PSL) at the dose of 60 mg (1 mg/kg) daily and cyclosporine A, the blood trough concentration of which was adjusted to 150–200 ng/mL, were orally administered after mPSL and IV-CsA therapy, resulting in improved fatigue, appetite loss, fever, edema of the hands, eruptions on the face and back, and arthralgia. Muscle weakness also recovered, and serum CK level normalized. Meanwhile, respiratory insufficiency persisted, and oxygenation support was ultimately required.

TABLE 1: Summarized clinical profiles in patients of anti-MDA5-antibody–positive DM with ILD who were treated with rituximab.

Ref. no.	Sex/age	Preceding manifestations Respiratory (ILD)	Preceding manifestations Muscular (CK levels)	Preceding manifestations Cutaneous	Preceding manifestations Others	Previous treatment	Admission/after RTX [maximum][1] Ferritin (ng/mL)	Admission/after RTX [maximum][1] KL-6 (U/mL)	RTX targeting lesion	Duration prior to RTX[2]	RTX dosage (cycles)	Therapy during or after RTX	Outcome
[14]	F/68	Cough, unusual dyspnea	Generalized weakness (normal)	Raynaud, erythema on the face, back, limbs, and hands	Fever, arthralgia, appetite loss	mPSL, PSL, IVIg, IVCY, MMF, CsA, Tac (topical), HCQ	805/n.d.	n.d./n.d.	Cutaneous lesion	About 2 years	1000 mg, per 15 days (×2)	n.d.	Improved[3]
[15]	F/58	n.d.	Weakness on the deltoids (normal)	Heliotrope rash, Gottron's papules	n.d.	PSL, Tac, IVCY	891.7/n.d.	613/2756 [4185]	ILD	About 3 months	500 mg, 375 mg/m² week (×4)	mPSL, PSL, IVCY, IVIg, PMX	Improved
[16]	F/55	Rapidly progressive shortness of breath	None (normal)	Raynaud, heliotrope rash, Gottron's papules, rash on the hands	Weight loss	mPSL	n.d./n.d.	n.d./n.d.	ILD	n.d.	n.d.	CPA, PE	Died
[17]	F/71	Rapid deterioration of respiratory status, hypoxia	None (211 U/L)	Heliotrope rash, Gottron's papules, ulcer on the buttocks, papules on the fingers and elbows	Appetite loss, fatigue	mPSL, PSL, IVCY, IVIg, PMX	1782.8/253.1 [3149.8]	666/[4]	ILD cutaneous lesion	102 days	525 mg, 350 mg/m² week (×4)	PSL, Tac	Improved
[18]	F/71	Dry cough, continuous deterioration of respiratory status	None (n.d.)	Purpura on the elbows, erythema on the anterior chest	Fever	mPSL, PSL, Tac, CsA, IVCY	507/1740 [1740]	991/n.d.	ILD	38 days	600 mg, 375 mg/m² week (×2)	mPSL, PSL, CsA, MMF, Tac	Died
[18]	F/69	Exertional dyspnea, respiratory distress with hypoxia	None (225 U/L)	Gottron's papules, rash on the extremities, hyperkeratosis on the palmer side of fingers	Arthralgia	mPSL, PSL, CsA	219/1930	922/1520	ILD	33 days	500 mg, 375 mg/m² week (×2)	mPSL, PSL, CsA, IVCY, tocilizumab, CHD	Died
This case	M/48	Exertional dyspnea with hypoxia, dry cough	Mild weakness on the lower limbs (278 U/L)	Heliotrope rash, Gottron's papules, mechanic's hands, palmar papules, erythema on the face and back, ulcer/erosion on the elbows	Fatigue, fever, appetite loss, arthralgia	mPSL, PSL, CsA, IVCY	781/186 [1437]	602/638 [1674]	ILD cutaneous lesion	125 days	700 mg, 375 mg/m² week (×4)	PSL, CsA	Improved

DM, dermatomyositis; ILD, interstitial lung disease; Ref, reference; CK, creatine kinase; n.d., not described; Raynaud, Raynaud phenomenon; RTX, rituximab; mPSL, methylprednisolone; PSL, prednisolone; IVIg, intravenous immunoglobulin; IVCY, intravenous cyclophosphamide; MMF, mycophenolate mofetil; CsA, cyclosporine A; Tac, tacrolimus; HCQ, hydroxychloroquine; CPA, cyclophosphamide; PMX, polymyxin B hemoperfusion treatment; PE, plasma exchange; CHD, continuous hemodiafiltration. [1]Maximum value if it was described in the report. [2]Duration prior to administering RTX since initiating hospitalization. [3]Remission of painful erythematous papules on the hands was obtained [14]. [4]Decrease of KL-6 levels after RTX administration was shown in the figure of the described report [17].

Therefore, IVCY was additionally administered at the dosage of 500 mg every 2 weeks for 6 cycles. However, his respiratory status was gradually worsening even after additional administration of 750 mg of IVCY. Moreover, further exacerbation of the chest CT finding was obviously demonstrated (Figure 3(b)). In addition, ulcerative and erosive eruptions on his hands and elbows also deteriorated (Figures 2(b) and 2(e)). On the 125th day since the initiation of the therapy, RTX was administered at the dosage of 700 mg (375 mg/m^2) weekly for total 4 weeks. Consequently, cutaneous involvements on his hands and elbows were remarkably improved (Figures 2(c) and 2(f)), and recovery from respiratory insufficiency and amelioration of the radiographic finding were also achieved (Figure 3(c)). Furthermore, serum levels of ferritin and anti-MDA5-Ab decreased to 186 ng/mL and 44 indexes, respectively (Figure 4).

3. Discussion

This patient was found to be in the severe stage of ILD associated with DM because of having some prognostic factors including not only hypoxemia with anti-MDA5-Ab positivity but also refractory ulcerative eruptions as well as palmer papules. In fact, it has been previously described that existing cutaneous ulceration and/or palmer papules are associated with acute progression of ILD in DM [6, 7]; furthermore, the positive correlation between severity of ulcerative cutaneous involvement and anti-MDA5-Ab has been demonstrated [6, 19, 20]. In addition, anti-MDA5-Ab positivity is associated with fever and arthritis [19, 20], which were also revealed prior to initiating treatment in the present case. Therefore, immediate and intensive immunosuppressive therapy was required in this patient in order to avoid a fatal situation. It has been recognized that the concomitant use of CsA or tacrolimus with PSL is indispensable to prevent the progression of ILD in DM [21–23]; furthermore, additional administration of IVCY should be required in the acute exacerbation of the disease [7, 9, 23]. However, initial combination therapy, including PSL, CsA, and IVCY, was eventually insufficient for healing both cutaneous involvement and ILD. On the other hand, RTX therapy obviously contributed to achieving a favorable outcome.

MDA5 plays a crucial role in inducing an innate immune response against viral infection and is also recognized as the specific autoantigen in DM, suggesting that upregulation of MDA5 in the innate immune system subsequently promotes anti-MDA5-Ab production [24]. The production of specific autoantibodies in autoimmune diseases is attributed to autoreactive B cells; furthermore, RTX is found to succeed in depleting the pathogenic autoreactive B cells which secrete a specific autoantibody in several autoimmune diseases [25]. Even though autoreactive B cells also play the roles in activating effector T cells or producing proinflammatory cytokines, RTX may be indirectly implicated in preventing these immunological factors from attacking the target organ [25–27]. Interestingly, the recent overviewed study demonstrated that favorable therapeutic efficacy of RTX could be obtained in majority of patients with inflammatory myositis who had disease-specific autoantibodies [28]. It was described

that high titer of anti-MDA5-Ab is associated with the severity of disease [29, 30]. On the other hand, subsequent reduction of anti-MDA5-Ab after starting the treatment means obviously predicting a successful outcome [20]. Although this patient initially had a level of anti-MDA5-Ab over the upper measurable limit, RTX administration reduced the levels of anti-MDA5-Ab and serum ferritin, which is also known as the prognostic factor in DM-related RP-ILD [31] (Figure 4), demonstrating that RTX therapy could correspondingly contribute to the recovery from severe clinical situations and suppress the production of anti-MDA5-Ab. Given the relationship between the therapeutic mechanism of RTX and autoantibodies including anti-MDA5-Ab, RTX therapy may be a reasonable option for achieving a favorable outcome, especially in RP-ILD related to anti-MDA5-Ab–positive DM.

To our knowledge, six cases treated with RTX in anti-MDA5-Ab–positive DM with ILD have been reported in the English literature to date [14–18] (Table 1). Their clinical characteristics were CADM or minimal muscular manifestations, the latter of which is consistent with the present case. One patient was also given RTX to treat the refractory cutaneous involvement even after ILD remission induced by the prior immunosuppressive therapy, whereas others required RTX because the preceding use of other immunosuppressive agents was ineffective in suppressing the exacerbation of ILD with or without cutaneous involvement. However, only half of them recovered from the RP-ILD, suggesting that it may be necessary to initiate effective therapy within the reversible state of disease even if RTX is a potential remedy in cases that are resistant to the prevalent immunosuppressive therapies.

Anti-MDA5-Ab–positive DM usually emerges with refractory cutaneous involvement and/or RP-ILD as a life-threatening complication. The present case demonstrated that RTX could be a useful therapy for achieving a favorable outcome. On the other hand, further clinical experiences must be accumulated to establish the therapeutic strategy using RTX for this disease.

References

[1] M. C. Dalakas and R. Hohlfeld, "Polymyositis and dermatomyositis," *Lancet*, vol. 362, no. 9388, pp. 971–982, 2003.

[2] P. Gerami, J. M. Schope, L. McDonald, H. W. Walling, and R. D. Sontheimer, "A systematic review of adult-onset clinically amyopathic dermatomyositis (dermatomyositis sine myositis): a missing link within the spectrum of the idiopathic inflammatory myopathies," *Journal of the American Academy of Dermatology*, vol. 54, no. 4, pp. 597–613, 2006.

[3] S. Sato, M. Hirakata, M. Kuwana et al., "Autoantibodies to a 140-kd polypeptide, CADM-140, in Japanese patients with clinically amyopathic dermatomyositis," *Arthritis and Rheumatism*, vol. 52, no. 5, pp. 1571–1576, 2005.

[4] T. Gono, Y. Kawaguchi, T. Satoh et al., "Clinical manifestation and prognostic factor in anti-melanoma differentiation-associated

gene 5 antibody-associated interstitial lung disease as a complication of dermatomyositis," *Rheumatology*, vol. 49, no. 9, pp. 1713–1719, 2010.

[5] Y. Muro, K. Sugiura, K. Hoshino, and M. Akiyama, "Disappearance of anti-MDA-5 autoantibodies in clinically amyopathic DM/interstitial lung disease during disease remission," *Rheumatology*, vol. 51, no. 5, pp. 800–804, 2012.

[6] H. Cao, M. Pan, Y. Kang et al., "Clinical manifestations of dermatomyositis and clinically amyopathic dermatomyositis patients with positive expression of anti-melanoma differentiation-associated gene 5 antibody," *Arthritis Care & Research*, vol. 64, no. 10, pp. 1602–1610, 2012.

[7] H. Kameda, H. Nagasawa, H. Ogawa et al., "Combination therapy with corticosteroids, cyclosporin A, and intravenous pulse cyclophosphamide for acute/subacute interstitial pneumonia in patients with dermatomyositis," *Journal of Rheumatology*, vol. 32, no. 9, pp. 1719–1726, 2005.

[8] Y. Matsuki, H. Yamashita, Y. Takahashi et al., "Diffuse alveolar damage in patients with dermatomyositis: a six-case series," *Modern Rheumatology*, vol. 22, no. 2, pp. 243–248, 2012.

[9] Y. Shimojima, W. Ishii, M. Matsuda, D. Kishida, and S. I. Ikeda, "Effective use of calcineurin inhibitor in combination therapy for interstitial lung disease in patients with dermatomyositis and polymyositis," *Journal of Clinical Rheumatology*, vol. 23, no. 2, pp. 87–93, 2017.

[10] C. V. Oddis, A. M. Reed, R. Aggarwal et al., "Rituximab in the treatment of refractory adult and juvenile dermatomyositis and adult polymyositis: a randomized, placebo-phase trial," *Arthritis and Rheumatism*, vol. 65, no. 2, pp. 314–324, 2013.

[11] R. Aggarwal, P. Loganathan, D. Koontz, Z. Qi, A. M. Reed, and C. V. Oddis, "Cutaneous improvement in refractory adult and juvenile dermatomyositis after treatment with rituximab," *Rheumatology*, vol. 56, no. 2, pp. 247–254, 2017.

[12] H. Andersson, M. Sem, M. B. Lund et al., "Long-term experience with rituximab in anti-synthetase syndrome-related interstitial lung disease," *Rheumatology*, vol. 54, no. 8, pp. 1420–1428, 2015.

[13] I. Marie, S. Dominique, A. Janvresse, H. Levesque, and J. F. Menard, "Rituximab therapy for refractory interstitial lung disease related to antisynthetase syndrome," *Respiratory Medicine*, vol. 106, no. 4, pp. 581–587, 2012.

[14] A. Clottu, E. Laffitte, C. Prins, and C. Chizzolini, "Response of mucocutaneous lesions to rituximab in a case of melanoma differentiation antigen 5-related dermatomyositis," *Dermatology*, vol. 225, no. 4, pp. 376–380, 2012.

[15] R. Watanabe, T. Ishii, K. Araki et al., "Successful multi-target therapy using corticosteroid, tacrolimus, cyclophosphamide, and rituximab for rapidly progressive interstitial lung disease in a patient with clinically amyopathic dermatomyositis," *Modern Rheumatology*, vol. 26, no. 3, pp. 465–466, 2016.

[16] B. Gil, L. Merav, L. Pnina, and G. Chagai, "Diagnosis and treatment of clinically amyopathic dermatomyositis (CADM): a case series and literature review," *Clinical Rheumatology*, vol. 35, no. 8, pp. 2125–2130, 2016.

[17] Y. Koichi, Y. Aya, U. Megumi et al., "A case of anti-MDA5-positive rapidly progressive interstitial lung disease in a patient with clinically amyopathic dermatomyositis ameliorated by rituximab, in addition to standard immunosuppressive treatment," *Modern Rheumatology*, vol. 27, no. 3, pp. 536–540, 2017.

[18] K. Tokunaga and N. Hagino, "Dermatomyositis with rapidly progressive interstitial lung disease treated with rituximab: a report of 3 cases in Japan," *Internal Medicine*, vol. 56, no. 11, pp. 1399–1403, 2017.

[19] D. Fiorentino, L. Chung, J. Zwerner, A. Rosen, and L. Casciola-Rosen, "The mucocutaneous and systemic phenotype of dermatomyositis patients with antibodies to MDA5 (CADM-140): a retrospective study," *Journal of the American Academy of Dermatology*, vol. 65, no. 1, pp. 25–34, 2011.

[20] S. Sato, A. Murakami, A. Kuwajima et al., "Clinical utility of an enzyme-linked immunosorbent assay for detecting anti-melanoma differentiation-associated gene 5 autoantibodies," *PLoS One*, vol. 11, no. 4, p. e0154285, 2016.

[21] T. Kotani, S. Makino, T. Takeuchi et al., "Early intervention with corticosteroids and cyclosporin A and 2-hour postdose blood concentration monitoring improves the prognosis of acute/subacute interstitial pneumonia in dermatomyositis," *Journal of Rheumatology*, vol. 35, no. 2, pp. 254–259, 2008.

[22] T. Kurita, S. Yasuda, K. Oba et al., "The efficacy of tacrolimus in patients with interstitial lung diseases complicated with polymyositis or dermatomyositis," *Rheumatology*, vol. 54, no. 1, pp. 39–44, 2015.

[23] T. Kurita, S. Yasuda, O. Amengual, and T. Atsumi, "The efficacy of calcineurin inhibitors for the treatment of interstitial lung disease associated with polymyositis/dermatomyositis," *Lupus*, vol. 24, no. 1, pp. 3–9, 2015.

[24] S. Sato, K. Hoshino, T. Satoh et al., "RNA helicase encoded by melanoma differentiation-associated gene 5 is a major autoantigen in patients with clinically amyopathic dermatomyositis: association with rapidly progressive interstitial lung disease," *Arthritis and Rheumatism*, vol. 60, no. 7, pp. 2193–2200, 2009.

[25] P. Engel, J. A. Gomez-Puerta, M. Ramos-Casals, F. Lozano, and X. Bosch, "Therapeutic targeting of B cells for rheumatic autoimmune diseases," *Pharmacological Reviews*, vol. 63, no. 1, pp. 127–156, 2011.

[26] R. Stasi, G. Del Poeta, E. Stipa et al., "Response to B-cell depleting therapy with rituximab reverts the abnormalities of T-cell subsets in patients with idiopathic thrombocytopenic purpura," *Blood*, vol. 110, no. 8, pp. 2924–2930, 2007.

[27] N. Jacob and W. Stohl, "Autoantibody-dependent and autoantibody-independent roles for B cells in systemic lupus erythematosus: past, present, and future," *Autoimmunity*, vol. 43, no. 1, pp. 84–97, 2010.

[28] S. Fasano, P. Gordon, R. Hajji, E. Loyo, and D. A. Isenberg, "Rituximab in the treatment of inflammatory myopathies: a review," *Rheumatology*, vol. 56, no. 1, pp. 26–36, 2017.

[29] T. Takada, A. Aoki, K. Asakawa et al., "Serum cytokine profiles of patients with interstitial lung disease associated with anti-CADM-140/MDA5 antibody positive amyopathic dermatomyositis," *Respiratory Medicine*, vol. 109, no. 9, pp. 1174–1180, 2015.

[30] S. Sato, M. Kuwana, T. Fujita, and Y. Suzuki, "Anti-CADM-140/MDA5 autoantibody titer correlates with disease activity and predicts disease outcome in patients with dermatomyositis and rapidly progressive interstitial lung disease," *Modern Rheumatology*, vol. 23, no. 3, pp. 496–502, 2013.

[31] T. Gono, Y. Kawaguchi, M. Hara et al., "Increased ferritin predicts development and severity of acute interstitial lung disease as a complication of dermatomyositis," *Rheumatology*, vol. 49, no. 7, pp. 1354–1360, 2010.

37

HIV Infection and Osteoarticular Tuberculosis: Strange Bedfellows

B. Hodkinson,[1] N. Osman,[2] and S. Botha-Scheepers[1]

[1]Department of Medicine, Division of Rheumatology, University of Cape Town and Groote Schuur Hospital,
Cape Town 7945, South Africa
[2]Division of Anatomical Pathology, National Health Laboratory Service, University of Cape Town and Groote Schuur Hospital,
Cape Town 7945, South Africa

Correspondence should be addressed to B. Hodkinson; drbridget@gmail.com

Academic Editor: Suleyman Serdar Koca

We report the case of a 47-year-old female patient with rheumatoid arthritis and HIV infection presenting with a 3-week history of a painful swollen knee, increased serum inflammatory markers, and a low CD4 lymphocyte count. The diagnosis of TB arthritis was made by synovial fluid culture, GeneXpert/PCR, and confirmed by histopathology of a synovial biopsy. A mini literature review suggests that although HIV infection is associated with extrapulmonary TB, osteoarticular TB is a relatively unusual presentation in an HIV positive patient. The diagnostic utility of the GeneXpert test is explored. We also describe the patient's good response to an intra-articular corticosteroid injection in combination with standard anti-TB therapy.

1. Introduction

Patients infected with human immunodeficiency virus (HIV) are at increased risk of tuberculosis (TB) coinfection. We describe an unusual presentation of HIV and TB coinfection in a patient with rheumatoid arthritis (RA). We present a mini literature review and discussion regarding 3 aspects of this case:

(i) the association between HIV and osteoarticular TB;

(ii) diagnostic tests;

(iii) adjuvant management.

2. Case Presentation

A 47-year-old female with seropositive RA was diagnosed 6 years previously with a 3-week history of a painful right knee. She reported no fever, night sweats, cough, or loss of weight and had received no recent intra-articular steroid injections. Two years earlier she was diagnosed with HIV infection and was initiated on combination antiretroviral (ARV) therapy (tenofovir/efavirenz/emtricitabine). Her RA therapy consisted of methotrexate (MTX) 15 mg weekly and prednisone 7.5 mg daily and the RA had been in remission for 24 months prior to this presentation. She had no history of previous TB.

Examination revealed a thin middle-aged female with a swollen tender right knee with a reduced range of motion. She was afebrile with clinically inactive RA, and there was no tenderness or swelling of her other joints. Blood investigations showed a normochromic anaemia (hemoglobin = 10.3 g/dL), leukocytosis (WCC = 19.3×10^9/L), and thrombocytosis (platelet = 486×10^9/L). Her C-reactive protein was elevated (340 mg/L) and CD4 cell count was low (199/mm^3). Chest and knee radiographs were normal. Pus was aspirated from the right knee and submitted for microbiology with Gram and Ziehl-Neelsen stain negative. GeneXpert on the fluid was positive. Culture was positive at 21 days for *Mycobacterium tuberculosis*. A synovial biopsy submitted for histology revealed necrotising granulomatous inflammation and the Ziehl-Neelsen stain was positive for acid-fast bacilli (Figures 1–3) confirming the diagnosis of osteoarticular TB/tubercular arthritis. MTX was discontinued, and combination antituberculous therapy was started. Due to the

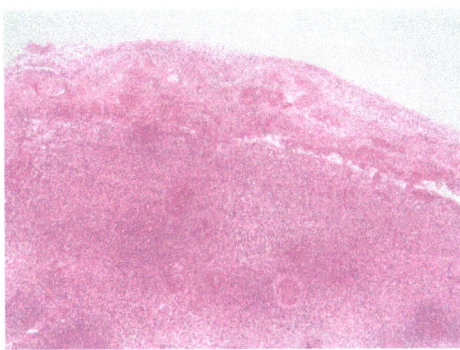

FIGURE 1: Haematoxylin and Eosin (H&E) stain of the synovial biopsy showing foci of granulomatous inflammation (20x magnification).

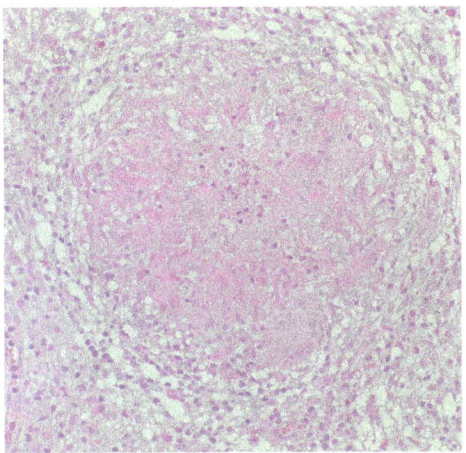

FIGURE 2: H + E stain of synovial biopsy showing granulomatous inflammation (400x magnification).

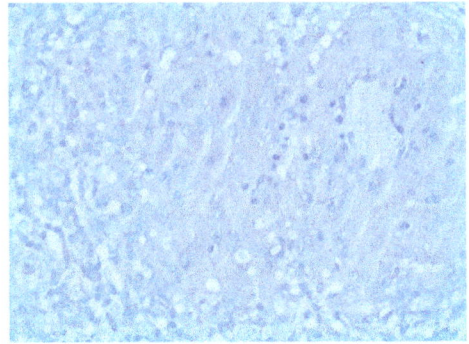

FIGURE 3: Ziehl-Neelsen stain of synovial biopsy showing acid-fast bacillus (arrow) (400x magnification).

ongoing symptoms of the arthritis, a single intra-articular corticosteroid injection (methylprednisolone acetate 80 mg) was administered. Clinical improvement and a good range of motion of the right knee were noted within 2 weeks. At her follow-up visit at 3 months she was symptom-free and had recovered the full range of motion of the joint. Her blood counts normalised, her CRP was 3, and the CD4 cell count improved to 410/mm^3.

3. Discussion

The single most important risk factor for contracting TB is HIV infection, particularly in Sub-Saharan Africa where HIV-related TB comprises 79% of TB cases [1]. In particular, extrapulmonary forms of TB (ExP-TB) are encountered in HIV positive patients with low CD4 lymphocyte counts. Skeletal TB is an uncommon form of ExP-TB and affects either the spine (comprising 5% of ExP-TB) or peripheral joints as "osteoarticular TB (OA-TB)" which constitutes a further 5% of ExP-TB. Usually presenting as a chronic monoarthritis, most often affecting the hip, knee, or wrist joint, OA-TB typically has an insidious onset without constitutional symptoms or features of pulmonary TB [2].

Many reports claim a strong association between OA-TB and HIV infection, including a review from Zambia that describes 60% of OA-TB cases as HIV-associated [3]. However, studies of OA-TB, including studies from areas of high HIV prevalence, report very few HIV positive cases (Table 1), suggesting that HIV infection may not be a risk factor for OA-TB. It has been shown in Soweto, South Africa, that although HIV is associated with ExP-TB, the relative frequency of OA-TB amongst HIV positive patients was significantly lower than in HIV negative patients [4]. A South African study of TB-associated skeletal changes revealed an increase in the number of cases with skeletal TB, from 28% in the pre-1985 era to 41% after 1985 [5]. In the case of TB spine, there may be more convincing evidence of an association with HIV, with 17–33% of cases testing HIV positive in areas with a high prevalence of HIV (such as South Africa, Nigeria, Morocco, and Spain) and a much lower incidence (0–8%) elsewhere [6]. A recent report from SA described 20 cases of TB spine with half of these patients coinfected with HIV [7]. HIV positive patients have been shown to have less vertebral body destruction and more abscess formation compared to HIV negative patients. Microscopic features between the two groups are similar but an inverted CD4 : CD8 lymphocyte ratio is seen within the granulomas of patients coinfected with HIV [8, 9].

The synovial fluid of our patient was GeneXpert positive. GeneXpert MTB/RIF (Cepheid, Sunnyvale, CA, USA) is a polymerase chain reaction (PCR) assay allowing rapid diagnosis of TB and detection of resistance to rifampicin. Sputum GeneXpert detects with a high specificity the majority of pulmonary TB cases and is a useful screening test for ExP-TB, in particular CSF and tissue specimens [10]. For the diagnosis of TB spine, PCR tests on pus or vertebral bone samples have a very high sensitivity and specificity (96% and 96–100%, resp.) [11, 12]. In the case of synovial fluid, PCR tests have shown moderate sensitivity (63%) but excellent specificity (92–100%) [13]. Thus PCR tests are a useful and very convenient test for OA-TB, but synovial biopsy should be performed in patients with a negative test. A recent study from Mexico demonstrated the excellent clinical utility of serum PCR in the diagnosis of spine and OA-TB, with sensitivity and specificity of 91% and 97%, respectively [14].

The patient described in this case study was on MTX, low dose oral corticosteroids, and ARV therapy. The safety of MTX in patients who are HIV positive is uncertain. In patients with low CD4 counts, MTX may predispose patients

TABLE 1: Case series of osteoarticular TB with HIV status.

Country	Duration of study	Number of HIV+ cases/no of OA-TB* cases (%)	Antiretroviral therapy
India [22]	2010–2012	0/13	—
India [23]	—	0/93	—
Thailand [24]	1997–2006	1/77	—
Nigeria [25]	1998–2009	0/97**	
France [26] (including 74% African immigrants)	1980–1994	1/206**	
United Kingdom [27] (including 89% South Asian immigrants)	1988–2005	0/44	—
Denmark [28] (including 50% Somalian refugees)	1993–1997	3/26**	—
US [29]	1999–2003	1/31 (3.2%)	All on ARV therapy
China [30]	2011-2012	0/43	—
Thailand [31]	1994–2002	1/27 (3.7%)	—

OA-TB: osteoarticular TB; ARV therapy: antiretroviral therapy.
*Extraspinal OA-TB cases only.
**Spine and extraspinal OA-TB cases combined.

further to opportunistic infections, including TB [15]. The use of MTX in HIV positive individuals may be acceptable in the setting of a CD4 count >200, particularly if ARV therapies are prescribed and if the patient is closely followed up.

We treated our patient with antituberculous therapy and an intra-articular corticosteroid injection, with a fairly dramatic resolution of signs and symptoms and restoration of joint function. The rationale for this management approach was based on the postulated role of the immune-mediated response to TB in the development of joint damage in OA-TB. Reducing inflammation may preserve the articular cartilage and joint space. In a study of rabbits with staphylococcal septic arthritis, intra-articular steroids reduced joint damage [16]. A similar approach in humans may be beneficial [17]. In two randomized placebo-controlled trials in children with bacterial arthritis, adjuvant intravenous corticosteroids in combination with antibiotic therapy reduced the clinical symptoms and improved outcomes without any adverse effects [18, 19].

Adjuvant corticosteroids reduce complications and improve survival in TB meningitis and in the case of TB pericarditis reduce the incidence of constrictive pericarditis, which may be analogous to joint destruction and contractures in the setting of OA-TB [20, 21]. Randomized controlled studies would establish the role of adjuvant intra-articular corticosteroids in the management of OA-TB.

In summary, this case is a relatively unusual presentation of ExP-TB in an HIV positive patient. The diagnosis was aided by a positive GeneXpert test, and an excellent outcome was achieved. Adjuvant intra-articular corticosteroids may have hastened resolution of the clinical symptoms and signs of infection.

Competing Interests

The authors declare that they have no competing interests.

References

[1] World Health Organisation, *Key indicators for the WHO African Region Global Tuberculosis Report 2014*, World Health Organization, Geneva, Switzerland, 2014.

[2] M. M. Madkour, A. J. Kudwah, and M. A. El Bagi, *Tuberculosis*, Springer, Berlin, Germany, 2004.

[3] J. E. Jellis, "Human immunodeficiency virus and osteoarticular tuberculosis," *Clinical Orthopaedics and Related Research*, no. 398, pp. 27–31, 2002.

[4] B. Hodkinson, E. Musenge, and M. Tikly, "Osteoarticular tuberculosis in patients with systemic lupus erythematosus," *Quarterly Journal of Medicine*, vol. 102, no. 5, pp. 321–328, 2009.

[5] M. Steyn, Y. Scholtz, D. Botha, and S. Pretorius, "The changing face of tuberculosis: trends in tuberculosis-associated skeletal changes," *Tuberculosis*, vol. 93, no. 4, pp. 467–474, 2013.

[6] M. Fuentes Ferrer, L. Gutierrez Torres, O. Ayala Ramírez, M. R. Zarzuelo, and N. Del Prado González, "Tuberculosis of the spine. A systematic review of case series," *International Orthopaedics*, vol. 36, no. 2, pp. 221–231, 2012.

[7] R. Dunn, A. van der Horst, and S. Lippross, "Tuberculosis of the spine—prospective neurological and patient reported outcome study," *Clinical Neurology and Neurosurgery*, vol. 133, pp. 96–101, 2015.

[8] C. Anley, A. Brandt, and R. Dunn, "Magnetic resonance imaging findings in spinal tuberculosis: comparison of HIV positive and negative patients," *Indian Journal of Orthopaedics*, vol. 46, no. 2, pp. 186–190, 2012.

[9] S. Danaviah, J. A. Sacks, K. P. S. Kumar et al., "Immunohistological characterization of spinal TB granulomas from HIV-negative and -positive patients," *Tuberculosis*, vol. 93, no. 4, pp. 432–441, 2013.

[10] L. Maynard-Smith, N. Larke, J. A. Peters, and S. D. Lawn, "Diagnostic accuracy of the Xpert MTB/RIF assay for extrapulmonary and pulmonary tuberculosis when testing non-respiratory samples: a systematic review," *BMC Infectious Diseases*, vol. 14, no. 1, article 709, 2014.

[11] M. Held, M. Laubscher, H. J. Zar, and R. N. Dunn, "GeneXpert polymerase chain reaction for spinal tuberculosis: an accurate and rapid diagnostic test," *Bone and Joint Journal*, vol. 96, no. 10, pp. 1366–1369, 2014.

[12] V. Pandey, K. Chawla, K. Acharya, S. Rao, and S. Rao, "The role of polymerase chain reaction in the management of osteoarticular tuberculosis," *International Orthopaedics*, vol. 33, no. 3, pp. 801–805, 2009.

[13] V. K. Aggarwal, D. Nair, G. Khanna, J. Verma, V. K. Sharma, and S. Batra, "Use of amplified Mycobacterium tuberculosis direct test (Gen-probe Inc., San Diego, CA, USA) in the diagnosis of tubercular synovitis and early arthritis of knee joint," *Indian Journal of Orthopaedics*, vol. 46, no. 5, pp. 531–535, 2012.

[14] G. García-Elorriaga, O. Martínez-Elizondo, G. Del Rey-Pineda, and C. González-Bonilla, "Clinical, radiological and molecular diagnosis correlation in serum samples from patients with osteoarticular tuberculosis," *Asian Pacific Journal of Tropical Biomedicine*, vol. 4, no. 7, pp. 581–585, 2014.

[15] M. Tikly, "The scourge of HIV infection in sub-Saharan Africa—a rheumatological perspective," *Journal of Rheumatology*, vol. 38, no. 6, pp. 973–974, 2011.

[16] A. J. Wysenbeek, J. Volchek, M. Amit, D. Robinson, I. Boldur, and Z. Nevo, "Treatment of staphylococcal septic arthritis in rabbits by systemic antibiotics and intra-articular corticosteroids," *Annals of the Rheumatic Diseases*, vol. 57, no. 11, pp. 687–690, 1998.

[17] S. E. Lane and P. Merry, "Intra-articular corticosteroids in septic arthritis: beneficial or barmy?" *Annals of the Rheumatic Diseases*, vol. 59, article 240, 2000.

[18] L. Harel, D. Prais, E. Bar-On et al., "Dexamethasone therapy for septic arthritis in children: results of a randomized double-blind placebo-controlled study," *Journal of Pediatric Orthopaedics*, vol. 31, no. 2, pp. 211–215, 2011.

[19] C. M. Odio, T. Ramirez, G. Arias et al., "Double blind, randomized, placebo-controlled study of dexamethasone therapy for hematogenous septic arthritis in children," *Pediatric Infectious Disease Journal*, vol. 22, no. 10, pp. 883–888, 2003.

[20] B. M. Mayosi, M. Ntsekhe, J. Bosch et al., "Prednisolone and *Mycobacterium indicus pranii* in tuberculous pericarditis," *The New England Journal of Medicine*, vol. 371, no. 12, pp. 1121–1130, 2014.

[21] S. Wasserman and G. Meintjes, "The diagnosis, management and prevention of HIV-associated tuberculosis," *South African Medical Journal*, vol. 104, no. 12, pp. 886–893, 2014.

[22] N. Arathi, F. Ahmad, and N. Huda, "Osteoarticular tuberculosis-a three years' retrospective study," *Journal of Clinical and Diagnostic Research*, vol. 7, no. 10, pp. 2189–2192, 2013.

[23] V. Agashe, S. Shenai, G. Mohrir et al., "Osteoarticular tuberculosis—diagnostic solutions in a disease endemic region," *Journal of Infection in Developing Countries*, vol. 3, no. 7, pp. 511–516, 2009.

[24] C. Foocharoen, R. Nanagara, T. Foocharoen, P. Mootsikapun, S. Suwannaroj, and A. Mahakkanukrauh, "Clinical features of tuberculous septic arthritis in Khon Kaen, Thailand: a 10-year retrospective study," *Southeast Asian Journal of Tropical Medicine and Public Health*, vol. 41, no. 6, pp. 1438–1446, 2010.

[25] E. Iyidobi, C. Nwadinigwe, and R. Ekwunife, "Management of musculoskeletal tuberculosis in enugu, Nigeria," *Tropical Medicine & Surgery*, vol. 1, pp. 1–3, 2013.

[26] E. Pertuiset, J. Beaudreuil, A. Horusitzky et al., "Epidemiologic patterns of bone and joint tuberculosis in adults. A retrospective study of 206 cases," *Presse Medicale*, vol. 26, no. 7, pp. 311–315, 1997.

[27] D. S. Sandher, M. Al-Jibury, R. W. Paton, and L. P. Ormerod, "Bone and joint tuberculosis: cases in Blackburn between 1988 and 2005," *The Journal of Bone & Joint Surgery—British Volume*, vol. 89, no. 10, pp. 1379–1381, 2007.

[28] S. Houshian, S. Poulsen, and P. Riegels-Nielsen, "Bone and joint tuberculosis in Denmark: increase due to immigration," *Acta Orthopaedica Scandinavica*, vol. 71, no. 3, pp. 312–315, 2000.

[29] J. Marquez, C. S. Restrepo, L. Candia, A. Berman, and L. R. Espinoza, "Human immunodeficiency virus-associated rheumatic disorders in the HAART era," *Journal of Rheumatology*, vol. 31, no. 4, pp. 741–746, 2004.

[30] S.-T. Chen, L.-P. Zhao, W.-J. Dong et al., "The clinical features and bacteriological characterizations of bone and joint tuberculosis in China," *Scientific Reports*, vol. 5, Article ID 11084, 2015.

[31] P. Lertsrisatit, K. Nantiruj, K. Totemchokchyakarn, and S. Janwityanujit, "Extraspinal tuberculous arthritis in HIV era," *Clinical Rheumatology*, vol. 26, no. 3, pp. 319–321, 2007.

38

The Case of Reactive Arthritis Secondary to *Echinococcus* Infestation

Bülent Alım,[1] **Sinan Çetinel,**[2] **M. Alperen Servi,**[2]
Fahrettin Bostancı,[2] **and Mehmet Ozan Bingöl**[2]

[1]*Clinic of Physical Medicine and Rehabilitation, Bayburt State Hospital, Bayburt, Turkey*
[2]*Clinic of Physical Medicine and Rehabilitation, Cumhuriyet University Hospital, Sivas, Turkey*

Correspondence should be addressed to Sinan Çetinel; drsinancetinel@gmail.com

Academic Editor: Remzi Cevik

Reactive arthritis is an inflammatory joint disease that develops after an infection and it usually occurs following a gastrointestinal or genitourinary system infection and it belongs to the family of arthritis called "spondyloarthritis." We wanted to represent a rare case of reactive arthritis secondary to *Echinococcus* infestation. Cyst hydatid disease is common in endemic regions like Turkey. Internal organ involvements, especially liver and lung, are most frequent involvements. Primary bone involvement is rare complication of *Echinococcus* infestation. In our case, the patient with *Echinococcus* infection developed right knee arthritis and sacroiliitis. Other reactive and oligoarthritis causes were excluded and diagnosis of reactive arthritis secondary to cyst hydatid infestation was done with the present findings. Cold pack and TENS treatment were applied as symptomatic treatment to the right knee of the patient. Acemetacin was given as medical treatment. On the 5th day of treatment, right knee and ankle arthritis were clinically regressed. In regions where the disease is seen as endemic, such as Turkey, patients with musculoskeletal symptoms should consider the possibility of musculoskeletal involvement due to the hydatid cyst.

1. Introduction

Reactive arthritis is usually described as nonseptic arthritis arising in the joint after a bacterial infection [1]. It usually occurs following a gastrointestinal or genitourinary system infection and it belongs to the family of arthritis called "spondyloarthritis." Cases of reactive arthritis that develops after many infections have been reported, although it often follows after classical agents like *Salmonella*, *Shigella*, *Campylobacter*, and *Yersinia* infections [2]. Reactive arthritis cases due to different parasitic infestations have also been reported. Most of these cases develop due to the infestation of *Giardia lamblia* parasites [3–8]. Although it is known that parasitic infestations lead to development of arthritis, there is little information in the literature on this topic [8]. Cyst hydatid disease is a parasitic infection that is seen all over the world and it is endemic in the southern parts of Middle East, Africa, South America, New Zealand, Australia, Turkey, India, and southern parts of Europe [9]. The disease most commonly occurs in liver (55–70%) and lungs (18–35%) resulting from

infestation of the parasite named *Echinococcus granulosus*. More rarely, other organs and systemic involvement can also be seen. Bone involvement is around 1% [9] and it has also been reported that this disease rarely causes arthritic diseases [10]. We also wanted to represent a rare case of reactive arthritis secondary to *Echinococcus* infestation.

2. Case Presentation

A 53-year-old female patient consulted physical medicine, rehabilitation and rheumatology department due to the pain radiating from the right inguinal region and the right hip to knee while she was being followed by general surgery clinic because of solid mass in the liver. During the assessment, patient complained of having an intermittent backache for a long time; she described a constant pain in her right hip and groin spreading to right knee that started 1 week ago and was increasing with rest. Patient also reported there was pain and slight swelling in the right ankle 10 days

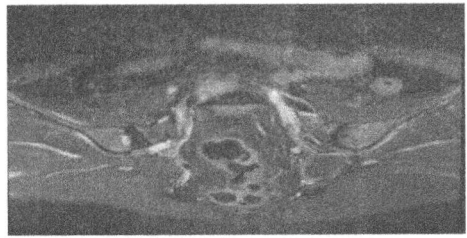

FIGURE 1: Signal enhancement consistent with the right iliac focal bone marrow edema adjacent to the right sacroiliac junction, T2 MRI sequences.

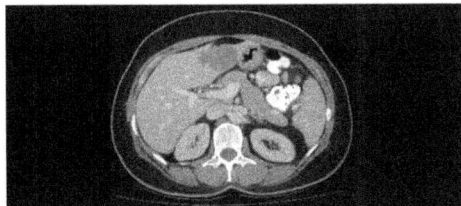

FIGURE 2: Liver hydatid cyst in abdomen tomography.

before that lasted for 3 days. In her background no previous illness is noted. Patient had an abdominal pain lasting for the last 6 months and abdominal ultrasound was performed; a solid mass was detected in the liver. We learned that the patient had no history of arthritis, gastroenteritis, urinary tract infection, psoriasis, or previous operation. She has not been using any medication except for analgesic. The patient had no relatives with history of inflammatory disease or malignancy in her family history. In the physical examination loss of lumbar lordosis was detected. Waist movement was slightly restricted to all directions due to pain, hand fingertip-to-floor distance was 10 cm, sacroiliac compression test was positive on the right, FABERE test was positive on the right, her right knee was warm and tender, there was no rash on the skin, local sensitivity was detected in the right upper quadrant with palpation, and other system evaluations were normal. Sacroiliac MRI was seen because of the suspicion of sacroiliitis. The sacroiliac MRI, which was assessed independently by radiology department, showed a signal enhancement consistent with the right iliac focal bone marrow edema adjacent to the right sacroiliac junction (Figure 1) and there were 2 cystic lesions at iliac front adjacent to the right hip joint. Abdomen tomography of our patient, which was requested by general surgery department, showed a well-defined 55×48 mm hypodense lesion with a superior calcification (lily symptom) in segment 3 (Figure 2). Hydatid cyst hemagglutination titer test was 1/320 and the patient was diagnosed as hydatid cyst disease. The patient was taken to our clinic because of development of right ankle arthritis and right knee arthritis.

In our clinic, the laboratory tests required for sacroiliitis and arthritis etiology were done. The results of these tests showed that RF was negative, anti-CCP was negative, anti-cardiolipin antibodies were negative, ds DNA was negative, ANA was negative, c-ANCA and p-ANCA were negative,

sedimentation was 38 m/h, CRP was 23 mg/L, WBC was 7,31 (103/12.7 g/dL), PLT was 364 (103/μL), tumor markers were negative. In addition, *Brucella* Wright and Coombs agglutination tests were negative. EBV VCA Ig M, EBV VCA Ig G, and Anti-CMV Ig G were detected as positive; EBV EA, Anti-CMV IG m were detected as negative. The right knee joint was punctured and 60 cc yellow clear liquid aspirated. At the examination of knee joint fluid Tbc DNA, tbc real time PCR, mycobacterial culture were detected as negative and there was no reproduction in cell culture; 8000 leucocytes (30% MNL, 70% PMNL) and 20 erythrocytes were detected in the cell analysis of aspiration fluid. Microscopic examination of the joint fluid showed no protoscolex and hook structures of the *Echinococcus* parasite. There was no reproduction in the blood culture. Anti-HCV, HBsAg, and Anti-HIV tests were negative. There was no evidence in the ECO for infective endocarditis. The patient consulted pulmonary medicine department. In the assessment PPD test was 5 mm and sputum culture and microscopic examination showed no Tbc *Bacillus*. HLA-B27 genetic assay was negative for spondyloarthropathy. The patient is diagnosed as reactive arthritis secondary to echinococcal infestation after all tests and no history of other diseases which can cause sacroiliitis and peripheral arthritis like SPA (spondyloarthropathy), familial Mediterranean fever, Behçet's disease, sarcoidosis, inflammatory bowel disease, and malignancy. Symptomatic treatment as 4×1 cold pack and TENS treatment were applied to the right knee of the patient. Acemetacin 60 mg capsule 2×1 was given as medical treatment. On the 5th day of treatment, right knee and ankle arthritis were clinically regressed and then patient was directed to the general surgery department for surgical treatment of hydatid cysts.

3. Discussion

Cyst hydatid disease is *Echinococcus granulosus* cestode larval phase infestation in tissues and it is a zoonotic parasitic disease that constitutes an important health problem in endemic regions like Turkey [11, 12]. Internal organ involvements, especially the liver and lung, are common. Primary bone involvement is rare but the incidence in the literature is 1–2.4%. Cases of femur, pelvic bone, humerus, and vertebrae involvement have been reported [13–15]. Hydatid cyst cases with bone involvement have also been reported in our country [16, 17]. In our case, 2 cysts were detected at iliac area adjacent to right sacroiliac joint and right hip joint.

In literature review, Küçükşen et al. reported that pelvic involvement of cyst hydatid disease may be confused with sacroiliitis. At the case of Küçükşen et al., patient was diagnosed with ankylosing spondylitis and followed up for 2 years. When the response was not obtained from the treatments, it was learned that patient had cystectomy operation due to hydatid disease in detailed anamnesis [18]. In our case, because of the interpretation of the lesion which was detected in the sacroiliac joint as bone marrow edema, sacroiliitis was considered in the first stage. However, as a result of further investigations, bone involvement of cyst hydatid disease was considered on detection of cystic lesions in other parts of the iliac wing. Clinical symptoms in hydatid cyst depend on depth of location and size of the cyst. The diagnosis must be with anamnesis, examination, and laboratory and radiological examinations. Lesion can be detected by ultrasonography and the diagnosis of cyst hydatid is confirmed by the appearance of the wheel pattern and the water-lily sign on the computed tomography. In our patient, abdominal ultrasonography was requested for abdominal pain and showed solid mass. Then computed tomography confirmed the diagnosis of hydatid cyst with the appearance of the wheel pattern and water-lily sign [19]. Abdomen tomography of our patient showed a well-defined 55 × 48 mm hypodense lesion with a superior calcification (lily symptom) in segment 3. In addition, various serological tests such as ELISA, immuno-electrophoresis, indirect hemagglutination, and latex agglutination tests can be used to evaluate the diagnosis, follow-up, and posttreatment relapse of the disease [20]. The indirect hemagglutination test in our patient was found positive at 1/320 titer.

The basic approach of hydatid cyst treatment is removing the cysts by open or laparoscopic operation methods and applying albendazole and praziquantel before and after operation. In addition, percutaneous approaches such as cyst puncture, aspiration, and hypertonic saline and alcohol injection to the cyst with chemotherapeutics and reaspiration are another treatment method. In some cases, albendazole monotherapy is used as a treatment modality [20–22]. In our case, for the development of arthritis in ankle and knee, surgical treatment was delayed and the patient was transferred to our clinic. Reactive arthritis and sacroiliitis were diagnosed and other etiological reasons of reactive and oligoarthritis were excluded. Diagnosis of reactive arthritis secondary to hydatid infestation was diagnosed with the present findings.

In the literature review, we did not find any case of reactive arthritis due to cyst hydatid. However, in a case reported by Sanchez Ibarrola et al., a temporal relationship between arthritic disease and cyst hydatid disease has been demonstrated. In this study, autoantibodies against cyst hydatid antigens in synovial fluid specimens were demonstrated by ELISA and immunofluorescence assessment of synovial tissue specimens showed vascular changes due to complement accumulation [10]. Protoscolex and hook structures of *Echinococcus* parasite were not observed in painted and unpainted microscopic examination of our patient's knee joint aspiration fluid. However, aspiration fluid was not examined by ELISA method and immunofluorescence examination could not be performed because synovial tissue biopsy could not be taken. The patient's clinical complaints regressed with symptomatic treatment and the patient was redirected to general surgery for the planning of surgical treatment.

4. Conclusion

Hydatid cyst is a parasitic disease with diffuse internal organ involvement but musculoskeletal involvement is rare. However, in regions where the disease is seen as endemic, such as Turkey, patients with musculoskeletal symptoms should consider the possibility of musculoskeletal involvement due to the hydatid cyst. Early diagnosis can prevent the secondary

problems that emerged with progress of the disease and prevent unnecessary health spending. For example, Abdelhakim et al. reported that the neural pressure due to the formation of the hydatid cystic bone erosions and giant dimensions in the sacral region caused a serious problem such as cauda equina syndrome at patient and radical surgery had to be performed in the treatment of this patient [23]. In the literature, many cases have been reported where no correct diagnosis was made at an early stage and due to incomplete or incorrect diagnosis, many cases were reported with more radical treatment methods applied when the diagnosis was made [24, 25]. Therefore, detailed anamnesis, detailed physical examination, imaging methods, and serological tests in areas where the disease is endemic will help us to diagnose cyst hydatid.

References

[1] J. Sieper, "Pathogenesis of reactive arthritis," *Current Rheumatology Reports*, vol. 3, no. 5, pp. 412–418, 2001.

[2] D. Morris and R. D. Inman, "Reactive arthritis: developments and challenges in diagnosis and treatment," *Current Rheumatology Reports*, vol. 14, no. 5, pp. 390–394, 2012.

[3] J. Goobar, "Joint symptoms in giardiasis," *The Lancet*, vol. 309, no. 8019, pp. 1010–1011, 1977.

[4] R. A. Shaw and M. B. Stevens, "The reactive arthritis of giardiasis: a case report," *The Journal of the American Medical Association*, vol. 258, no. 19, pp. 2734-2735, 1987.

[5] J. J. Barton, J. P. Burke, and E. B. Casey, "Reactive arthritis—giardia lamblia, another new pathogen?" *Irish Medical Journal*, vol. 79, no. 8, p. 223, 1986.

[6] M. I. Arman, "Arthritis bei lambliasis intestinalis (giardiasis) des erwachsenen," *Zeitschrift Fur Rheumatologie*, vol. 50, pp. 216–218, 1991.

[7] M. Bassiouni and M. Kamel, "Bilharzial arthropathy," *Annals of the Rheumatic Diseases*, vol. 43, no. 6, pp. 806–809, 1984.

[8] D. Karakuş, N. K. O. Gökkaya, F. Oktay, and H. Uçan, "A rare cause of reactive arthritis: Giardia Lamblia," *Turkish Journal of Rheumatology*, vol. 24, no. 1, pp. 51-52, 2009.

[9] S. Goyal, S. Goyal, S. Sangwan, and S. Sachar, "Uncommon locations and presentations of hydatid cyst," *Annals of Medical and Health Sciences Research*, vol. 4, no. 3, pp. 447–452, 2014.

[10] A. Sanchez Ibarrola, J. Guisantes, J. Tunon, M. L. Subira, and J. P. Valtuena, "Deposits of complement in synovial vessels in Reiters syndrome. Arole for hydatid antigen?" *Allergologia et Immunopathologia (Madr)*, vol. 11, no. 4, pp. 273–275, 1983.

[11] O. Akhan, M. N. Özmen, A. Dinçer, I. Sayek, and A. Göçmen, "Liver hydatid disease: long-term results of percutaneous treatment," *Radiology*, vol. 198, no. 1, pp. 259–264, 1996.

[12] F. Arslan, K. Zengin, A. Mert, R. Ozaras, and F. Tabak, "Pelvic and retroperitoneal hydatid cysts superinfected with Brucella sp. and review of infected hydatid cysts," *Tropical Biomedicine*, vol. 30, no. 1, pp. 92–96, 2013.

[13] I. Sayek, M. B. Tirnaksiz, and R. Dogan, "Cystic hydatid disease: current trends in diagnosis and management," *Surgery Today*, vol. 34, no. 12, pp. 987–996, 2004.

[14] A. J. Alldred and N. W. Nisbet, "Hydatid disease of bone in australasia," *The Journal of Bone and Joint Surgery. British Volume*, vol. 46, pp. 260–267, 1964.

[15] E. Kizilkaya, E. Silit, C. Basekim, and A. F. Karsli, "Hepatic, extrahepatic soft tissue and bone involvement in hydatid disease," *Turkish Journal of Diagnostic and Interventional Radiology*, vol. 8, pp. 101–104, 2002.

[16] Y. Ekinci, F. Duygulu, F. Vatansever, and K. Gürbüz, "A giant hydatid cyst localized in pelvis and thigh," *Eklem Hastaliklari ve Cerrahisi*, vol. 25, no. 2, pp. 121–124, 2014.

[17] S. Işlekel, Y. Erşahin, M. Zileli et al., "Spinal hydatid disease," *Spinal Cord*, vol. 36, no. 3, pp. 166–170, 1998.

[18] S. Küçükşen, B. K. Kaçira, S. Bağcaci, İ. Albayrak, and O. Yaşar, "Sacroiliac joint hydatidosis mimicking ankylosing spondylitis: a case report," *Archives of Rheumatology*, vol. 29, no. 2, pp. 138–142, 2014.

[19] L. Thambidurai, R. Santhosham, and B. Dev, "Hydatid cyst: anywhere, everywhere," *Radiology Case Reports*, vol. 6, no. 3, p. 486, 2011.

[20] M. Mushtaque, M. F. Mir, A. A. Malik, S. H. Arif, S. A. Khanday, and R. A. Dar, "Atypicallocalizations of hydatid disease: experience from a single institute," *Nigerian Journal of Surgery*, vol. 18, pp. 2–7, 2012.

[21] J. Eckert and P. Deplazes, "Biological, epidemiological, and clinical aspects of echinococcosis, a zoonosis of increasing concern," *Clinical Microbiology Reviews*, vol. 17, no. 1, pp. 107–135, 2004.

[22] Z. Pawlowski, S. J. Eckert, D. A. Vuitton et al., "Echinococcosis in humans: clinical aspects, diagnosis and treatment," in *WHO/OIE Manual on Echinococcus in Humans and Animals: A Public Health Problem of Global Concern*, J. Eckert, M. A. Germmell, F. X. Meslin, and Z. S. Pawlowski, Eds., pp. 20–66, World Organisation for Animal Health, Paris, France, 2011.

[23] K. Abdelhakim, A. Khalil, B. Haroune, M. Oubaid, and M. Mondher, "A case of sacral hydatid cyst," *International Journal of Surgery Case Reports*, vol. 5, no. 7, pp. 434–436, 2014.

[24] H. Diktas, S. Cakmak, V. Turhan et al., "Hydatid cyst presenting with multiple recurrence and pelvic involvement: case report," *Turkish Journal of Parasitology*, vol. 35, no. 3, pp. 178–180, 2011.

[25] M. De Lavaissiere, C. Voronca, I. Ranz, M. Pirame, H. Hounieu, and M. Carreiro, "Pelvic hydatid cyst: differential diagnosis with a bacterial abscess with cutaneous fistula," *Bulletin de la Societe de Pathologie Exotique*, vol. 105, no. 4, pp. 256–258, 2012.

39

Hepatitis E during Tocilizumab Therapy in a Patient with Rheumatoid Arthritis

Hidekazu Ikeuchi[ID],[1] Kana Koinuma,[1] Masao Nakasatomi[ID],[1] Toru Sakairi,[1] Yoriaki Kaneko,[1] Akito Maeshima,[1] Yuichi Yamazaki,[2] Hiroaki Okamoto,[3] Toshihide Mimura[ID],[4] Satoshi Mochida,[5] Yoshihisa Nojima,[6] and Keiju Hiromura[ID][1]

[1]Department of Nephrology and Rheumatology, Gunma University Graduate School of Medicine, Maebashi, Japan
[2]Department of Medicine and Molecular Science, Gunma University Graduate School of Medicine, Maebashi, Japan
[3]Division of Virology, Department of Infection and Immunity, Jichi Medical University School of Medicine, Shimotsuke, Japan
[4]Department of Rheumatology and Applied Immunology, Faculty of Medicine, Saitama Medical University, Saitama, Japan
[5]Division of Gastroenterology and Hepatology Internal Medicine, Saitama Medical University, Saitama, Japan
[6]Department of Rheumatology and Nephrology, Japan Red Cross Maebashi Hospital, Maebashi, Japan

Correspondence should be addressed to Hidekazu Ikeuchi; hikeuchi@gunma-u.ac.jp

Academic Editor: Shigeko Inokuma

Hepatitis E is an acute self-limiting disease caused by hepatitis E virus (HEV). Recent reports show that HEV can induce chronic hepatitis or be reactivated in immunocompromised hosts. We report a 63-year-old woman with rheumatoid arthritis (RA) who developed hepatitis E during treatment with tocilizumab. Analysis of serially stocked serum samples confirmed that hepatitis was caused by primary infection with HEV and not by viral reactivation. Her liver function improved after discontinuing tocilizumab and remained within the normal range without reactivation of HEV for >5 years after restarting tocilizumab. We also reviewed the published cases of hepatitis E that developed during RA treatment.

1. Introduction

Hepatic disorders are some of the most common complications that arise during rheumatoid arthritis (RA) treatment. Routine liver enzyme testing is recommended to detect the side effects of disease-modifying antirheumatic drugs (DMARDs) as well as the reactivation of viruses such as hepatitis type B (HBV), hepatitis type C (HCV), and cytomegalovirus [1, 2].

Hepatitis E is a disease of the liver that is caused by hepatitis type E virus (HEV) infection. HEV usually induces acute self-limiting hepatitis in healthy individuals. However, HEV is known to induce chronic hepatitis in immunocompromised hosts, including patients with HIV infection, chemotherapy recipients, and organ transplant recipients [3, 4]. In addition, HEV deterioration has been reported in patients after allogenic stem cell transplantation [5, 6], despite low risk of deterioration [7].

Here, we report a case of hepatitis E that developed during tocilizumab therapy for RA. In this case, we sequentially determined the serum titers of HEV antibodies and RNA before and after the onset of hepatitis using stocked serum samples. In addition, we reviewed the published cases of hepatitis E that occurred during RA treatment with DMARDs.

2. Case Presentation

A 63-year-old woman visited our outpatient clinic because of general malaise that lasted 6 days. She developed RA at the age of 60 years and had been treated with 400 mg monthly intravenous tocilizumab for the past 10 months and 3 mg/day prednisolone. She had no history of blood transfusion, alcohol use, travel abroad, or raw meat intake, and her joints were not tender or swollen. Disease Activity Score 28-joint count C reactive protein was 1.13. Laboratory

TABLE 1: Sequential changes of liver enzymes and laboratory tests for hepatitis E.

Time after admission	AST (13–33 IU/L[*])	ALT (6–27 IU/L[*])	Anti-HEV IgG (OD$_{450}$ < 0.175[*])	Anti-HEV IgM (OD$_{450}$ < 0.440[*])	Anti-HEV IgA (OD$_{450}$ < 0.642[*])	HEV RNA (−)
−30 months	17	9	0.046	0.043	0.042	−
−20 months	16	14	0.047	0.05	0.035	−
−10 months	19	14	0.035	0.088	0.04	−
0	338	523	2.563	2.845	2.93	+
1 week	44	137	2.822	>3.000	>3.000	+
2 weeks	32	37	>3.000	2.894	2.296	+
3 weeks	22	18	2.748	2.771	1.499	+
6 weeks	27	25	2.956	2.661	1.113	−
10 weeks	22	15	>3.000	2.303	1.019	−
14 weeks	27	19	>3.000	1.863	0.799	−
22 weeks	43	28	>3.000	1.022	0.536	−
26 weeks	31	26	NA	NA	NA	NA
57 months	24	17	1.659	0.176	0.115	−

[*]Normal range. HEV, hepatitis E virus; IgG, immunoglobulin G; IgM, immunoglobulin M; IgA, immunoglobulin A; NA, not available.

data revealed elevated liver enzyme levels: AST, 338 IU/L; ALT, 523 IU/L; ALP, 377 IU/L; and γ-GTP, 68 IU/L. Blood counts, total protein, albumin, total bilirubin, electrolytes, renal tests, C reactive protein, and coagulation test results were almost within normal ranges. Her serum HBV nucleic acid levels were monitored regularly to detect HBV reactivation because she tested positive for antibodies to HBV surface and core antigens without HBs antigen before the initiation of tocilizumab. At admission, HBV DNA levels were within normal range. Tests to detect antibodies to hepatitis A and C were negative. Tests to detect antibodies to Epstein–Barr virus and cytomegalovirus were both negative for immunoglobulin M (IgM) but positive for immunoglobulin G (IgG). Abdominal ultrasound revealed normal liver morphology.

The patient was diagnosed with HEV infection (genotype 3) because tests to detect anti-HEV immunoglobulin A (IgA) antibody and HEV RNA in her sera were both positive. Tocilizumab, pregabalin, eldecalcitol, and teriparatide were discontinued, and stronger neo-minophagen C and urso-deoxycholic acid were administered. Liver enzyme levels decreased and returned to normal 3 weeks after admission, and she was discharged from our hospital. Results of HEV RNA tests were negative 6 weeks after admission. Tocilizumab and eldecalcitol were reinitiated 4 weeks after liver enzyme normalization. RA remained in remission, and liver enzymes remained stable for the subsequent 5 years under tocilizumab therapy.

Because she had been a participant in a prospective clinical study to investigate the incidence of HBV reactivation in patients receiving immunosuppressive and/or anticancer therapies [8], her sera that was collected prior to hepatitis E onset had been stored. The use of serially stocked sera for HEV detection was approved by the Ethics Committee of Gunma University Hospital (#15-61). We examined her serum for anti-HEV antibodies and HEV RNA before and after admission (Table 1). Neither anti-HEV antibodies nor HEV RNA was detected in the preadmission samples. In contrast, all of them were positive at admission. Anti-HEV IgM and IgA antibody levels peaked 1 week after admission and declined thereafter. Anti-HEV IgG antibody

levels remained elevated until the final observation at 57 months. HEV RNA was detected at 0, 2, and 3 weeks after admission and was undetectable thereafter.

3. Discussion

HEV was previously believed to cause acute hepatitis but not chronic hepatitis. However, Kamar et al. first reported that chronic HEV infection was observed in patients after organ transplantation [3]. They further reported that HEV infection caused chronic hepatitis in >60% of solid-organ transplant recipients [9]. Chronic HEV infection was also reported in patients with HIV infection and in a patient with malignant lymphoma treated with rituximab [4, 10]. In addition, HEV persistent infection has been reported in recipients of bone marrow transplant under severe immunosuppression [5–7]. Recently, biological DMARDs (bDMARDs) or targeted synthetic DMARDs (tsDMARDs) are frequently used in RA treatment. Treatment with bDMARDs is reported to increase the risk of hepatitis B virus reactivation in patients with RA [11]. Therefore, chronic transformation of hepatitis E may occur in patients with RA who are treated with bDMARDs or tsDMARDs. In our case, sequential analysis of anti-HEV antibodies and HEV RNA using stocked serum samples clearly confirmed that our patient developed hepatitis as a result of primary acute HEV infection, but not recurrence or chronic infection of HEV. The clinical course of our patient was self-limiting, and the virus was eradicated from the serum without chronic transformation. In addition, there was neither recurrence of hepatitis nor persistent infection of HEV infection during the following 5 years, even after the reintroduction of tocilizumab.

The case reports of hepatitis E infection in patients with RA are accumulating [12–21]. Table 2 summarizes published cases of hepatitis E developed during the treatment of RA with DMARDs. Of 26 cases including ours, 20 were treated with bDMARDs or tsDMARDs with or without conventional synthetic DMARDs (csDMARDs) and 6 cases were treated with csDMARDs alone. Low-dose steroids were used in 16 cases. In most cases, DMARDs were discontinued for

TABLE 2: Summary of cases of hepatitis E during treatment of rheumatoid arthritis.

Number	First author	Year	Reference	Sex	Age	bDMARDs /tsDMARDs	Stopping bDMARDs /tsDMARDs	csDMARDs	Stopping csDMARDs	PSL (mg/day)	HEV genotype	Ribavirin	Periods for disappearance of HEV RNA	Prognosis
1	Sugawara	2009	[12]	M	60	IFX	NA	MTX, BUC		(+)*	4	(−)	NA	Died due to fulminant hepatitis
2	Bauer	2013	[13]	F	68	ABA	Yes	LEF	Yes	5	3	(−)	NA	Improved
3	Roux	2013	[14]	M	55	RTX	Yes	MTX	Yes	(+)*	3	(+)	3 months	Improved
4	Bauer	2015	[15]	F	62	IFX	Yes	MTX	Yes	(−)	NA	(−)	4 weeks	Improved
5	Bauer	2015	[15]	M	72	RTX	No	MTX, LEF	Yes	(−)	NA	(−)	NA	Improved
6	Bauer	2015	[15]	F	49	TCZ	Yes	(−)	Yes	3	3f	(−)	6 weeks	Improved
7	Bauer	2015	[15]	F	69	ABA	Yes	LEF	Yes	5	3f	(−)	6 weeks	Improved
8	Bauer	2015	[15]	M	69	RTX	No	MTX	No	(−)	NA	(+)	10.5 weeks	Improved
9	Bauer	2015	[15]	M	61	RTX	No	LEF	Yes	3	NA	(−)	8 weeks	Improved
10	Bauer	2015	[15]	F	53	ABA	Yes	MTX	Yes	(−)	NA	(−)	9 weeks	Improved
11	Bauer	2015	[15]	F	44	RTX	Yes	MTX	Yes	(−)	3c	(−)	9.5 weeks	Improved
12	Bauer	2015	[15]	F	55	ETN	Yes	MTX	Yes	(−)	NA	(−)	4 weeks	Improved
13	Bauer	2015	[15]	F	60	ADA	Yes	MTX	Yes	4	3f	(−)	8 weeks	Improved
14	Bauer	2015	[15]	M	59	TCZ	Yes	MTX	Yes	7	NA	(−)	4 weeks	Improved
15	Schultze	2015	[16]	F	68	(−)	Yes	MTX	Yes	5**	NA	(−)	40 days	Improved
16	Leloy	2015	[17]	F	33	TCZ	Yes	(−)		(−)	NA	(−)	NA	Improved
17	Kanda	2015	[18]	F	64	(−)		MTX, BUC	NA	(−)	3	(−)	NA	Improved
18	Kanda	2015	[18]	F	74	TOF	Yes	(−)		(+)*	3	(−)	NA	Improved
19	Kanda	2015	[18]	F	52	(−)		MTX	NA	(−)	3	(−)	NA	Improved
20	Verhoeven	2016	[19]	F	51	RTX	Yes	(−)		(−)	NA	(+)	2 months	Improved
21	Kobayashi	2017	[20]	F	58	(−)		BUC, MIZ, ACT	No	5	NA	(−)	NA	Improved
22	Kobayashi	2017	[20]	M	61	ETN	Yes	MTX	Yes	3	NA	(−)	NA	Improved
23	Kobayashi	2017	[20]	M	67	(−)		MTX, TAC	Yes	5	NA	(−)	NA	Improved
24	Kobayashi	2017	[20]	F	52	(−)		MTX, MIZ, TAC	Yes	4	NA	(−)	NA	Improved
25	van Bijnen	2017	[21]	M	63	ADA	Yes	MTX	Yes	3	3	(+)	42 days after ribavirin	Chronic infection→improved
26	Our case			F	63	TCZ	Yes	(−)		3	3e	(−)	6 weeks	Improved

DMARDs, disease-modifying antirheumatic drugs; bDMARDs, biologic DMARDs; csDMARDs, conventional synthetic DMARDs; PSL, prednisolone/prednisone; HEV, hepatitis E virus; IFX, infliximab; RTX, rituximab; TCZ, tocilizumab; ABA, abatacept; ETN, etanercept; TOF, tofacitinib; MTX, methotrexate; BUC, bucillamine; LEF, leflunomide; MIZ, mizoribine; ACT, actarit; TAC, tacrolimus; NA, not available. *Dose is not available; **weekly dosage.

a certain period after the diagnosis of hepatitis. Temporal withdrawal of DMARDs may help the immune system to recover and eliminate HEV. In most patients, liver function was normalized without antiviral therapy. However, 1 patient (case 1) died of fulminant hepatitis, despite treatment with plasma exchange and continuous hemofiltration [12]. The HEV genotype detected in this patient was genotype 4, which is known to be more virulent than genotype 3. In addition, a male patient (case 25) who was administered adalimumab and methotrexate developed chronic hepatitis E [21]. The routine testing revealed elevated liver enzyme levels, and methotrexate, but not adalimumab, was discontinued. Eight months later, he was diagnosed with HEV infection, and adalimumab was discontinued. However, serum HEV RNA remained positive for more than 5 months; therefore, he was treated with ribavirin for 42 days until the test results for serum HEV RNA were negative [21].

In transplant recipients with chronic HEV infection, antiviral therapy with interferon-α and ribavirin as monotherapy or in combination is recommended if immunosuppressive therapy has to be continued or viral clearance is difficult to achieve even after weakening immunosuppression [22, 23]. In patients with RA who are treated with DMARDs as listed above, only 4 cases were treated with ribavirin and 3 of them had been treated with rituximab. Another patient had been treated with adalimumab before and after notification of elevated liver enzymes for several months and ultimately developed chronic hepatitis E, as described above [14, 15, 19, 21]. Based on these results, antiviral therapy may be considered only in high-risk patients: patients with HEV (genotype 4), those who had been treated with long-lasting and immunosuppressive DMARDs such as rituximab, and those with severe or chronic hepatitis. Further investigation is to clarify the adequate use of ribavirin in acute hepatitis E patients taking DMARDs.

In summary, we presented a case of RA with hepatitis E that developed during tocilizumab therapy, and we reviewed published cases of hepatitis E among patients with RA on DMARDs treatment. In RA patients whose liver dysfunction was detected at routine examination, the possibility of HEV infection should be considered. In a case of hepatitis E, discontinuation of bDMARDs or tsDMARDs is recommended, and administration of ribavirin may be necessary in high-risk patients. In addition, in our case, tocilizumab was safely used after normalization of liver function for a long term without persistent infection of HEV.

Disclosure

Parts of this manuscript were reported in *Kanto Riumachi* (2016; 1: 96–102) in Japanese, from the proceedings of the 47th Kanto Riumachi Conference (Tokyo, Japan).

References

[1] K. G. Saag, G. G. Teng, N. M. Patkar et al., "American College of Rheumatology 2008 recommendations for the use of nonbiologic and biologic disease-modifying antirheumatic drugs in rheumatoid arthritis," *Arthritis and Rheumatism*, vol. 59, no. 6, pp. 762–784, 2008.

[2] J. A. Singh, K. G. Saag, S. L. Bridges Jr. et al., "2015 American College of Rheumatology Guideline for the Treatment of Rheumatoid Arthritis," *Arthritis and Rheumatology*, vol. 68, no. 1, pp. 1–26, 2016.

[3] N. Kamar, J. Selves, J. M. Mansuy et al., "Hepatitis E virus and chronic hepatitis in organ-transplant recipients," *New England Journal of Medicine*, vol. 358, no. 8, pp. 811–817, 2008.

[4] H. R. Dalton, R. P. Bendall, F. E. Keane, R. S. Tedder, and S. Ijaz, "Persistent carriage of hepatitis E virus in patients with HIV infection," *The New England Journal of Medicine*, vol. 361, no. 10, pp. 1025–1027, 2009.

[5] P. le Coutre, H. Meisel, J. Hofmann et al., "Reactivation of hepatitis E infection in a patient with acute lymphoblastic leukaemia after allogeneic stem cell transplantation," *Gut*, vol. 58, no. 5, pp. 699–702, 2009.

[6] J. Versluis, S. D. Pas, H. J. Agteresch et al., "Hepatitis E virus: an underestimated opportunistic pathogen in recipients of allogeneic hematopoietic stem cell transplantation," *Blood*, vol. 122, no. 6, pp. 1079–1086, 2013.

[7] F. Abravanel, J. M. Mansuy, A. Huynh et al., "Low risk of hepatitis E virus reactivation after haematopoietic stem cell transplantation," *Journal of Clinical Virology*, vol. 54, no. 2, pp. 152–155, 2012.

[8] S. Mochida, M. Nakao, N. Nakayama et al., "Nationwide prospective and retrospective surveys for hepatitis B virus reactivation during immunosuppressive therapies," *Journal of Gastroenterology*, vol. 51, no. 10, pp. 999–1010, 2016.

[9] N. Kamar, C. Garrouste, E. B. Haagsma et al., "Factors associated with chronic hepatitis in patients with hepatitis E virus infection who have received solid organ transplants," *Gastroenterology*, vol. 140, no. 5, pp. 1481–1489, 2011.

[10] L. Ollier, N. Tieulie, F. Sanderson et al., "Chronic hepatitis after hepatitis E virus infection in a patient with non-Hodgkin lymphoma taking rituximab," *Annals of Internal Medicine*, vol. 150, no. 6, pp. 430-431, 2009.

[11] Y. Urata, R. Uesato, D. Tanaka et al., "Prevalence of reactivation of hepatitis B virus replication in rheumatoid arthritis patients," *Modern Rheumatology*, vol. 21, no. 1, pp. 16–23, 2011.

[12] N. Sugawara, A. Yawata, K. Takahashi, N. Abe, and M. Arai, "The third case of fulminant hepatitis associated with "Kitami/Abashiri strain" of hepatitis E virus genotype 4," *Kanzo*, vol. 50, no. 8, pp. 473-374, 2009.

[13] H. Bauer, J. Sibilia, P. Moreau, and L. Messer, "Acute hepatitis E during biotherapy," *Joint Bone Spine*, vol. 80, no. 1, pp. 91-92, 2013.

[14] C.H. Roux, R. Anty, S. Patouraux, and L. Euller-Ziegler, "Hepatitis E: are rheumatic patients at risk?," *Journal of Rheumatology*, vol. 40, no. 1, p. 99, 2013.

[15] H. Bauer, C. Luxembourger, J. E. Gottenberg et al., "Outcome of hepatitis E virus infection in patients with inflammatory arthritides treated with immunosuppressants: a French retrospective multicenter study," *Medicine*, vol. 94, no. 14, p. e675, 2015.

[16] D. Schultze, B. Mani, G. Dollenmaier, R. Sahli, A. Zbinden, and P. A. Krayenbuhl, "Acute Hepatitis E Virus infection with coincident reactivation of Epstein-Barr virus infection in an

immunosuppressed patient with rheumatoid arthritis: a case report," *BMC Infectious Diseases*, vol. 15, no. 1, p. 474, 2015.

[17] M. Leroy, G. Coiffier, C. Pronier, L. Triquet, A. Perdriger, and P. Guggenbuhl, "Macrophage activation syndrome with acute hepatitis E during tocilizumab treatment for rheumatoid arthritis," *Joint Bone Spine*, vol. 82, no. 4, pp. 278-279, 2015.

[18] T. Kanda, S. Yasui, M. Nakamura et al., "Recent trend of hepatitis E virus infection in Chiba area, Japan: 3 of 5 cases with rheumatoid arthritis," *Case Reports in Gastroenterology*, vol. 9, no. 3, pp. 317–326, 2015.

[19] F. Verhoeven, D. Weil-Verhoeven, V. Di Martino, C. Prati, T. Thevenot, and D. Wendling, "Management of acute HVE infection in a patient treated with rituximab for rheumatoid arthritis," *Joint Bone Spine*, vol. 83, no. 5, pp. 577-578, 2016.

[20] D. Kobayashi, S. Ito, C. Takai et al., "Type-E hepatitis in rheumatoid arthritis patients," *Modern Rheumatology Case Reports*, vol. 1, no. 2, pp. 30–34, 2017.

[21] S. T. van Bijnen, M. Ledeboer, and H. A. Martens, "Chronic hepatitis E in a patient with rheumatoid arthritis treated with adalimumab and methotrexate," *Rheumatology*, vol. 56, no. 3, pp. 497-498, 2017.

[22] N. Kamar, R. Bendall, F. Legrand-Abravanel et al., "Hepatitis E," *The Lancet*, vol. 379, no. 9835, pp. 2477–2488, 2012.

[23] N. Kamar, J. Izopet, S. Tripon et al., "Ribavirin for chronic hepatitis E virus infection in transplant recipients," *New England Journal of Medicine*, vol. 370, no. 12, pp. 1111–1120, 2014.

40

Recurrent Interstitial Pneumonitis in a Patient with Entero-Behçet's Disease Initially Treated with Mesalazine

Akihiro Nakamura,[1,2] **Tomoya Miyamura,**[1] **Brian Wu,**[2] **and Eiichi Suematsu**[1]

[1]Department of Internal Medicine and Rheumatology, Clinical Research Institute, National Hospital Organization, Kyushu Medical Center, 1-8-1 Jigyohama, Chuo-ku, Fukuoka 810-8563, Japan
[2]Department of Genetics and Development, Krembil Research Institute, Toronto Western Hospital, 60 Leonard Avenue, Toronto, ON, Canada M5T 2S8

Correspondence should be addressed to Akihiro Nakamura; anakamur@uhnresearch.ca

Academic Editor: Suleyman Serdar Koca

A 65-year-old man with entero-Behçet's disease (BD) being treated with mesalazine was presented to our hospital complaining of dyspnea. Computed tomography (CT) of the chest showed ground-glass opacities and he was initially diagnosed with mesalazine-induced interstitial pneumonitis (IP). Besides the discontinuation of mesalazine, a high dose of oral prednisolone was administered and the patient seemed to recover. However, four months later, dyspnea recurred and repeated CT revealed more extensive pulmonary infiltration despite steroid therapy. After the exclusion of infections, we suspected either a recurrence of mesalazine-induced IP or BD-related IP as a clinical manifestation of BD. The patient was treated with intravenous methylprednisolone and cyclophosphamide, followed by orally administered azathioprine, based on the assumption of underlying vasculitis. Thereafter, his condition improved. BD-related IP is an extremely rare condition with limited reports in the literature. Mesalazine-induced IP is also uncommon but the prognosis is generally good after discontinuation of mesalazine with or without steroid therapy. We discuss an extremely rare case, especially focusing on BD-related IP and mesalazine-induced IP as a potential cause of recurrent IP in a patient with entero-BD.

1. Introduction

Entero-Behçet's disease (BD) is a particular type of BD according to the diagnostic criteria of BD from the Japanese Ministry of Health, Labour and Welfare. It is characterized by intestinal aphthae, typically located at the ileocecal lesion, as a prominent manifestation leading to recurrent abdominal pain, diarrhea, and melena. Large aphthae may cause intestinal perforations which often require emergency surgery due to panperitonitis. Although the exact pathogenesis of entero-BD remains unclear, inflammation of vessels (vasculitis) is considered a main culprit of intestinal involvement in patients with BD.

Chronic interstitial lung disease (ILD) is characterized by diffuse lung interstitial wall inflammation, often resulting in severe pulmonary fibrosis and impaired gas exchange. Although pulmonary involvement is uncommon in patients with BD, pulmonary artery aneurysm (PAA), pulmonary infarction, hemorrhage, thrombosis, bronchiolitis, and pleurisy have been reported [1]. More than 200 cases of BD with pulmonary involvement have been reported in the literature [2]; however, interstitial pneumonitis (IP) associated with BD is extremely rare with few existing reports [3–8].

Aminosalicylates have been generally used in mild-to-moderate entero-BD. One of the serious side effects arising from the use of these agents is lung toxicity. Mesalazine is a newer drug with less frequent adverse events due to the lack of sulfapyridine moiety, but there have been rare reports of mesalazine-induced lung toxicity.

Here we report the case of recurrent IP in a patient with entero-BD initially treated with mesalazine. Despite the discontinuation of mesalazine and use of steroid, dyspnea persisted and computed tomography (CT) deteriorated.

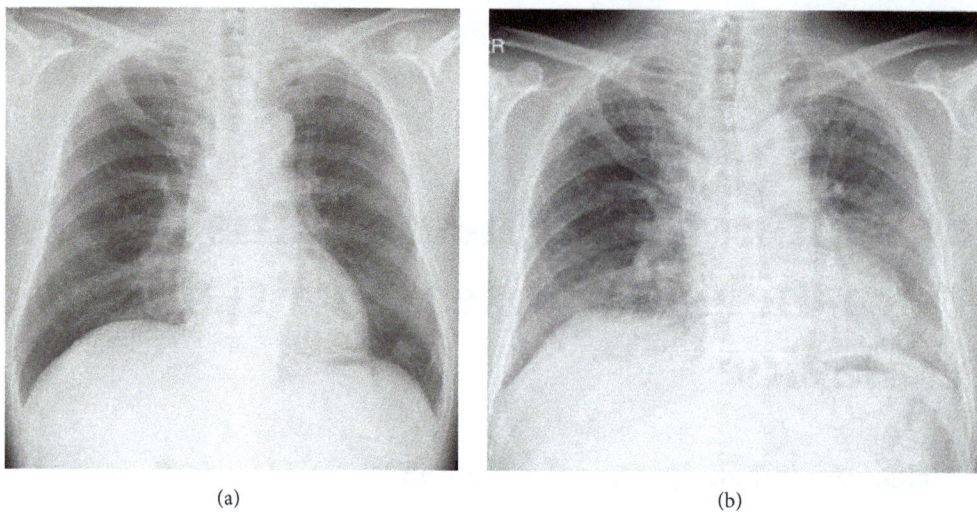

(a)   (b)

FIGURE 1: Chest X-ray images at the time of diagnosis with BD (a) and at the first time appearance of dyspnea (b).

The patient's condition eventually improved on high dose oral prednisolone (PSL) in combination with monthly intravenous cyclophosphamide (IVCY) followed by azathioprine (AZA).

2. Case Report

A 55-year-old Japanese man was admitted for refractory stomatitis and persistent low-grade pyrexia. Four weeks prior to admission, he consulted a primary care physician and was diagnosed with acute bronchitis, but the fever persisted despite treatment with oral antibiotics. On admission, his symptoms had become more extensive and he was complaining of mild watery diarrhea without hematochezia. His vital signs were as follows: pulse of 75 beats per minute, blood pressure of 102/63 mmHg, respiratory rate of 16 breaths per minute, temperature of 38.0°C, and oxygen saturation of 97% on room air. Several areas of painful stomatitis were found in his mouth. On auscultation both lung fields were clear. Erythema nodosum was present on both lower limbs and arthritis was evident in bilateral knee and ankle joints. No genital ulcers were observed. Ophthalmologist did not detect any visual abnormalities including uveitis. Laboratory findings on admission revealed a white blood cell count of 13.4×10^9/L with 86% of neutrophils, hemoglobin of 10.3 g/dL with a mean corpuscular volume of 99.6 fL, and reticulocyte count of 1.8%. Platelet count was within the normal range. Serum iron level was low (14 μg/dL), unbound iron-binding capacity was normal (93 μg/dL), and ferritin was elevated (619 ng/dL). Serum inflammatory markers were elevated, including C-reactive protein (85 mg/L), serum amyloid A (756 μg/mL), and erythrocyte sedimentation rate (91 mm/h). Urinalysis revealed no significant findings. The result of HIV test was negative. HLA typing was positive for the B51 haplotype. Cultures of blood, urine, and sputum obtained on admission were sterile, and chest X-ray showed no significant findings (Figure 1(a)). An electrocardiogram revealed sinus rhythm at a rate of 68 beats per minute with normal intervals.

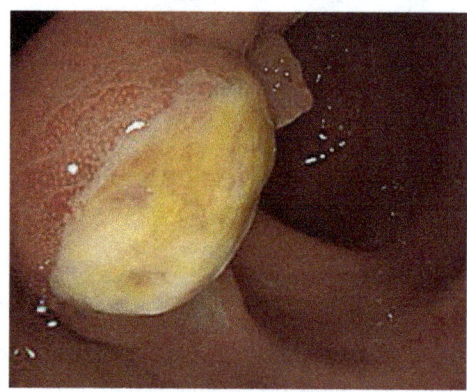

FIGURE 2: An ulcer on the ileum identified by colonoscopy.

On the fourteenth day of admission, the patient found watery diarrhea with abdominal discomfort. Colonoscopy revealed ulceration of the ileum, cecum, and ascending colon (Figure 2). An ileocecal biopsy showed mucosal atrophy and marked lymphocytic infiltration with a formation of lymph follicle. According to the criteria for BD from Ministry of Health, Labor and Welfare in Japan (chronic stomatitis, EN, arthralgia, and ileum ulcers), the patient was diagnosed with BD, specifically a type of entero-BD based on prominent intestinal manifestations. Treatment with prednisolone (PSL) (45 mg/day, 1 mg/kg/day), mesalazine (500 mg/day), and colchicine (1.0 mg/day) was initiated, and the symptoms of fever, arthralgia, and watery diarrhea subsided over the subsequent few weeks, and he was discharged.

Three months later, he was readmitted to our hospital complaining of subacute onset of exertional dyspnea, fever, and dry cough. Chest X-ray showed diffuse infiltrates (Figure 1(b)) and CT of the chest without contrast medium showed diffuse ground-glass opacities (GGO) in both lung fields (Figure 3(a)). We considered differential diagnoses of bacterial, viral, or fungal pneumonia, congestive cardiac

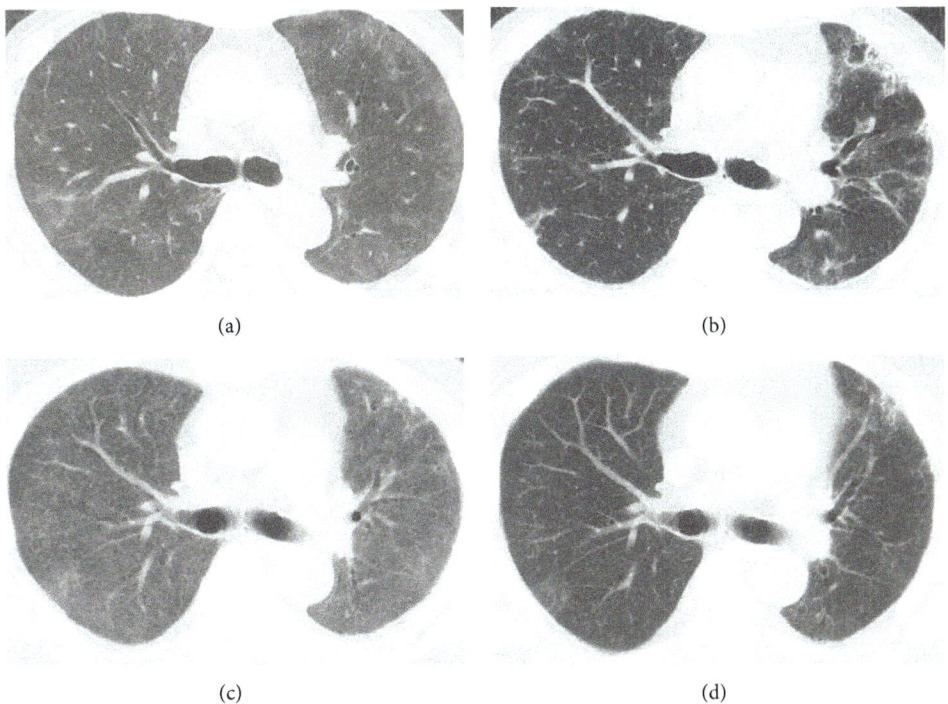

(a)   (b)

(c)   (d)

FIGURE 3: Computed tomography of the chest at the first time appearance of dyspnea (a), after treatment with prednisone 40 mg/day (b), at recurrence of dyspnea (c), and after treatment with methylprednisolone pulse and cyclophosphamide pulse therapy (d).

failure, or IP associated with drug associated IP or BD activity. Laboratory data showed high levels of CRP (39.5) and ESR (66 mm/h) but no elevation of β-D glucan as well as negative results of cytomegalovirus (CMV) antigen (C7-HRP) and IgM antibody. We excluded congestive cardiac failure on the basis of an unremarkable cardiovascular examination, a normal result of brain natriuretic peptide (BNP), and essentially no dyskinetic movement of his heart assessed by echocardiography. Bronchoscopy, lavage, and culture found a predominance of CD8-positive T-lymphocytes over CD4-positive ones (CD4/CD8 ratio 0.62), with no bacterial growth. Additionally, polymerase chain reaction (PCR) for *Pneumocystis jirovecii* in bronchoalveolar lavage (BAL) was negative. Similarly, blood and sputum cultures were sterile. Transbronchial lung biopsy (TBLB) revealed nonspecific intestinal inflammation with fibrosis and no signs of vasculitis including lymphocyte infiltration around vessels or vascular occlusion (Figure 4). As a result of these findings, a drug-induced acute lung injury was suspected, with mesalazine as a potential trigger. Mesalazine was withdrawn and PSL increased to 40 mg/day (0.8 mg/kg). Thereafter, his symptoms and the GGO appearance on chest CT both improved compared with admission, although a small amount of fibrosis remained visible (Figure 3(b)). He was discharged after approximately 6 weeks in hospital and continued taking steroids.

After another three months the patient was readmitted with worsening dyspnea. On examination, although body temperature and blood pressure were 37.5°C and 150/70 mmHg, respectively, respiratory rate was 28/min, and

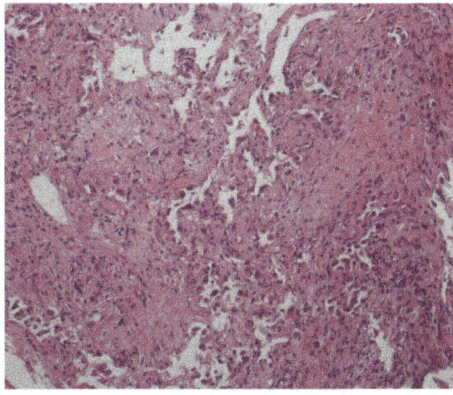

FIGURE 4: The result of transbronchial lung biopsy. Hematoxylin and eosin (HE) stain revealed diffuse lymphocytes infiltration without any findings of vasculitis (magnification: 100x).

the oxygen saturation was 85% on room air. Chest CT without contrast revealed more widespread interstitial infiltration than the examination performed on the previous admission (Figure 3(c)). After exclusion of infections, we suspected either the diagnosis of persistent mesalazine-induced IP or IP secondary to BD. The patient was treated with a pulse of methylprednisolone (mPSL) 1 g/day for 3 days followed by PSL 50 mg/day orally and six doses of monthly IVCY (1000 mg/month). By the 7th day of admission, the symptoms improved and supplemental oxygen was no longer required. Since there was the possibility of BD-related IP despite steroid

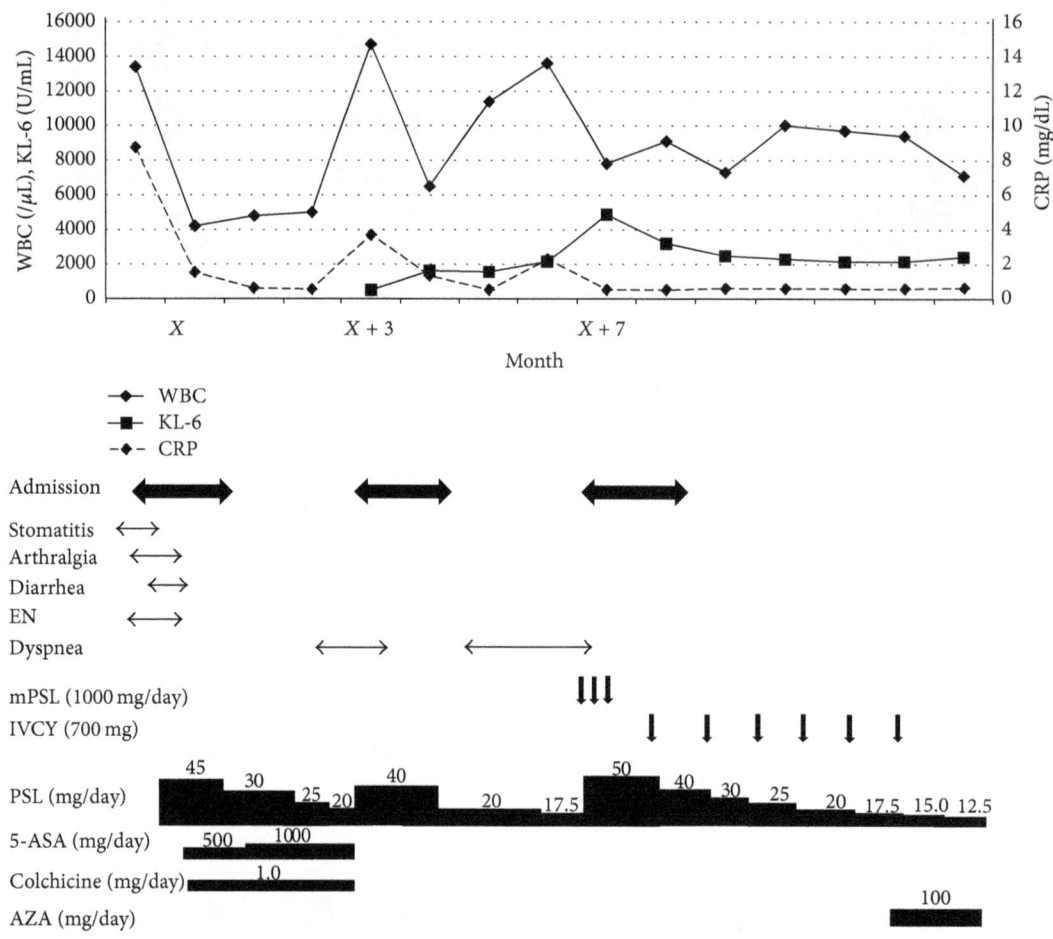

FIGURE 5: Clinical course of the patient. mPSL: methylprednisolone; IVCY: intravenous cyclophosphamide; 5-ASA: mesalazine; AZA: azathioprine; EN: erythema nodosum.

therapy, AZA was added to PSL as maintenance therapy. The appearance of unenhanced chest CT also improved (Figure 3(d)). He has since remained asymptomatic and the BD has been well controlled for 15 months to date (Figure 5).

3. Discussion

This is an extremely rare case of IP in a patient with entero-BD. Pulmonary findings have been reported in BD including PAA, pulmonary infarction, hemorrhage, and both organizing and eosinophilic pneumonias [1], but they are uncommon. There are several reports that have estimated the prevalence of pulmonary manifestations of BD to be between 1% and 7.7% [9, 10]. Among the pulmonary complications associated with BD, PAA is the most frequently occurring, as a consequence of vasculitis affecting the small pulmonary vessels [11]. The pulmonary arteries are the second most common site of arterial involvement after the aorta in patients with BD [2]. The interstitial pneumonia related to BD is also considered to be secondary to vasculitis of pulmonary vessels.

The most controversial point in the current case is whether the interstitial infiltration is due to BD or not:

ILD associated with BD is certainly extremely rare. Furthermore, since there was no other systemic sign of BD at the time of respiratory dysfunction, it could be argued that BD was not the cause. However, only three months had passed since he was diagnosed with established entero-BD, so it was considered that the activity of BD might be still high. Particularly, as the central feature of entero-BD is vasculitis, it would not be surprising if vasculitis coexisted in lung and intestine. Furthermore, the IP occurred under the treatment of moderate dose of PSL (20 mg/day) and his condition responded well to immunosuppressant therapies including pulsed mPSL and IVCY, followed by PSL and AZA, demonstrating the existence of underlying vasculitis.

We also considered that mesalazine was a likely cause of his acute illness as lung damage is rarely seen soon after the drug has been administered [12–15], and TBLB showed nonspecific interstitial inflammation without any findings of vasculitis. In our case, the dyspnea began 3 months after the mesalazine had been started, and the finding of predominantly CD8-positive cells in the BAL was suggestive of drug-induced lung injury. However, dyspnea and more extensive infiltrates recurred three months after mesalazine had been withdrawn. In general, the mesalazine-induced

TABLE 1: Previous reports of interstitial pneumonia in patients with Behçet's disease and our case.

Author	Year published	Number of patients	CXR/CT findings	Pathological findings	Treatment
Efthimiou et al. [3]	1986	5	Opacities	Thrombosis, infarction, hemorrhage, fibrosis	N/A
Akoglu et al. [4]	1987	1	Diffuse reticulonodular infiltration	Interstitial pneumonia	PSL
Gül et al. [5]	1999	1	Mural thrombosis, GGO	Organizing pneumonia	mPSL pulse, IVCY monthly
Rutherford et al. [6]	2004	1	Patchy infiltration	Nonspecific interstitial pneumonia	PSL, IVCY monthly
Ning-Sheng et al. [7]	2004	1	GGO, multiple patchy consolidation	Organizing pneumonia	mPSL pulse, IVCY monthly
Nanke et al. [8]	2007	2	GGO, peripheral nodular opacities	Organizing pneumonia	PSL
Our case		1	GGO, patchy infiltration	Nonspecific interstitial inflammation	mPSL pulse, IVCY monthly

CXR: chest X-ray; GGO: ground-glass opacities; PSL: prednisolone; mPSL: methylprednisolone; IVCY: intravenous cyclophosphamide; N/A: not available.

lung injury only improves by discontinuing the drug. To our knowledge, there was no report that the immunosuppressants were needed in combination with steroid therapy to cure the mesalazine-induced IP. Although the efficacy of steroid therapy for mesalazine-induced IP is controversial, it may facilitate the recovery if discontinuing the drug is not sufficient [13].

We initially suspected the possibility of infection because the GGO and interstitial infiltration are often seen in patients with pneumonia caused by many pathogens. *Pneumocystis jirovecii*, fungi, *Cytomegalovirus*, and *Mycobacterium* are frequently implicated as major causative organisms in immunosuppressed patients with acute progressive GGO. However, none of these organisms were identified on BAL or sputum culture and the results of serum β-D glucan and cytomegalovirus antigen and IgM antibody were not detected. Taken together, the possibility of infection was excluded in this patient. Indeed, immunosuppressive therapy did not deteriorate the patient's condition.

It was true that bronchoscopy and TBLB were not performed on the third admission, since the patient's respiratory function was substantially compromised and he was hypoxemic. If we could identify some evidence of vasculitis, the making diagnosis would be easier. In previous reports (Table 1), pathological examination found that GGO and patchy infiltration like those seen in this case were consequences of organizing pneumonia or nonspecific IP. In these 6 previous reports, four reports described that the PAA coexisted with IP implying the presence of vasculitis; however, Ning and Nanke reported cases of IP in patients with BD without association with vasculitis as our case. The pathology on why interstitial pneumonia occurred in those patients has not been revealed, but it might be an omen of vasculitis.

Our first-line treatments were pulsed mPSL and IVCY for induction and PSL and AZA for maintenance therapy, based on the assumption at the time that the interstitial infiltration had been caused by vasculitis. Although the TBLB did not show the presence of vasculitis, the tissue obtained by

TBLB was very tiny. Therefore, we considered that vasculitis could not be excluded. There have been reports of IP being caused by secondary vasculitis, which were also treated with IVCY followed by oral AZA [5–7]. One report states that parenchymal abnormalities including IP are usually associated with areas of infarction and lung hemorrhage caused by *in situ* thrombosis of pulmonary vessels and leaking aneurysms caused by vasculitis [9]. These may be forerunners of more serious complications, such as PAA formation. Histological examination of infiltrates is rarely performed, as an open approach would be warranted because of the risk of hemorrhage. Therefore the true incidence of interstitial lung involvement in BD may be underestimated.

In conclusion, this case is an exclusively rare case of recurrent IP in a patient with entero-BD. It is crucial to rule out the possibility of pulmonary infections and drug-induced lung injury when investigating the cause of IP, but BD-related interstitial infiltration caused by vasculitis should also be considered. Although pulmonary abnormalities are uncommon in patients with BD, the diffuse interstitial infiltration on both lungs in this case showed a good response to immunosuppressants including PSL, IVCY, and AZA. As relatively little is known about IP in BD, further research into the incidence and pathophysiology is needed.

Competing Interests

The authors declare that they have no competing interests.

References

[1] O. Uzun, L. Erkan, I. Akpolat, S. Findik, A. G. Atici, and T. Akpolat, "Pulmonary involvement in Behçet's disease," *Respiration*, vol. 75, no. 3, pp. 310–321, 2008.

[2] F. Erkan, A. Gül, and E. Tasali, "Pulmonary manifestations of Behçet's disease," *Thorax*, vol. 56, no. 7, pp. 572–578, 2001.

[3] J. Efthimiou, C. Johnston, S. G. Spiro, and M. Turner-Warwich, "Pulmonary disease in Behçet's syndrome," *Quarterly Journal of Medicine*, vol. 58, no. 227, pp. 259–280, 1986.

[4] T. Akoglu, S. Paydas, and S. Sarpel, "Incomplete Behcet's syndrome with unusual manifestations," *Annals of the Rheumatic Diseases*, vol. 46, no. 8, pp. 632–633, 1987.

[5] A. Gül, D. Yilmazbayhan, N. Büyükbabani et al., "Organizing pneumonia associated with pulmonary artery aneurysms in Behcet's disease," *Rheumatology*, vol. 38, no. 12, pp. 1285–1289, 1999.

[6] R. M. Rutherford, D. O'Keeffe, and J. J. Gilmartin, "An unusual case of non-specific interstitial pneumonitis," *Respiration*, vol. 71, no. 2, pp. 202–205, 2004.

[7] L. Ning-Sheng, L. Chun-Liang, and L. Ray-Sheng, "Bronchiolitis obliterans organizing pneumonia in a patient with Behçet's disease," *Scandinavian Journal of Rheumatology*, vol. 33, no. 6, pp. 437–440, 2004.

[8] Y. Nanke, T. Kobashigawa, T. Yamada, N. Kamatani, and S. Kotake, "Cryptogenic organizing pneumonia in two patients with Behçet's disease," *Clinical and Experimental Rheumatology*, vol. 25, no. 4, pp. S103–S106, 2007.

[9] F. Erkan, "Pulmonary involvement in Behcet disease," *Current Opinion in Pulmonary Medicine*, vol. 5, pp. 314–318, 1999.

[10] J. Castillo, M. Lema, A. Alvarez-Prechous et al., "Behçet's disease: report of ten cases and of a new clinical manifestation (portal vein thrombosis) (author's transl)," *Medicina Clinica*, vol. 75, no. 7, pp. 279–283, 1980.

[11] E. Seyahi, M. Melikoglu, C. Akman et al., "Pulmonary artery involvement and associated lung disease in Behçet disease: a series of 47 patients," *Medicine*, vol. 91, no. 1, pp. 35–48, 2012.

[12] T. Lamsiah, K. Moudden, M. Baaj, and L. Hadri, "Interstitial pneumonia related to mesalamine," *Gastroenterologie Clinique et Biologique*, vol. 34, no. 3, pp. 224–226, 2010.

[13] R. A. Foster, D. S. Zander, P. J. Mergo, and J. F. Valentine, "Mesalamine-related lung disease: clinical, radiographic, and pathologic manifestations," *Inflammatory Bowel Diseases*, vol. 9, no. 5, pp. 308–315, 2003.

[14] J. F. Pascual-Lledo, J. Calvo-Bonachera, F. Carrasco Miras, and H. Sanchez-Martinez, "Interstitial pneumonitis due to mesalamine," *Annals of Pharmacotherapy*, vol. 31, article 499, 1997.

[15] E. Alskaf, A. Aljoudeh, and F. Edenborough, "Mesalazine-induced lung fibrosis," *BMJ Case Reports*, vol. 2013, 2013.

41

A Rare but Fascinating Disorder: Case Collection of Patients with Schnitzler Syndrome

Maaman Bashir⬛,[1] Brittany Bettendorf⬛,[2] and Richard Hariman⬛[1]

[1]Division of Rheumatology, Department of Medicine, Medical College of Wisconsin, Milwaukee, WI 53226, USA
[2]Division of Rheumatology, Department of Medicine, University of Iowa, Iowa City, IA 52242, USA

Correspondence should be addressed to Maaman Bashir; maamanbashir@gmail.com

Academic Editor: Mehmet Soy

Background. Schnitzler syndrome is a rare disorder characterized by a chronic urticarial rash and monoclonal gammopathy (IgM in more than 90% of the cases). It is difficult to distinguish from other neutrophilic urticarial dermatoses, and diagnosis is based on the Strasbourg criteria. Interleukin-1 is considered the key mediator, and interleukin-1 inhibitors are considered first line treatment. Here, we present two cases of Schnitzler syndrome, both successfully treated with anakinra. *Objectives.* To increase awareness regarding clinical presentation, diagnosis, and treatment of this rare disorder. *Cases.* We describe the clinical features and disease course of two patients with Schnitzler syndrome, diagnosed using the Strasbourg criteria. Both were treated with anakinra with remarkable response to therapy. *Conclusion.* Schnitzler syndrome is a rare and underdiagnosed disorder. High suspicion should be maintained in patients with chronic urticaria-like dermatoses, intermittent fevers, and arthralgias. A serum protein electrophoresis and immunofixation should be performed in these patients. The diagnosis is important to recognize as Schnitzler syndrome is associated with malignancy. A lymphoproliferative disorder develops in about 20% of patients at an average of 7.6 years after onset of symptoms. Thus, patients warrant long-term follow-up. IL-1 inhibitors are extremely effective in relieving symptoms and are considered first line therapy.

1. Introduction

Schnitzler syndrome is a rare disorder in the family of neutrophilic urticarial dermatoses with fewer than 300 reported cases [1]. The syndrome can often be difficult to recognize, and the diagnosis can easily be confused with one of the other NUD counterparts, including adult-onset Still's disease, lupus erythematosus, and cryopyrin-associated periodic syndromes [2]. Initially described in 1972 by the French dermatologist Liliane Schnitzler [3, 4], the disorder is diagnosed when patients meet the Strasbourg criteria. This includes two obligate criteria: recurrent, nonpruritic urticaria and monoclonal gammopathy (IgM kappa light chain in >90%) [1]. At least two of the following minor criteria are also required: recurrent fever, objective findings of abnormal bone remodeling with or without bone pain (assessed by bone scintigraphy, MRI, or elevation of bone alkaline phosphatase), neutrophilic dermal infiltrate on skin biopsy, and elevated CRP and/or leukocytosis (CRP > 30 mg/L and/or neutrophils > 10,000/mm^3) [4]. The diagnosis is considered definite if the two obligate criteria and at least two minor criteria are met if the patient has IgM monoclonal gammopathy. The two obligate criteria and three minor criteria are required if there is IgG monoclonal gammopathy.

Skin biopsy from patients with the disorder is categorized as a neutrophilic urticarial dermatosis with histopathology demonstrating perivascular and interstitial neutrophilic inflammation with leukocytoclasia but without leukocytoclastic vasculitis [2, 5]. The pathogenesis of the disease remains unknown although it is thought to be autoinflammatory [2]. The disorder is best treated with medications that inhibit IL-1 such as anakinra, canakinumab, and rilonacept, but additional medications of symptomatic benefit have been identified including corticosteroids, rituximab, and cyclophosphamide [2]. A small case series also reported effectiveness of the anti-IL-6 receptor monoclonal antibody, tocilizumab, in patients who did not tolerate IL-1 inhibitors [6].

The diagnosis is important to recognize as Schnitzler syndrome is associated with malignancy. A lymphoproliferative disorder develops in about 20% of patients [2] at an average of 7.6 years after onset of symptoms and signs of Schnitzler syndrome [2].

2. Case 1

2.1. Presenting Concerns. The patient is a 56-year-old female with a past medical history of hypertension, hyperlipidemia, and ulcerative colitis who presented with complaints of joint pains for over 30 years. Her symptoms started with pain in the back radiating down the leg which later progressed to involve her shoulders, arms, wrists, and legs. She also described occasional swelling in her ankles, nonrefreshing sleep, and joint stiffness.

Eight years before presenting to our clinic, she was given a diagnosis of chronic Lyme disease based on non-CDC-approved testing and received IV ceftriaxone. However, repeat Lyme testing with IgG and IgM antibody by our facility was negative. MRI of her tibia and fibula two years prior to presenting in our clinic had revealed marrow edema, but a biopsy of her bone marrow was normal.

Upon initial presentation to our clinic, she was felt to have inflammatory arthritis and was treated with prednisone taper starting at 40 mg daily and weaned off slowly over several months. This helped her joint pain but did not resolve her symptoms completely. She was then trialed on treatment with hydroxychloroquine, methotrexate, and pregabalin without significant improvement.

2.2. Clinical Findings. At the time of diagnosis, exam revealed raised erythematous papules and plaques consistent with urticaria. They were distributed over the neck, upper back, and some on the arms. There were no signs of palpable purpura or necrosis. On joint exam, she had tenderness and swelling on palpation of bilateral 3rd PIPs. There was also tenderness in both shoulders, elbows, forearms, pretibial regions, and ankles without any swelling, erythema, or warmth. There was no evidence of synovitis or dactylitis in the feet.

2.3. Diagnostic Focus and Assessment. A detailed workup was performed (including ANA, ENA panel, RF, ANCA, serum protein electrophoresis and immunofixation, Lyme serology, muscle enzymes, ESR, CRP, ferritin, and cryoglobulins). She was found to have elevated inflammatory markers, with ESR 48 mm/hr, CRP 4.3 mg/dL, and ferritin 320.2 ng/mL. The electrophoresis and immunofixation revealed an IgM kappa monoclonal gammopathy. The rest of the blood work was negative. A bone survey of all long bones and a bone scan were also performed which showed diffuse osteitis and remodeling of long bones. Based on the urticarial rash, IgM kappa monoclonal gammopathy, abnormal bone

remodeling, and elevated acute phase reactants, she fulfilled the Strasbourg criteria for diagnosis of Schnitzler syndrome.

2.4. Therapeutic Focus and Assessment. She was started on anakinra 100 mg subcutaneous daily. The patient also tested quantiferon positive and was started on isoniazid and vitamin B-6 simultaneously for treatment of latent tuberculosis.

2.5. Follow-Up and Outcome. The patient noticed significant improvement in her urticarial rash within days after initiating the anakinra. Shortly after that, she also had progressive decline in her musculoskeletal pain and gradually became symptom free. The improvement was also reflected in her inflammatory markers. Her CRP dropped from 4.3 mg/dL to 0.7 mg/dL, and ESR dropped from 48 mm/hr to 4 mm/hr.

3. Case 2

3.1. Presenting Concerns. The patient is a 44-year-old male with a past medical history of HIV and Burkitt's lymphoma who presented to clinic with daily nocturnal fevers and rash for 3 months. He also complained of bilateral ankle swelling and pain for 1 month. The fevers initially occurred once a week but gradually increased in frequency. The rash typically became more prominent with the fever but not always. He denied any other joint pains.

He was initially evaluated by dermatology, where a biopsy revealed perivascular and interstitial mixed dermal inflammation, including neutrophils. The dermatologist suggested a trial of prednisone 60 mg daily, dapsone, and colchicine for possible Sweet's syndrome. However, there was no improvement.

He denied any foreign travel in years and did not have a history of tick or unusual animal exposures. His HIV was appropriately treated, and he had a negligible viral load. He had completed therapy for Burkitt's lymphoma 1 year ago and was in complete remission.

3.2. Clinical Findings. On initial exam in our clinic, pink, blanching, tender, warm, nonpruritic wheals were seen on his shoulders, arms, chest, and back. He also had bilateral ankle synovitis.

3.3. Diagnostic Focus and Assessment. Labs revealed elevated inflammatory markers, including CRP (17 mg/dL), ESR (95 mm/hr), and ferritin (625 ng/mL). White blood cell count was elevated to 12,700/mm³. His ANA, RF, SS-A, SS-B, and ANCA were negative. Repeat skin biopsy of the left shoulder revealed superficial and deep perivascular interstitial mixed inflammation with scattered neutrophils. The electrophoresis and immunofixation revealed monoclonal bands with faint IgM lambda.

Based on his chronic urticarial rash, IgM lambda monoclonal gammopathy, recurrent fever, neutrophilic infiltrate on skin biopsy, elevated inflammatory markers, and leukocytosis, a diagnosis of Schnitzler syndrome was made.

3.4. Therapeutic Focus and Assessment. After an extensive literature search regarding the safety and efficacy of anakinra use in patients with HIV and Burkitt lymphoma, anakinra was initiated. Prednisone was tapered off over a 2-month period.

3.5. Follow-Up and Outcome. The patient's rash improved within hours of the first anakinra injection. He did not have any further fevers once anakinra was initiated. His arthritis resolved over 1-2 months. Marked improvement was also noted in his inflammatory markers; 1 month after beginning treatment, his CRP improved from 17 mg/dL to 0.2 mg/dL, and ESR improved from 95 mm/hr to 8 mm/hr. The patient has continued to do well on daily anakinra.

4. Discussion

Schnitzler syndrome is likely underrecognized with an average delay to diagnosis of 5-6 years [2, 7] because of the nonspecific nature of the presentation with intermittent fever and rash. Urticarial rash is often the first symptom to appear in Schnitzler syndrome [8]. The similarities between Schnitzler syndrome and adult-onset Still's disease (AOSD), including urticarial rash, fever, joint pain, and leukocytosis, can make the two disease entities difficult to distinguish from each other. However, there are a few unique features that can be helpful in differentiating between the two. AOSD often presents with an initial pharyngitis, which is absent in Schnitzler syndrome. Additionally, ferritin in AOSD is very high whereas it rarely exceeds 1200 ng/mL in Schnitzler syndrome. [4, 8, 9]. Of course, the diagnosis of Schnitzler syndrome also requires monoclonal IgM or IgG, further differentiating this from AOSD. Urticarial vasculitis can also mimic Schnitzler syndrome; however, with urticarial vasculitis, skin biopsy should reveal features of true vasculitis with fibrinoid necrosis of small vessel walls, which should not be present in Schnitzler syndrome. Additionally, patients with urticarial vasculitis often have complement consumption and anti-C1q antibodies not observed in patients with Schnitzler syndrome [4].

It is difficult to draw direct conclusions about pathogenesis of Schnitzler syndrome due to the small number of biopsy-proven patients with available direct immunofluorescence studies. However, it has been proposed that the skin lesions seen in Schnitzler syndrome may be triggered by deposition of IgM in the epidermis and at the dermoepidermal junction [7]. Mutations in the *NLRP3* gene (nucleotide-binding oligomerization domain leucine-rich repeats containing pyrin domain 3) have also been proposed to play a role. No germline *NLRP3* mutation has been reported; however, somatic mosaicism of *NLRP3* mutations in the myeloid lineage has been previously reported in 2 patients with Schnitzler syndrome [10]. It is possible that infections such as HIV and tuberculosis may also play a causative role in the development of Schnitzler syndrome, as both HIV [11] and tuberculosis [12] are known to activate the *NLRP3* inflammasome, which induces IL-1-beta production. Interestingly, both patients in the case scenarios above had one of these infections. Systemic overproduction of interleukin-1-beta in patients with Schnitzler syndrome is thought to result in a profound loss of anti-inflammatory Th17 cell functionalities [13], consistent with the well-described excellent response to IL-1 receptor blockade in patients with Schnitzler syndrome. The response to anakinra is so immediate and striking, that it has been proposed that response to anakinra be added as a diagnostic criterion [14].

There have been successful case reports and small clinical trials with other IL-1-blocking medications as well, including canakinumab [15–17] and rilonacept [18]. A recent placebo-controlled study involving 20 patients with Schnitzler syndrome had promising results. 7 days after treatment, significantly more patients (5/7) in the canakinumab group showed complete clinical response as compared to those in the placebo group (0/13), highlighting its potential as a treatment option for this disease [19]. A small number of patients have also achieved long-term remission with the use of anakinra [20, 21], and some authors have proposed that after 2 years of complete remission, treatment can be stopped to assess whether symptoms persist [4]. However, other authors have noted that symptoms always recur after treatment is stopped [22], with one small study of patients on canakinumab demonstrating a median time to relapse of 72 days after the last canakinumab dose [15]. Flares can take several days to resolve after IL-1 blockade is restarted.

The overall prognosis for the disease is dependent on whether the patient develops a lymphoproliferative disorder. Lymphoma or Waldenstrom disease occurs in 15–20% of patients [20, 23–25]. Other less frequently associated lymphoproliferative disorders include lymphoplasmacytic lymphoma, chronic lymphocytic leukemia, splenic marginal zone lymphoma, multiple myeloma, and marginal zone B-cell lymphoma [2, 8, 9].

Although Schnitzler syndrome requires the presence of monoclonal gammopathy to establish the diagnosis, the significance of the type of monoclonal protein is unclear. In the study by Sokumbi et al., 2 of 3 patients (66%) with IgG monoclonal gammopathy went on to develop malignancy, whereas 7 of 17 patients (41%) with IgM gammopathy developed malignancy. Because Schnitzler syndrome is so rare, there are no large case series studying this association. This may present an opportunity for future study as it would provide prognostic information to patients and clinicians.

Other diseases associated with Schnitzler syndrome include AA amyloidosis in untreated patients, sensorimotor neuropathy, severe anemia of chronic inflammation, and even hearing loss [8]. Proposed criteria for monitoring patients with Schnitzler syndrome include clinical evaluation, CBC, and CRP every 3 months. Monitoring of MGUS should be as usually recommended, based on its serum level (once yearly if under 10 g/L, twice yearly if less than 30 g/L, and every 3 months if more than 30 g/L) [4]. This monitoring should include CBC with differential, SPEP, creatinine, calcium (if mIgG), LDH, and urine protein [4]. Providers should remain vigilant for increases in the monoclonal Ig level or new lymphadenopathy which should prompt further appropriate testing such as bone marrow or lymph node biopsy. Once the patient is successfully treated, parameters should be monitored twice per year [4].

References

[1] H. de Koning, "Schnitzler's syndrome: lessons from 281 cases," *Clinical and Translational Allergy*, vol. 4, no. 1, p. 41, 2014.

[2] O. Sokumbi, L. A. Drage, and M. S. Peters, "Clinical and histopathologic review of Schnitzler syndrome: The Mayo Clinic experience (1972–2011)," *Journal of the American Academy of Dermatology*, vol. 67, no. 6, pp. 1289–1295, 2012.

[3] H. Barriere, L. Schnitzler, G. Moulin, and Y. Grolleau, "Chronic urticarial lesions and macroglobulinemia. Apropos of 5 cases," *La Semaine des Hôpitaux*, vol. 52, pp. 221–227, 1976.

[4] A. Simon, B. Asli, M. Braun-Falco et al., "Schnitzler's syndrome: diagnosis, treatment, and follow-up," *Allergy*, vol. 68, no. 5, pp. 562–568, 2013.

[5] C. Kieffer, B. Cribier, and D. Lipsker, "Neutrophilic urticarial dermatosis: a variant of neutrophilic urticaria strongly associated with systemic disease: report of 9 new cases and review of the literature," *Medicine*, vol. 88, no. 1, pp. 23–31, 2009.

[6] K. Krause, E. Feist, M. Fiene, T. Kallinich, and M. Maurer, "Complete remission in 3 of 3 anti-IL-6-treated patients with Schnitzler syndrome," *Journal of Allergy and Clinical Immunology*, vol. 129, no. 3, pp. 848–850, 2012.

[7] D. Lipsker, D. Spehner, R. Drillien et al., "Schnitzler syndrome: heterogeneous immunopathological findings involving IgM-skin interactions," *British Journal of Dermatology*, vol. 142, no. 5, pp. 954–959, 2000.

[8] H. D. de Koning, E. J. Bodar, and J. W. van der Meer, "Schnitzler syndrome study group. Schnitzler syndrome: beyond the case reports: review and follow-up of 94 patients with an emphasis on prognosis and treatment," *Seminars in Arthritis and Rheumatism*, vol. 37, no. 3, pp. 137–148, 2007.

[9] D. Lipsker, Y. Veran, F. Grunenberger, B. Cribier, E. Heid, and E. Grosshans, "The Schnitzler syndrome. Four new cases and review of the literature," *Medicine*, vol. 80, no. 1, pp. 37–44, 2001.

[10] H. D. De Koning, M. E. Van Gijn, M. Stoffels et al., "Myeloid lineage-restricted somatic mosaicism of NLRP3 mutations in patients with variant Schnitzler syndrome," *Journal of Allergy and Clinical Immunology*, vol. 135, no. 2, pp. 561–564, 2015.

[11] H. Guo, J. Gao, D. J. Taxman et al., "HIV-1 infection induces interleukin-1β production via TLR8 protein-dependent and NLRP3 inflammasome mechanisms in human monocytes," *Journal of Biological Chemistry*, vol. 289, no. 31, pp. 21716–21726, 2014.

[12] V. Briken, S. E. Ahlbrand, and S. Shah, "Mycobacterium tuberculosis and the host cell inflammasome: a complex relationship," *Frontiers in Cellular and Infection Microbiology*, vol. 3, p. 62, 2013.

[13] R. Noster, H. D. de Koning, E. Maier et al., "Dysregulation of proinflammatory versus anti-inflammatory human TH17 cell functionalities in the autoinflammatory Schnitzler syndrome," *Journal of Allergy and Clinical Immunology*, vol. 138, no. 4, pp. 1161–1169, 2016.

[14] A. Kolivras, A. Theunis, A. Ferster et al., "Cryopyrin-associated periodic syndrome: an autoinflammatory disease manifested as neutrophilic urticarial dermatosis with additional perieccrine involvement," *Journal of Cutaneous Pathology*, vol. 38, pp. 202–208, 2011.

[15] H. D. De Koning, J. Schalkwij, J. Van der Ven-Jongerkriig et al., "Sustained efficacy of the monoclonal anti-interleukin-1 beta antibody canakinumab in a 9-month trial in Schnitzler's syndrome," *Annals of the Rheumatic Diseases*, vol. 72, no. 10, pp. 1634–1638, 2013.

[16] S. Vanderschueren and D. Knockaert, "Canakinumab in Schnitzler syndrome," *Seminars in Arthritis and Rheumatism*, vol. 42, no. 4, pp. 413–416, 2013.

[17] R. Pesek and R. Fox, "Successful treatment of Schnitzler syndrome with canakinumab," *Cutis*, vol. 94, pp. E11–E12, 2014.

[18] K. Krause, K. Weller, R. Stefaniak et al., "Efficacy and safety of the interleukin-1 antagonist rilonacept in Schnitzler syndrome: an open-label study," *Allergy*, vol. 67, no. 7, pp. 943–950, 2012.

[19] K. Krause, A. Tsianakas, N. Wagner et al., "Efficacy and safety of canakinumab in Schnitzler syndrome: a multicenter randomized placebo-controlled study," *Journal of Allergy and Clinical Immunology*, vol. 139, no. 4, pp. 1311–1320, 2017.

[20] D. Lipsker, "The Schnitzler syndrome," *Orphanet Journal of Rare Diseases*, vol. 5, no. 1, p. 38, 2010.

[21] B. Asli, J. C. Brouet, and J. P. Fernand, "Spontaneous remission of Schnitzler syndrome," *Annals of Allergy, Asthma & Immunology*, vol. 107, no. 1, pp. 87-88, 2011.

[22] L. Gusdorf and D. Lipsker, "Schnitzler syndrome: a review," *Current Rheumatology Reports*, vol. 19, no. 8, p. 46, 2017.

[23] E. Tinazzi, A. Puccetti, G. Patuzzo, M. Sorleto, A. Barbieri, and C. Lunardi, "Schnitzler syndrome, an autoimmune-autoinflammatory syndrome: report of two new cases and review of the literature," *Autoimmunity Reviews*, vol. 10, no. 7, pp. 404–409, 2011.

[24] R. A. Kyle, T. M. Therneau, S. V. Rajkumar et al., "Long-term follow-up of IgM monoclonal gammopathy of undetermined significance," *Blood*, vol. 102, no. 10, pp. 3759–3764, 2003.

[25] W. Lim, K. H. Shumak, M. Reis et al., "Malignant evolution of Schnitzler's syndrome: chronic urticaria and IgM monoclonal gammopathy: report of a new case and review of the literature," *Leukemia & Lymphoma*, vol. 43, no. 1, pp. 181–186, 2002.

42

Improvement of Arterial Wall Lesions in Parallel with Decrease of Plasma Pentraxin-3 Levels in a Patient with Refractory Takayasu Arteritis after Treatment with Tocilizumab

Shiho Iwagaitsu[1,2] and Taio Naniwa[1,2]

[1]*Division of Rheumatology, Department of Internal Medicine, Nagoya City University Hospital, Nagoya, Japan*
[2]*Department of Respiratory Medicine, Allergy and Clinical Immunology, Nagoya City University Graduate School of Medical Sciences, Nagoya, Japan*

Correspondence should be addressed to Taio Naniwa; tnaniwa@med.nagoya-cu.ac.jp

Academic Editor: Gregory J. Tsay

A 19-year-old Japanese woman with active Takayasu arteritis despite multiple conventional immunosuppressive therapies with glucocorticoids in combination with intravenous cyclophosphamide, azathioprine, or infliximab with methotrexate and tacrolimus was successfully treated by switching from infliximab to intravenous tocilizumab. Worsening of claudication of the legs and elevated acute phase reactants, including plasma pentraxin-3 levels, were observed during combination therapy with infliximab. Computed tomography demonstrated increased wall thickening with contrast enhancement in the preexisting lesion of the descending aorta and the femoral arteries. After switching from infliximab to tocilizumab, plasma pentraxin-3 levels gradually decreased to the normal range in parallel with the improvement of claudication. Follow-up computed tomographic scans confirmed the marked improvement of these arterial lesions. Moreover, plasma pentraxin-3 level was increased in response to the worsening of claudication that occurred just after switching to a subcutaneous tocilizumab injection. Measurements of plasma pentraxin-3 might be useful for evaluation of the vascular wall inflammation and therapeutic efficacy even during biologic therapy targeting tumor necrosis factor α and interleukin-6.

1. Introduction

Takayasu arteritis (TAK) is an idiopathic vasculitis mainly involving the aorta and its main branches. Glucocorticoids and conventional immunosuppressants are the mainstays of the treatment of TAK. Methotrexate and azathioprine are widely used, and cyclophosphamide is reserved for severe cases. Mycophenolate mofetil, cyclosporine, tacrolimus, and leflunomide have been tried in selected cases with successful results [1]. Proinflammatory cytokines, such as tumor necrosis factor- (TNF-) α and interleukin-6 (IL-6) have been shown to play a pivotal role in perpetuating disease activity of TAK [2–6], and biologics selectively targeting TNF-α and IL-6 signaling have been successfully used to treat refractory cases [7, 8].

Disease activity of large vessel vasculitis including TAK is usually estimated using clinical features, inflammatory markers, and imaging characteristics. As for inflammatory markers, C-reactive protein (CRP) and erythrocyte sedimentation rate (ESR), which reflect systemic inflammation, are commonly used to estimate disease activity of TAK. On the other hand, pentraxin-3, which belongs to a long pentraxin and is produced by various cells, such as macrophages, dendritic cells, fibroblasts, smooth muscle cells, adipocytes, vascular endothelial cells, and neutrophils, has been reported to correlate with vascular wall inflammation [9, 10]. Pentraxin-3 is induced by inflammatory cytokines, particularly by TNF-α, but not directly by IL-6. Thus, it can be assumed that anti-TNF therapy might mitigate the response of pentraxin-3 to vascular wall inflammation, as observed in CRP and ESR levels during anti-IL-6 therapy.

Here, we report on a patient with refractory TAK despite treatment with infliximab, who was successfully treated with tocilizumab. The effects on the arterial lesions were evaluated by computed tomography as well as of inflammatory markers including plasma pentraxin-3. Written informed consent was obtained from the patient for publication of this case report and accompanying images.

2. Case Presentation

A 19-year-old Japanese woman with active TAK refractory to combination therapy with conventional immunosuppressants and infliximab was given tocilizumab therapy. She was diagnosed as having TAK at age 15 when she developed abdominal pain, right carotidynia, low-grade fever, and claudication in both legs and the left arm. Contrast-enhanced computed tomography (CT) revealed wall thickening and stenosis of the descending aorta near of the aortic hiatus and main branches of the aorta. The thickened wall of the affected portion of the aorta was enhanced by contrast material. CRP and ESR were elevated at 6.03 mg/dl and 122 mm/hour, respectively. She was initially treated with 40 mg per day of prednisolone. She developed reversible cerebral vasoconstriction syndrome in the initial treatment course of TAK, which was described in our previous report on this patient [11]. She relapsed on prednisolone 15 mg per day, was given azathioprine with no remarkable response, and required dose increments of prednisolone up to 40 mg per day. Following that, therapy with intravenous cyclophosphamide and methotrexate was instituted but failed to control her disease activity. One year before starting tocilizumab, she started infliximab, whose dose was increased to 6 mg per kilogram of body weight, every four weeks after week 10, in addition to prednisolone 6 mg per day and methotrexate 17.5 mg per week. Six months later, CT showed exacerbation of the preexisting lesion of the descending aorta and newly emerged lesions in both femoral arteries. Then prednisolone dose was increased to 20 mg per day, and tacrolimus 3 mg per day was added. Three months before starting tocilizumab, she again developed claudication in both legs and the left arm (Figure 1). CRP and ESR levels had been 0.08 to 1.3 mg/dl and 10 to 20 mm/hour, respectively. Plasma pentraxin-3 levels measured using the Human Pentraxin3/TSG-14 ELISA System, by Perseus Proteomics Inc. Tokyo, Japan, had remained high ranging from 5.00 to 7.35 ng/ml during the last three months of infliximab therapy. The geometric mean [confidence intervals] of plasma pentraxin-3 levels in healthy Japanese woman was reported to be 2.12 [2.05, 2.19] ng/ml [12]. We switched from infliximab to tocilizumab, 8 mg per kilogram of body weight, every four weeks. Improvement of claudication of symptoms was observed in four weeks and continued over six months. Contrary to CRP and ESR, which were decreased to <0.03 mg/dl and 3 mm/hour at four weeks, pentraxin-3 levels had decreased with fluctuation over five months after starting tocilizumab. By her wish, we switched from intravenous tocilizumab to subcutaneous form, 162 mg per body, every other week, at 35 weeks, and

when pentraxin-3 levels were 1.59 ng/ml. Four weeks later, claudication in the left arm was worsened when we switched the form of tocilizumab back to intravenous form. CRP and ESR had remained unchanged, but pentraxin-3 levels were slightly increased to 2.77 ng/ml. Four weeks after resuming intravenous tocilizumab, pentraxin-3 levels were decreased to 1.22 ng/ml. Just after switching to subcutaneous tocilizumab, the transient decrease of serum IL-6 and subsequent increase of IL-6 were observed. CT obtained one year after starting tocilizumab revealed normalization of the appearance of both femoral arteries and improvement of the arterial wall thickening in the lesion of the descending aorta (Figure 2). Tocilizumab treatment could allow tapering off prednisolone over 27 months. No serious adverse events were observed during tocilizumab treatment.

3. Discussion

Previous reports have shown that anti-TNF and anti-IL-6 therapies were equally efficacious in patients with active TAK refractory to conventional therapies [7]. Although there are limited data on the efficacy of tocilizumab in patients with active TAK, despite anti-TNF therapy, the efficacy of tocilizumab was observed in more than half of the reported cases of refractory to anti-TNF-α therapy [13, 14]. In the present case, marked improvement in the clinical and radiographic signs of TAK was observed after switching from infliximab to tocilizumab.

We measured serial plasma pentraxin-3 levels, which are reported to correlate with vascular wall inflammation of TAK [15], as well as CRP and ESR during infliximab and tocilizumab therapy. During the last three months of infliximab therapy, which was clinically and radiographically ineffective, serum CRP and ESR levels remained normal to slightly positive, 0.08 to 1.3 mg/dl and 10 to 20 mm/hour, respectively. Although pentraxin-3 is induced by inflammatory cytokines, particularly by TNF-α, plasma pentraxin-3 levels remained high, 5.00 to 7.35 ng/ml in the presence of active vascular wall lesions despite treatment with anti-TNF therapy. These findings suggest that plasma pentraxin-3 could reflect vascular wall inflammation during anti-TNF therapy.

Tocilizumab, an IL-6 receptor antagonist, directly inhibits the production of downstream acute phase reactants, including CRP, and it may normalize CRP and ESR, irrespective of the disease activity of inflammatory diseases. Thus, these classic markers might be of limited value as surrogate markers for estimating disease activity in TAK in patients receiving tocilizumab. In the present case, CRP and ESR levels promptly decreased to and remained in undetectable quantities and near the minimum of the normal range, respectively, after starting the tocilizumab therapy. On the other hand, plasma pentraxin-3 had decreased with the fluctuations but normalized within five months of starting tocilizumab. A marked improvement of claudication was observed during the first four weeks of the tocilizumab treatment, while further improvements of claudication continued for the following six months. Furthermore, plasma pentraxin-3 levels increased during a symptomatic flare, which increased the Indian Takayasu Activity Score (ITAS2010) [16], directly

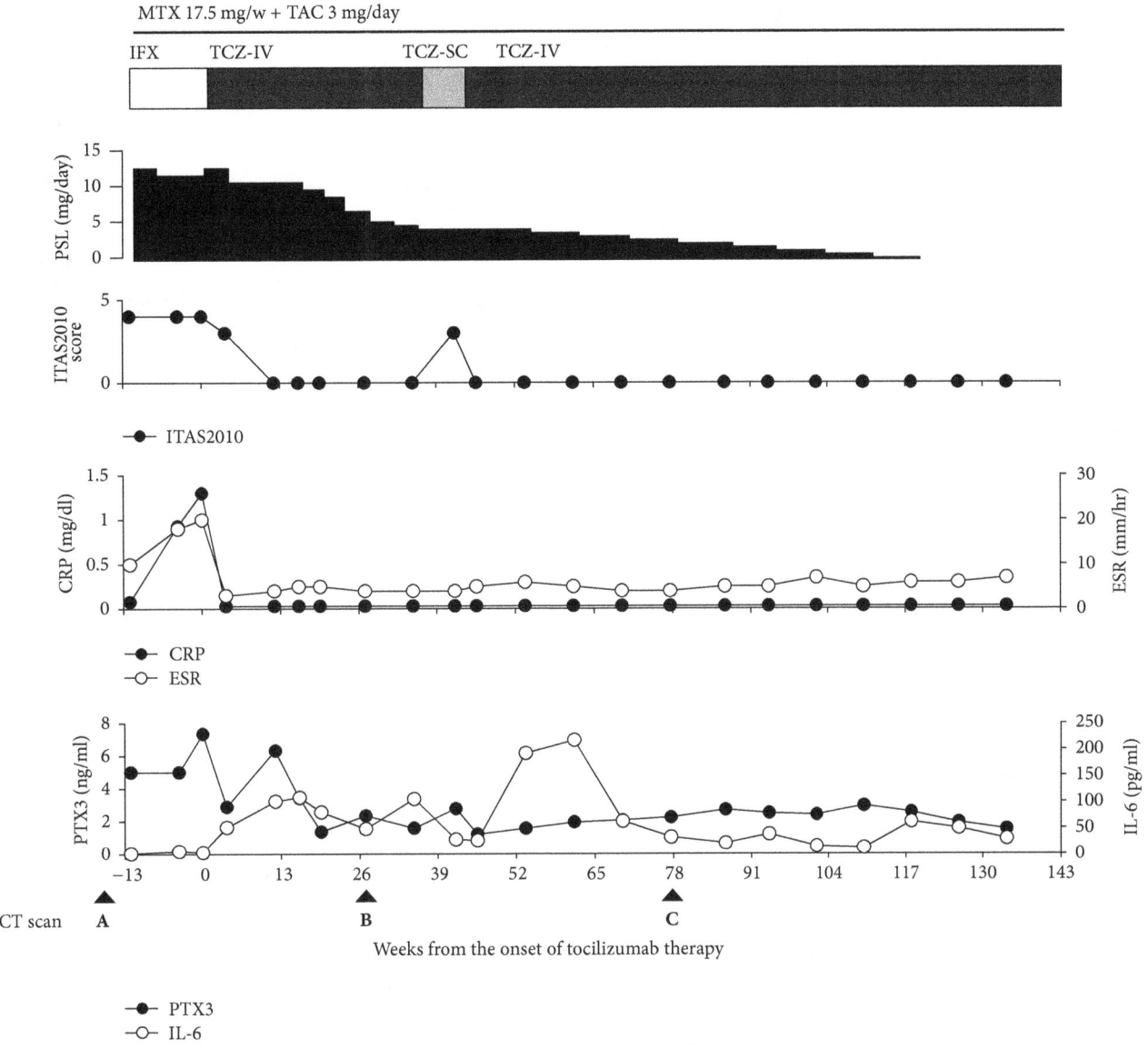

FIGURE 1: Changes in disease activity, biomarkers, and treatment during anticytokine biologic therapy. Infliximab (IFX) was administered at a dose of 6 mg per kilogram of body weight every four weeks (white bar). Intravenous tocilizumab (TCZ-IV) was administered at a dose of 8 mg per kilogram of body weight every four weeks (black bar), and subcutaneous tocilizumab (TCZ-SC) was administered at a dose of 162 mg per body weight every other week (gray bar). CRP, C-reactive protein; ESR, erythrocyte sedimentation rate; IL-6, interleukin-6; ITAS2010, The Indian Takayasu Activity Score 2010; PSL, prednisolone; PTX3, pentraxin-3.

after temporarily switching to a subcutaneous tocilizumab injection. At the same time, a temporary decrease in serum IL-6 levels and a subsequent increase in IL-6 levels were observed after resuming intravenous tocilizumab infusion. Serum IL-6 levels in the course of tocilizumab therapy with sufficient doses will reflect the actual endogenous IL-6 production that correlates with the true disease activity, while inflammatory symptoms are ameliorated by the inhibition of IL-6 signaling through IL-6 receptors [17]. It can be assumed that temporal change of IL-6 levels after switching to subcutaneous tocilizumab might be due to decreased saturated ratio of IL-6 receptor with tocilizumab caused by

lower blood concentration of tocilizumab, which made room for free IL-6 to bind to IL-6 receptor and might cause less sufficient inhibition of IL-6 signaling that contributes to worsening of disease activity of TAK.

Previous literature has shown that plasma pentraxin-3 levels were similar in patients with active or inactive disease defined by clinical disease activity measures, such as National Institute of Health criteria and ITAS2010 [18]. On the other hand, plasma pentraxin-3 levels were increased in the presence of vascular wall enhancement by contrast-enhanced magnetic resonance imaging and ^{18}F-Fluorodeoxyglucose Uptake by Positron Emission Tomography, which could

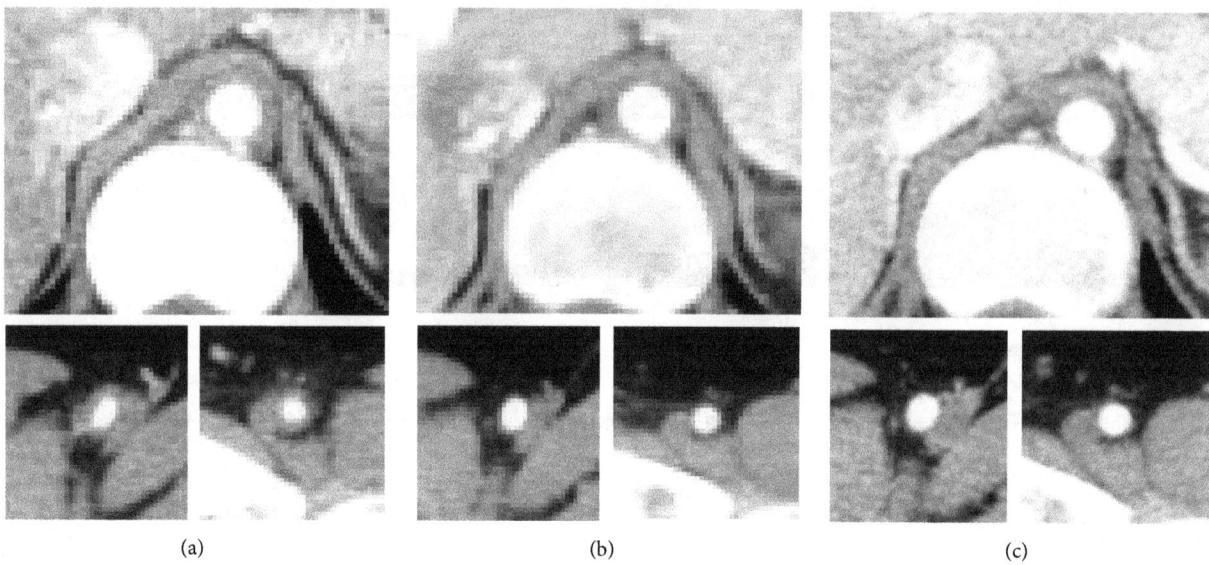

(a)	(b)	(c)

FIGURE 2: Changes in the computed tomographic findings of arterial lesions of Takayasu arteritis before and after starting tocilizumab therapy. Contrast-enhanced CT of the descending aorta (the upper), the right femoral artery (the bottom left), and the left femoral artery (the bottom right) was performed. Three months before starting tocilizumab therapy, while on the treatment with infliximab, arterial wall thickening of the femoral arteries was observed (a). After six months of tocilizumab therapy, there was a significant decrease in the wall thickness of the descending aorta and the femoral arteries (b). After 17 months of tocilizumab therapy, there was a further decrease in arterial wall thickness and an increase in the intraluminal diameter of the descending aorta and the femoral arteries (c).

reflect ongoing arterial wall inflammation [19]. In the present case, plasma pentraxin-3 levels seemed to correlate well with clinical manifestation related to active arterial lesions, which were confirmed by serial assessments with CT. Thus, plasma pentraxin-3 might be a useful biomarker for evaluation of the vascular wall inflammation and therapeutic efficacy even in patients receiving anti-TNF and anti-IL-6 biologic therapy, especially in those receiving the latter, which could normalize CRP and ESR irrespective of inflammatory disease activity.

In summary, our most important observation from the present case is that serial change of plasma pentraxin-3 levels could reflect vascular wall inflammation and the core pathology of TAK under treatment with these anticytokine biologics. This observation implicates the need for further exploration of plasma pentraxin-3 as a biomarker for estimating disease activity of TAK under treatment with these anticytokine biologics in a larger clinical study. Furthermore, the remission-inducing efficacy of tocilizumab in this patient with active TAK despite treatment with anti-TNF biologics highlights a crucial role of interleukin-6 in perpetuating disease activity of TAK.

References

[1] G. Keser, H. Direskeneli, and K. Aksu, "Management of Takayasu arteritis: a systematic review," *Rheumatology*, vol. 53, no. 5, Article ID ket320, pp. 793–801, 2014.

[2] J. Marquez, D. Flores, L. Candia, and L. R. Espinoza, "Granulomatous vasculitis," *Current Rheumatology Reports*, vol. 5, no. 2, pp. 128–135, 2003.

[3] M. Noris, E. Daina, S. Gamba, S. Bonazzola, and G. Remuzzi, "Interleukin-6 and RANTES in Takayasu arteritis: a guide for therapeutic decisions?" *Circulation*, vol. 100, no. 1, pp. 55–60, 1999.

[4] M. C. Park, S. W. Lee, Y. B. Park, and S. K. Lee, "Serum cytokine profiles and their correlations with disease activity in Takayasu's arteritis," *Rheumatology*, vol. 45, no. 5, pp. 545–548, 2006.

[5] C. Salvarani, F. Cantini, L. Boiardi, and G. G. Hunder, "Laboratory investigations useful in giant cell arteritis and Takayasu's arteritis," *Clinical and Experimental Rheumatology*, vol. 21, Supplement 32, no. 6, pp. S23–S28, 2003.

[6] Y. Seko, O. Sato, A. Takagi et al., "Restricted usage of T-cell receptor Vα-Vβ genes in infiltrating cells in aortic tissue of patients with Takayasu's arteritis," *Circulation*, vol. 93, no. 10, pp. 1788–1790, 1996.

[7] A. Mekinian, C. Comarmond, M. Resche-Rigon et al., "Efficacy of biological–targeted treatments in takayasu arteritis: multicenter, retrospective study of 49 patients," *Circulation*, vol. 132, no. 18, pp. 1693–1700, 2015.

[8] E. Tombetti, S. Franchini, M. Papa, M. G. Sabbadini, and E. Baldissera, "Treatment of refractory Takayasu arteritis with tocilizumab: 7 Italian patients from a single referral center," *The Journal of Rheumatology*, vol. 40, no. 12, pp. 2047–2051, 2013.

[9] B. Bottazzi, A. Doni, C. Garlanda, and A. Mantovani, "An integrated view of humoral innate immunity: pentraxins as a paradigm," *Annual Review of Immunology*, vol. 28, pp. 157–183, 2010.

[10] T. Ishihara, G. Haraguchi, T. Kamiishi, D. Tezuka, H. Inagaki, and M. Isobe, "Sensitive assessment of activity of takayasu's arteritis by pentraxin3, a new biomarker," *Journal of the American College of Cardiology*, vol. 57, no. 16, pp. 1712-1713, 2011.

[11] Y. Uchida, N. Matsukawa, T. Oguri et al., "Reversible cerebral vasoconstriction syndrome in a patient with Takayasu's arteritis," *Internal Medicine*, vol. 50, no. 15, pp. 1611–1614, 2011.

[12] K. Yamasaki, M. Kurimura, T. Kasai, M. Sagara, T. Kodama, and K. Inoue, "Determination of physiological plasma pentraxin 3 (PTX3) levels in healthy populations," *Clinical Chemistry and Laboratory Medicine*, vol. 47, no. 4, pp. 471–477, 2009.

[13] C. Salvarani, L. Magnani, M. Catanoso et al., "Rescue treatment with tocilizumab for takayasu arteritis resistant to TNF-α blockers," *Clinical and Experimental Rheumatology*, vol. 30, no. 70, pp. S90–S93, 2012.

[14] M. Bredemeier, C. M. Rocha, M. V. Barbosa, and E. H. Pitrez, "One–year clinical and radiological evolution of a patient with refractory Takayasu's arteritis under treatment with tocilizumab," *Clinical and Experimental Rheumatology*, vol. 30, no. 70, pp. S98–S100, 2012.

[15] L. Dagna, F. Salvo, M. Tiraboschi et al., "Pentraxin-3 as a marker of disease activity in takayasu arteritis," *Annals of Internal Medicine*, vol. 155, no. 7, pp. 425–433, 2011.

[16] R. Misra, D. Danda, S. M. Rajappa et al., "Development and initial validation of the Indian Takayasu Clinical Activity Score (ITAS '10)," *Rheumatology*, vol. 52, no. 10, pp. 1795–1801, 2013.

[17] N. Nishimoto, K. Terao, T. Mima, H. Nakahara, N. Takagi, and T. Kakehi, "Mechanisms and pathologic significances in increase in serum interleukin-6 (IL-6) and soluble IL-6 receptor after administration of an anti-IL-6 receptor antibody, tocilizumab, in patients with rheumatoid arthritis and Castleman disease," *Blood*, vol. 112, no. 10, pp. 3959–3964, 2008.

[18] F. Alibaz-Oner, K. Aksu, S. P. Yentur, G. Keser, G. Saruhan-Direskeneli, and H. Direskeneli, "Plasma pentraxin-3 levels in patients with Takayasu's arteritis during routine follow–up," *Clinical and Experimental Rheumatology*, vol. 34, pp. S73–S76, 2016.

[19] D. Tezuka, G. Haraguchi, T. Ishihara et al., "High Standardized Uptake Value of 18F-Fluorodeoxyglucose-Positron Emission Tomography/Computed Tomography was correlated with Disease Activity in Patients with Takayasu Arteritis," *Circulation*, vol. 122, article A15229, 2010.

43

The Foot That Broke Both Hips: A Case Report and Literature Review of Tumor-Induced Osteomalacia

Sara Beygi,[1] Alfred Denio,[2] and Tarun S. Sharma[3]

[1]Internal Medicine Department, Allegheny Health Network, Pittsburgh, PA, USA
[2]Rheumatology Department, Geisinger Medical Center, Danville, PA, USA
[3]Rheumatology Department, Allegheny Health Network, Pittsburgh, PA, USA

Correspondence should be addressed to Tarun S. Sharma; tsharma@wpahs.org

Academic Editor: Remzi Cevik

Tumor-induced osteomalacia (TIO) is a rare paraneoplastic syndrome characterized by hypophosphatemia and clinical symptoms of osteomalacia. Only discussed as case reports, there is still limited knowledge of this condition as a potentially curable cause of osteomalacia among clinicians and pathologists. In this article, we present a case of tumor-induced osteomalacia in a 59-year-old gentleman followed by an up-to-date review of the existing literature on TIO.

1. Introduction

Tumor-induced osteomalacia (TIO) or oncogenic osteomalacia is an underrecognized paraneoplastic syndrome presenting with hypophosphatemia and typical manifestations of osteomalacia [1]. The clinical syndrome of osteomalacia and associated biochemical abnormalities including low phosphate and 1,25-dihydroxyvitamin D levels are blamed on the production of phosphate-regulating substances, most notably fibroblast growth factor 23 (FGF23), by tumor cells [2, 3]. Since the FGF23-producing tumors tend to be small and hard to detect on physical exam, symptoms of osteomalacia, including bone pain and muscle weakness, sometimes precede the diagnosis of the tumor by years. The fact that surgical resection of the tumor is usually curative highlights the importance of raising awareness of this condition among clinicians and pathologists.

In this article, we present a case of TIO followed by a review of the current literature.

2. Case Presentation

A 59-year-old gentleman was hospitalized in May 2013 for elective repair of a stress fracture of the medial midshaft of the right femur. Orthopedic surgeons planned to perform an elective surgery. A routine rheumatology consult as a part of the fracture liaison service was requested. Upon further questioning, he admitted to a minor fall while carrying a heating unit up a flight of stairs a few months prior to admission. Since then, he had persistent discomfort in the right thigh and was complaining of difficulty walking, loss of balance, and leg "giving out on him" for a few months. His past medical history was only remarkable for hypertension and cervical spinal stenosis, and his social/family history was noncontributory.

Physical examination revealed a man of normal stature with normal-appearing limbs. He had tenderness to palpation of the right medial midthigh region. In addition, some mild tenderness in the left midthigh was noted. The remainder of the exam including testicles, sclera, and skin elasticity was unremarkable.

Preoperative workup included an AP pelvis X-ray which revealed a left subtrochanteric femur stress fracture in addition to the known right femur fracture (Figure 1).

An intramedullary device was placed bilaterally.

Laboratory parameters obtained prior to surgery are as follows:

(i) Calcium: 9.4 mg/dL (*n*: 8.3–10.5)

(ii) Alkaline phosphatase: 135 U/L (*n*: 0–153)

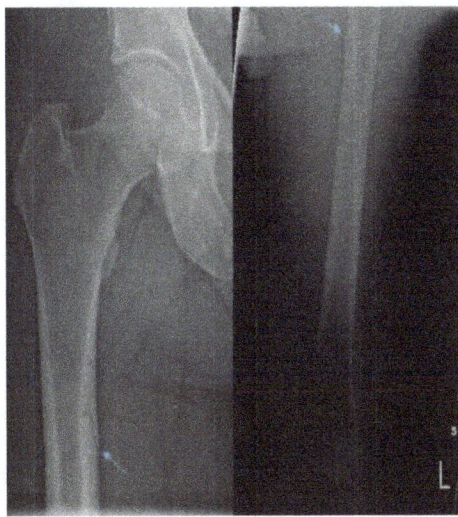

FIGURE 1: Radiographic image of both femurs with arrows pointing towards the fracture lines (the right femur on the left side and the left femur on the right side).

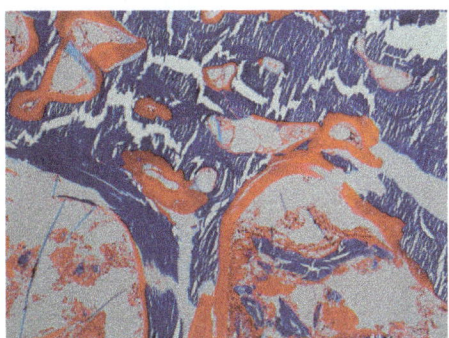

FIGURE 2: Plastic-embedded trichrome-stained pictures of the bone with 20x magnification. The trichrome staining shows wide seams of unmineralized osteoid (red) that covers virtually all trabecular surfaces, suggesting a severe mineralization defect.

(iii) 25-Hydroxyvitamin D level: 22 ng/mL (*n*: 30–100)

(iv) 24-hour urine calcium: 0.223 g/24 hours (*n*: 0.05–0.3)

(v) TSH: 2.24 uIU/mL (*n*: 0.27–4.2)

(vi) Creatinine: 1.0 mg/dL (*n*: 0.7–1.5)

(vii) iPTH: 50 pg/mL (*n*: 10–65)

(viii) *Phosphate: 1.5 mg/dL (n: 2.5–4.8)*

(ix) 24-hour urine phosphate: 0.821 g/24 hours (*n*: 0.3–1)

(x) *Plasma fibroblast growth factor 23 (FGF23): 211 RU/mL (n < 180)*

An iliac crest bone biopsy with trichrome staining (Figure 2) and tetracycline labeling (Figure 3) revealed marked osteomalacia and a severe mineralization defect.

A whole body PET/CT revealed uptake within a soft tissue nodule in the plantar surface of the left foot, at the level of the 2nd and 3rd metatarsophalangeal joints (Figure 4).

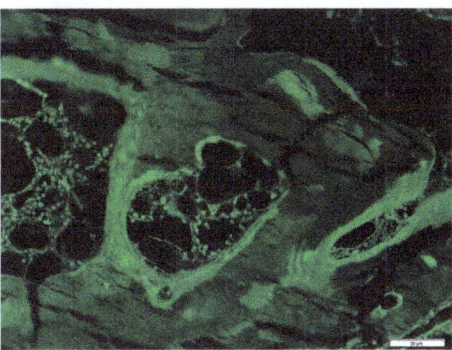

FIGURE 3: Fluorescence microscopic pictures of the tetracycline-labeled bone with 20x magnification. A severe mineralization defect is confirmed by an unstained section of the bone under fluorescence microscopy looking for tetracycline labeling which reveals faint fluorescence with a blurred pattern and no evidence of the typical double labeling of the bone matrix.

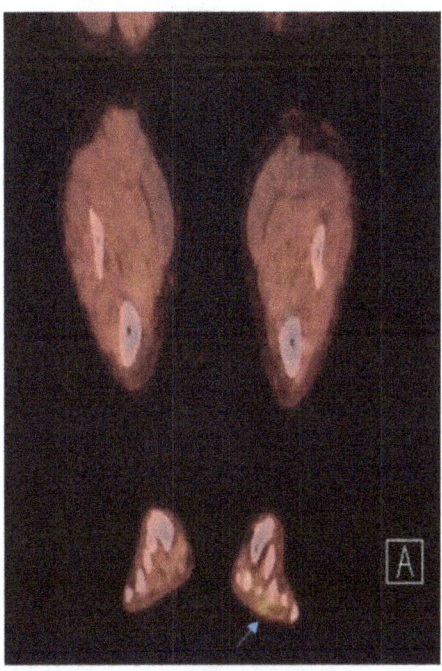

FIGURE 4: Positron emission tomographic image of the lower extremities showcasing a fluorodeoxyglucose (FDG) avid spot on the plantar surface of the left foot (arrow).

Excisional biopsy of the left plantar foot nodule revealed a benign mesenchymal tumor consisting of small vessels admixed with fibrocartilage foci (Figures 5–7).

The tumor was resected, and the patient's FGF23 and phosphate levels returned to normal soon after the surgery (phosphate: 4.6 mg/dL day 11 post-op, FGF23: 76 RU/mL 4 months post-op). The patient has been following up with an orthopedic oncologist every 6 months. The FGF23 and phosphate values continue to be within normal limits during the follow-up period, and the patient remains asymptomatic with no indications of recurrence (phosphate: 2.8 mg/dL, FGF23: 83 RU/mL at 14-month follow-up).

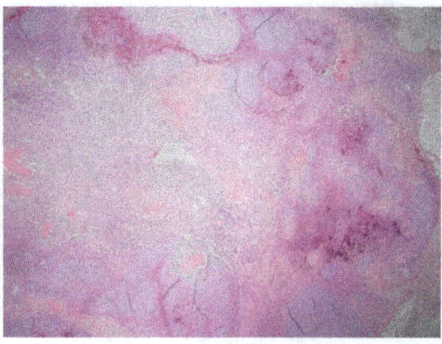

FIGURE 5: Low-power microscopic image (2x) showing a well-delineated tumor consisting of variegated mesenchymal components rich in small vessels with focal myxoid stroma.

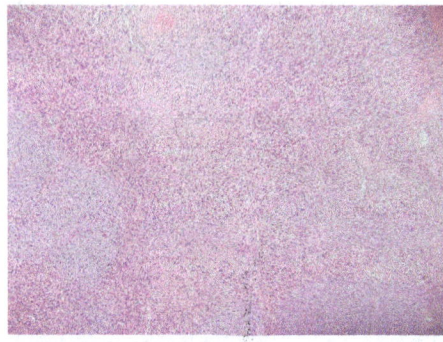

FIGURE 6: Low-power microscopic image (10x) showing a tumor consisting of prominent small vessels, myxoid stroma, and scattered osteoclast-type giant cells.

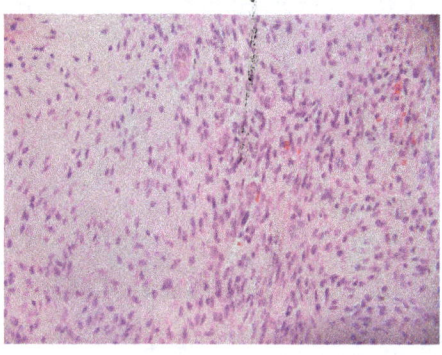

FIGURE 7: High-power microscopic image (40x) showing a tumor consisting of bland spindle cells sitting in slightly myxoid stroma with an osteoclast-type giant cell.

3. Literature Review Method

A PubMed search was performed on January 1, 2017, using the following search strategy:

(((((((oncogenic osteomalacia[Title/Abstract]) OR oncogenic hypophosphatemia[Title/Abstract]) OR tumor induced osteomalacia[Title/Abstract]) OR tumor induced hypophosphatemia[Title/Abstract]) OR tumor-induced hypophosphatemia[Title/Abstract]) OR tumor-induced osteomalacia[Title/Abstract]) OR phosphaturic mesenchymal tumor[Title/Abstract].

A total of 490 articles were retrieved and reviewed.

4. Background

For the first time in 1947, McCance reported a 15-year-old patient with weakness, gait disturbances, and low phosphate level whose symptoms completely resolved after resection of a tumor found in her femur [4]. However, her condition was inaccurately attributed to vitamin D resistance. As it is inferred from the literature, back in those days vitamin D resistance was believed to be the mechanism of what was eventually recognized as FGF23-induced phosphate-wasting disorder [5]. The first person who blamed the disease on the production of a "rachitogenic" substance by tumor cells was Prader [6]. He described severe rickets in an 11-year-old girl who was found to have a giant cell granuloma of the rib. Complete resolution of her rickets was achieved following resection of the tumor. Prader clearly delineated the association between resolution of the symptoms and tumor resection and proposed that the granuloma might have released a rachitogenic mediator. Since recognition of the condition, around 350 cases have been reported in the literature, most of them being published over the last 10 years.

It was repeatedly noted by different experts that TIO-associated tumors share distinctive morphological features, favoring an unidentified histopathological entity [7]. The term "phosphaturic mesenchymal tumor" (PMT) was introduced by Weidner and Santa Cruz [8], and PMT was eventually added to the 2013 WHO classification of tumors of the soft tissue and bone [9].

5. Clinical Characteristics

Tumor-induced osteomalacia typically occurs in adults, with equal gender distribution [10]. Patients usually present with progressive musculoskeletal symptoms including pain, proximal muscle weakness, and fractures. Due to general unawareness of this condition, there is usually a significant lag between the onset of symptoms and diagnosis. Therefore, it is not uncommon for patients to present with multiple fractures occasionally leading to height loss and a debilitated state [11].

The classic biochemical profile is characterized by normal calcium and parathormone levels, low or inappropriately normal 1,25-dihydroxyvitamin D levels, and elevated alkaline phosphatase levels [12].

Differentiating TIO from acquired and hereditary disorders that could present with hypophosphatemic osteomalacia would be of paramount importance. The acquired causes include nutritional deficiencies of vitamin D or phosphate as well as renal tubular abnormalities due to a variety of causes such as burns, heavy metal exposure, certain medications, and paraproteinemia [1, 13]. The inherited causes of hypophosphatemic osteomalacia include X-linked hypophosphatemic rickets (XLH), autosomal dominant hypophosphatemic rickets (ADHR), autosomal recessive hypophosphatemic rickets (ARHR), and hereditary hypophosphatemic rickets with hypercalciuria (HHRH) which are biochemical equivalents of TIO with high or inappropriately normal levels of FGF23 [1, 13].

Phosphaturic mesenchymal tumors tend to be small and not easily detectable on physical exam [10]. In fact, it is the osteomalacia and associated metabolic abnormalities which usually raise suspicion for an underlying tumor. TIO has been reported in association with other types of tumors as well, most notably small cell carcinoma and neurofibromatosis [14], although this is usually a feature of PMTs. However, unlike PMTs, in the case of TIO associated with other tumors, the primary tumor is usually known at the time of presentation. This type of presentation is sometimes referred to as secondary TIO [13]. Interestingly, few cases of TIO secondary to colon adenocarcinoma and ovarian cancer have also been reported [15, 16].

Reviewing the reported cases of TIO to date reveals that 50–55% of the tumors have been reported to arise from soft tissues and 40–45% in bones. Thigh and femur tend to be the most common anatomical sites (22.7%), followed by the craniofacial region (20.7%), ankle and foot (8.8%), pelvis (8.2%), tibia and fibula (6.5%), and arms (6.5%) [17]. In the head and neck region, three-fourths of the cases were noted in extraoral sites, with paranasal sinuses being the most common location [10]. There has not been a single report of the retroperitoneum or parenchymal organ as the primary site of the tumor [18].

6. Histopathological Features

The classic histological appearance of phosphaturic mesenchymal tumors consists of a background of spindle- to stellate-shaped neoplastic cells with a "smudgy" appearance which are generally normochromic with small nuclei and indistinct nucleoli [1]. The nuclear grade and mitotic activity are characteristically low. The cells are typically nested within a myxochondroid matrix with so-called "grungy" calcifications resembling the cartilage or osteoid tissue. Osteoclast-appearing giant cells are a common finding while mature lamellar bone may also be noted. A prominent feature of these tumors is an elaborate microvascular network with vessels of various sizes and patterns resembling a "staghorn" [13]. Microcytic changes have also been frequently described. Lately, immunostaining with D2-40, an antibody against a lymphatic marker, has proven to be positive in analysis of the fluids from microcysts, suggesting a partial differentiation toward lymphatic endothelial cells [19]. Initially, four different histological variants of PMTs were described: mixed connective tissue variant (PMTMCT), osteoblastoma-like variant, nonossifying fibroma-like variant, and ossifying fibroma-like variant [20]. However, later on, Folpe et al. [21] demonstrated that almost all previously identified mesenchymal tumors would fall under the single category of PMTMCT, debating the previous notion of 4 different histological subtypes. Of all the immunohistochemical markers investigated so far, only 2 have been tested positive, smooth muscle actin and FGF23, in 10 and 70% of the cases, respectively [21]. Of note, only proliferating cells within the tumor were noted to stain for FGF23 [21]. Somatostatin receptors have also been consistently detected in TIO tumors [22]. Therefore, it has been suggested that a positive staining for both FGF23 and somatostatin receptors

would be a sensitive test for PMTs, though probably not specific enough [22].

PMTMCT also manifests ultrastructural features of neuroendocrine tumors [23]. However, typical immunohistochemical markers of neurosecretory tumors including S-100, neuron-specific enolase, chromogranin, and synaptophysin have not been detected [13]. Perhaps, vimentin is the only neurosecretory marker that has consistently been noted positive [24]. Interestingly, there are reported instances of tumors with histopathological features consistent with PMTMCT, though not associated with the clinical syndrome of osteomalacia. These tumors are sometimes classified as nonphosphaturic variant [21, 25].

Although characteristically benign, malignant behavior and metastases have occasionally been reported [26, 27]. Similarly, there have been rare instances of locally aggressive lesions as well as multifocal lesions [18]. It is worth noting that, even in the case of metastasizing tumors, the histopathological appearance of the tumor tends to be benign. On the other hand, microscopic infiltration of the surrounding soft tissue is often noted in the margins of an otherwise benign-appearing lesion [18].

7. Pathogenesis

Overexpression of phosphate-regulating factors has been consistently implicated in the pathogenesis of tumor-induced osteomalacia. Among all, FGF23 has perhaps the most established role. FGF23 was identified as the culprit phosphaturic substance after mutations in FGF23 gene were recognized in the pathophysiology of ADHR [28]. FGF23 is physiologically produced by normal bone cells [29] and, aside from its phosphaturic action, is thought to act directly on the bone and suppress differentiation of osteoblasts [30]. There is some evidence that the phosphaturic effect of FGF23 is somewhat PTH dependent. The notion is supported by the observation that in the presence of low to undetectable PTH levels, as occurs in hypoparathyroidism, FGF23 does not lead to hypophosphatemia [31].

To date, several other phosphate-regulating factors including matrix extracellular phosphoglycoprotein (MEPE) [30], secreted frizzled related protein-4 (sFRP-4) [32], and dentin matrix protein 1 (DMP1) [33] have been identified. However, their precise pathogenicity remains to be elucidated. Of note, despite a strong expression of messenger ribonucleic acid (mRNA) of the aforementioned factors by tumor cells, elevated plasma levels have not yet been reported in the setting of TIO. More recently, Lee et al. [34] identified a fibronectin 1–fibroblast growth factor receptor 1, FN1–FGFR1, fusion in 42% of the studied phosphaturic mesenchymal tumors (21/50). Additionally, a novel FN1–FGF1 fusion gene was reported in 6% of the cases (3/50) [34]. Lately, a case of TIO with elevated venous levels of both FGF7 and FGF23 has been reported, suggesting a possible phosphaturic role for FGF7 as well [35]. The phosphate-regulating factors act primarily on the proximal renal tubules, causing redistribution of sodium phosphate cotransporters and therefore impairing reabsorption of phosphate [36]. Moreover, as a secondary mechanism, FGF23 and sFRP-4 decrease

TABLE 1: Differential diagnoses of hypophosphatemia.

Decreased absorption	Increased excretion	Intercellular shifts
Poor dietary intake	Hyperparathyroidism: primary and secondary	Insulin effect, i.e., during refeeding syndrome
Inhibition of absorption due to medications including phosphate binders, anticonvulsants, antacids, etc.	Hereditary hypophosphatemic rickets: XLHR (mutations in PHEX gene), ADHR (mutations in FGF23 gene), ARHR (mutations in DMP1 gene), HHRH (mutations in sodium phosphate transporter 2c)	Respiratory alkalosis
Malabsorption syndromes, i.e., celiac disease, Crohn's, nontropical sprue, etc.	Fanconi syndrome: inherited versus acquired, i.e., heavy metal induced, chemotherapeutic agents, monoclonal gammopathies, etc.	Hungry bone syndrome
Vitamin D deficiency or resistance: dietary, lack of sunlight, excess fluoride, etc.	Tumor-induced osteomalacia	Increased metabolism: blast crisis, thyrotoxicosis

FGF23, fibroblast growth factor 23; XLHR, X-linked hypophosphatemic rickets; ADHR, autosomal dominant hypophosphatemic rickets; ARHR, autosomal recessive hypophosphatemic rickets; HHRH, hereditary hypophosphatemic rickets with hypercalciuria.

vitamin D levels presumably through downregulation of 1α-hydroxylase and upregulation of 24-hydroxylase [32, 36].

8. Diagnosis

Diagnosis of TIO should always be suspected in case of hypophosphatemia and excessive phosphaturia. Some of the notable causes of hypophosphatemia are listed in Table 1. A thorough history including family history of genetic phosphate abnormalities along with a complete biochemical testing is recommended as the next step (Table 2). A typical patient with TIO manifests low serum phosphate, normal to low calcium, normal PTH, normal 25-hydroxyvitamin D, normal to low 1,25-dihydroxyvitamin D, elevated bone alkaline phosphatase, and high FGF23 levels.

After a biochemical profile supports the diagnosis of TIO, an exhaustive physical exam is warranted to locate the tumor. However, as discussed earlier, these tumors tend to be obscure and typically very hard to detect on physical exam, therefore prompting the use of functional and anatomical imaging modalities. On the other hand, precise localization of the tumor is of paramount importance since resection of the tumor is usually curative [1]. Overall, F-18 fluorodeoxyglucose positron emission tomography, coupled with computed tomography (FDG-PET/CT), is thought to be the most sensitive method for localizing TIO tumors [37]. However, poor specificity limits the value of this modality. Indium-111 octreotide scintigraphy is another useful functional modality which takes advantage of the high affinity of indium octreotide for somatostatin receptors, especially subtype 2 which is most frequently detected in PMTMCT [38]. One important consideration would be to ensure coverage of the entire body as opposed to the standard frame of PET/CT and octreotide scanning which excludes distal extremities as well as parts of the head [39]. A sensitivity of 60–80% has been suggested for octreotide scintigraphy [40] and PET/CT [37] for detection of the PMTs in small case series. Somatostatin receptor PET tracers, Ga68-DOTANOC [41] and Ga68-DOTATATE [42], have emerged as potential agents for localization of PMTs. Labeling a modified octreotide molecule, with high affinity for both somatostatin receptors 2 and 5 [43] with Ga68, a positron emitter, allows

TABLE 2: Laboratory tests recommended in cases of suspected TIO.

Serum phosphorus

Serum calcium

25-Hydroxyvitamin D

1,25-Dihydroxyvitamin D

Parathyroid hormone

Alkaline phosphatase (bone-specific form if available)

24-hour urine collection for phosphorus, calcium, and creatinine

Fibroblast growth factor 23

Serum protein electrophoresis and immunofixation

Urine monoclonal proteins, kappa and lambda chains

for an admixture of PET sensitivity and octreotide specificity. Recent reports have supported superiority of Ga68-DOTATATE to FDG-PET/CT in the diagnosis of TIO [42], as well as in the case of nonrevealing prior indium-111 octreotide scan [44].

Once a suspicious tumor is identified through functional studies, anatomical imaging needs to be pursued to confirm the location and further characterize the lesion. Magnetic resonance imaging (MRI) is the most frequently utilized anatomical modality [45]. The most typical radiographic appearance of PMTs is a well-defined lytic lesion on computed tomography (CT) and a T2 hyperintense and enhancing lesion on MRI. However, occasionally lesions expanding beyond the bone, resembling a primary bone malignancy, have also been noted [18].

Overall, different diagnostic approaches have been recommended in the current literature. Some authors advocate a multistep approach starting with functional modalities, most notably PET/CT [13]; however, other experts prefer to use MRI as the initial step [32]. If imaging studies fail to localize a suspected lesion, venous sampling could be the next step. However, blind venous sampling in the absence of a previously identified suspicious lesion on functional or anatomical imaging has not led to promising results [46]. Aspiration of the suspected lesion and measuring FGF23 levels in the aspirate along with microscopic evaluation of the floating cells may be of diagnostic value [47]. Finally, if tumor localization efforts are unsuccessful, serial imaging with 1-2-year interval may be a reasonable course of action. Once the tumor is localized and resected, microscopic evaluation of the lesion allows for an accurate diagnosis of the PMT. FGF23 expression can be confirmed by the reverse transcription polymerase chain reaction (RT-PCR) technique on the tissue and also by anti-FGF23 antibodies which are still not widely available [48]. It is worth noting that the exquisite sensitivity of the molecular method in detection of FGF23 may lead to false-positive results in the case of non–phosphaturic mesenchymal tumors producing trace amounts of FGF23 including fibrous dysplasia, chondromyxoid fibroma [29], and aneurysmal bone cyst [49].

9. Management

Resection of the tumor is the ultimate definitive treatment of tumor-induced osteomalacia. Maintaining a wide surgical margin cannot be emphasized enough to prevent the recurrence of the tumor which has been reported in several instances [27]. A 10 mm margin for extremity lesions and 5 mm for trunk lesions have been proposed. Since FGF23 has a short half-life of 45–58 minutes [50], a rapid resolution of symptoms upon surgical removal is expected.

Surgical cure is evidenced by normalization of the serum biochemical abnormalities including serum phosphate level. It is important to note that reversal of phosphate levels after surgical resection is required to confirm the diagnosis of TIO [13]. Late recurrence happens in a small percentage of patients [21, 27]; therefore, long-term follow-up is warranted after the surgery. Should metastasis occur, the lung is the most common site [21, 25–27]. In a review of 32 Japanese cases of PMTMCT, metastases were found in 4 patients (12.5%) on follow-up and 2 patients eventually died of the disease [25]. Radiofrequency ablation (RFA) has also received attention as a possible treatment modality which still needs further investigation [51]. Adjuvant radiotherapy, even though not well studied, has been recommended in cases of recurrence where repeat surgery would lead to significant disability such as losing a limb. Positive margins after surgery may also justify the use of postoperative radiotherapy.

If the tumor cannot be localized or surgically removed, medical therapy is recommended with phosphate supplementation and calcitriol [32]. The typical treatment regimen would be 15–60 mg/kg per day of elemental phosphate divided into 4–6 doses for 1–3 days. Calcitriol is given at 15–60 ng/kg per day, with a usual starting dose of 1.5 mg/day for an adult. Cinacalcet, an agonist of calcium-sensing receptors, has also led to promising outcomes, by lowering blood parathormone levels. Geller et al. [31] observed a significant bone-healing effect following treatment of two cases of TIO with 30 mg/day cinacalcet. Of note, despite the presence of somatostatin receptors on the cell surface of phosphaturic mesenchymal tumors, octreotide has not demonstrated significant clinical success [52].

Interestingly, the results of a phase I clinical trial on efficacy of a humanized anti-FGF23 antibody in adults with X-linked hypophosphatemic rickets (XLHR) indicated the safety and effectiveness of this novel treatment [53]. Given the similarity of pathogenesis, this antibody might be of therapeutic value for TIO as well.

10. Conclusion and Future Direction

In conclusion, TIO is a rare paraneoplastic syndrome caused by release of phosphate- and vitamin D-regulating mediators, most notably FGF23, from tumor cells. A distinct category of tumors, phosphaturic mesenchymal tumors, is responsible for majority of the cases. Excision of the culprit neoplasm is usually curative. Although these tumors are small and hard to locate on physical exam, a stepwise diagnostic approach involving functional and anatomical imaging studies and, if needed, selective venous sampling or aspiration of the lesion tends to be successful. Resection of the tumor is typically followed by a rapid decline in FGF23 levels and resolution of symptoms. Although characteristically benign, PMTs with aggressive features such as local invasion, metastasis, and late recurrence have also been described. When the tumor cannot be identified or resected, medical treatment with phosphate supplements, calcitriol, and cinacalcet is recommended.

Various aspects of TIO, ranging from pathogenesis to treatment, are yet to be understood. In terms of pathogenesis, the phosphaturic role of FGF7, which has recently been proposed, needs to be further elaborated in the future studies. From a diagnostic point of view, comparison between emerging modalities including somatostatin receptor PET tracers and more traditional imaging techniques such as MRI and PET/CT warrants further investigation. Finally, humanized anti-FGF23 antibody as a potential medical treatment for TIO is an area that is certainly worth exploring.

Disclosure

The authors would like to declare that this manuscript was presented as a poster at Allegheny Health Network's Internal Medicine Research Day in May 2016 and won the first prize in the clinical vignette category.

Acknowledgments

The authors would like to thank Dr. David Hicks and Dr. Jinhong Li for their kind help with procurement of high-quality pathology images and their expert interpretation.

References

[1] R. Kumar, A. L. Folpe, and B. P. Mullan, "Tumor-induced osteomalacia," *Translational Endocrinology and Metabolism*, vol. 7, no. 3, 2015.

[2] S. Fukumoto and T. Yamashita, "FGF23 is a hormone-regulating phosphate metabolism—unique biological characteristics of FGF23," *Bone*, vol. 40, no. 5, pp. 1190–1195, 2007.

[3] K. B. Jonsson, R. Zahradnik, T. Larsson et al., "Fibroblast growth factor 23 in oncogenic osteomalacia and X-linked

hypophosphatemia," *New England Journal of Medicine*, vol. 348, no. 17, pp. 1656–1663, 2003.

[4] R. A. McCance, "Osteomalacia with Looser's nodes (Milkman's syndrome) due to a raised resistance to vitamin D acquired about the age of 15 years," *Quarterly Journal of Medicine*, vol. 16, no. 1, pp. 33–46, 1947.

[5] F. Albright, A. M. Butler, and E. Bloomberg, "Rickets resistant to vitamin D therapy," *American Journal of Diseases of Children*, vol. 54, no. 3, pp. 529–547, 1937.

[6] A. Prader, R. Illig, E. Uehlinger, and G. Stalder, "Rickets following bone tumor," *Helvetica Paediatrica Acta*, vol. 14, pp. 554–565, 1959.

[7] D. J. Evans and J. G. Azzopardi, "Distinctive tumours of bone and soft tissue causing acquired vitamin-D-resistant osteomalacia," *Lancet*, vol. 299, no. 7746, pp. 353-354, 1972.

[8] N. Weidner and D. Santa Cruz, "Phosphaturic mesenchymal tumors. A polymorphous group causing osteomalacia or rickets," *Cancer*, vol. 59, no. 8, pp. 1442–1454, 1987.

[9] V. Y. Jo and C. D. M. Fletcher, "WHO classification of soft tissue tumours: an update based on the 2013 (4th) edition," *Pathology*, vol. 46, no. 2, pp. 95–104, 2014.

[10] H. Qari, A. Hamao-Sakamoto, C. Fuselier, Y. S. Cheng, H. Kessler, and J. Wright, "Phosphaturic mesenchymal tumor: 2 new oral cases and review of 53 cases in the head and neck," *Head and Neck Pathology*, vol. 10, no. 2, pp. 192–200, 2016.

[11] W. H. Chong, S. Yavuz, S. M. Patel, C. C. Chen, and M. T. Collins, "The importance of whole body imaging in tumor-induced osteomalacia," *Journal of Clinical Endocrinology and Metabolism*, vol. 96, no. 12, p. 3599, 2011.

[12] M. K. Drezner, "Tumor-induced osteomalacia," *Reviews in Endocrine and Metabolic Disorders*, vol. 2, no. 2, pp. 175–186, 2001.

[13] W. H. Chong, A. A. Molinolo, C. C. Chen, and M. T. Collins, "Tumor-induced osteomalacia," *Endocrine-Related Cancer*, vol. 18, no. 3, pp. R53–R77, 2011.

[14] V. Jagtap, V. Sarathi, A. R. Lila et al., "Tumor-induced osteomalacia: a single center experience," *Endocrine Practice*, vol. 17, no. 2, pp. 177–184, 2011.

[15] D. E. Leaf, R. C. Pereira, H. Bazari, and H. Jüppner, "Oncogenic osteomalacia due to FGF23-expressing colon adenocarcinoma," *Journal of Clinical Endocrinology & Metabolism*, vol. 98, no. 3, pp. 887–891, 2013.

[16] H.-A. Lin, S.-R. Shih, Y.-T. Tseng et al., "Ovarian cancer-related hypophosphatemic osteomalacia—a case report," *Journal of Clinical Endocrinology & Metabolism*, vol. 99, no. 12, pp. 4403–4407, 2014.

[17] J. Dadoniene, M. Miglinas, D. Miltiniene et al., "Tumour-induced osteomalacia: a literature review and a case report," *World Journal of Surgical Oncology*, vol. 14, no. 1, p. 4, 2016.

[18] M. Higley, B. Beckett, S. Schmahmann, E. Dacey, and E. Foss, "Locally aggressive and multifocal phosphaturic mesenchymal tumors: two unusual cases of tumor-induced osteomalacia," *Skeletal Radiology*, vol. 44, no. 12, pp. 1825–1831, 2015.

[19] S. Tajima and M. Fukayama, "Possibility of D2-40 as a diagnostic and tumor differentiation-suggestive marker for some of phosphaturic mesenchymal tumors," *International Journal of Clinical and Experimental Pathology*, vol. 8, no. 8, p. 9390, 2015.

[20] N. Weidner, "Review and update: oncogenic osteomalacia-rickets," *Ultrastructural Pathology*, vol. 15, no. 4-5, pp. 317–333, 1991.

[21] A. L. Folpe, J. C. Fanburg-Smith, S. D. Billings et al., "Most osteomalacia-associated mesenchymal tumors are a single histopathologic entity: an analysis of 32 cases and a comprehensive review of the literature," *American Journal of Surgical Pathology*, vol. 28, no. 1, pp. 1–30, 2004.

[22] M. Houang, A. Clarkson, L. Sioson et al., "Phosphaturic mesenchymal tumors show positive staining for somatostatin receptor 2A (SSTR2A)," *Human Pathology*, vol. 44, no. 12, pp. 2711–2718, 2013.

[23] G. E. Wilkins, S. Granleese, R. G. Hegele, J. Holden, D. W. Anderson, and G. P. Bondy, "Oncogenic osteomalacia: evidence for a humoral phosphaturic factor," *Journal of Clinical Endocrinology & Metabolism*, vol. 80, no. 5, pp. 1628–1634, 1995.

[24] A. Angeles-Angeles, A. Reza-Albarrán, F. Chable-Montero, J. C. Cordova-Ramón, J. Albores-Saavedra, and B. Martinez-Benitez, "Phosphaturic mesenchymal tumors. Survey of 8 cases from a single Mexican medical institution," *Annals of Diagnostic Pathology*, vol. 19, no. 6, pp. 375–380, 2015.

[25] R. Honda, Y. Kawabata, S. Ito, and F. Kikuchi, "Phosphaturic mesenchymal tumor, mixed connective tissue type, non-phosphaturic variant: report of a case and review of 32 cases from the Japanese published work," *Journal of Dermatology*, vol. 41, no. 9, pp. 845–849, 2014.

[26] T. Morimoto, S. Takenaka, N. Hashimoto, N. Araki, A. Myoui, and H. Yoshikawa, "Malignant phosphaturic mesenchymal tumor of the pelvis: a report of two cases," *Oncology Letters*, vol. 8, no. 1, pp. 67–71, 2014.

[27] A. Ogose, T. Hotta, I. Emura et al., "Recurrent malignant variant of phosphaturic mesenchymal tumor with oncogenic osteomalacia," *Skeletal Radiology*, vol. 30, no. 2, pp. 99–103, 2001.

[28] M. J. Econs and M. K. Drezner, "Tumor-induced osteomalacia—unveiling a new hormone," *New England Journal of Medicine*, vol. 330, no. 23, pp. 1679–1681, 1994.

[29] M. Riminucci, M. T. Collins, N. S. Fedarko et al., "FGF-23 in fibrous dysplasia of bone and its relationship to renal phosphate wasting," *The Journal of Clinical Investigation*, vol. 112, no. 5, pp. 683–692, 2003.

[30] Y. Imanishi, J. Hashimoto, W. Ando et al., "Matrix extracellular phosphoglycoprotein is expressed in causative tumors of oncogenic osteomalacia," *Journal of Bone and Mineral Metabolism*, vol. 30, no. 1, pp. 93–99, 2012.

[31] J. L. Geller, A. Khosravi, M. H. Kelly, M. Riminucci, J. S. Adams, and M. T. Collins, "Cinacalcet in the management of tumor-induced osteomalacia," *Journal of Bone and Mineral Research*, vol. 22, no. 6, pp. 931–937, 2007.

[32] T. Berndt, T. A. Craig, A. E. Bowe et al., "Secreted frizzled-related protein 4 is a potent tumor-derived phosphaturic agent," *Journal of Clinical Investigation*, vol. 112, no. 5, pp. 785–794, 2003.

[33] S. Toyosawa, Y. Tomita, M. Kishino et al., "Expression of dentin matrix protein 1 in tumors causing oncogenic osteomalacia," *Modern Pathology*, vol. 17, no. 5, pp. 573–578, 2004.

[34] J.-C. Lee, S. Y. Su, C. A. Changou et al., "Characterization of FN1–FGFR1 and novel FN1–FGF1 fusion genes in a large series of phosphaturic mesenchymal tumors," *Modern Pathology*, vol. 29, no. 11, pp. 1335–1346, 2016.

[35] S. Bansal, K. Khazim, R. Suri, D. Martin, S. Werner, and P. Fanti, "Tumor induced osteomalacia: associated with elevated circulating levels of fibroblast growth factor-7 in addition to fibroblast growth factor-23," *Clinical Nephrology*, vol. 85, no. 1, pp. 57–62, 2016.

[36] T. Shimada, M. Kakitani, Y. Yamazaki et al., "Targeted ablation of FGF23 demonstrates an essential physiological role of FGF23 in phosphate and vitamin D metabolism," *Journal of Clinical Investigation*, vol. 113, no. 4, pp. 561–568, 2004.

[37] J.-L. Dupond, H. Mahammedi, N. Magy, O. Blagosklonov, N. Meaux-Ruault, and B. Kantelip, "Detection of a mesenchymal tumor responsible for hypophosphatemic osteomalacia using FDG-PET," *European Journal of Internal Medicine*, vol. 16, no. 6, pp. 445-446, 2005.

[38] M. Duet, S. Kerkeni, R. Sfar, C. Bazille, F. Lioté, and P. Orcel, "Clinical impact of somatostatin receptor scintigraphy in the management of tumor-induced osteomalacia," *Clinical Nuclear Medicine*, vol. 33, no. 11, pp. 752–756, 2008.

[39] Y. Kaneuchi, M. Hakozaki, H. Yamada, O. Hasegawa, T. Tajino, and S. Konno, "Missed causative tumors in diagnosing tumor-induced osteomalacia with (18)F-FDG PET/CT: a potential pitfall of standard-field imaging," *Hellenic Journal of Nuclear Medicine*, vol. 19, no. 1, pp. 46–48, 2016.

[40] C. A. Garcia and R. P. Spencer, "Bone and In-111 octreotide imaging in oncogenic osteomalacia: a case report," *Clinical Nuclear Medicine*, vol. 27, no. 8, pp. 582-583, 2002.

[41] C. von Falck, T. Rodt, H. Rosenthal et al., "68Ga-DOTANOC PET/CT for the detection of a mesenchymal tumor causing oncogenic osteomalacia," *European Journal of Nuclear Medicine and Molecular Imaging*, vol. 35, no. 5, p. 1034, 2008.

[42] K. Agrawal, S. Bhadada, B. R. Mittal et al., "Comparison of 18F-FDG and 68Ga DOTATATE PET/CT in localization of tumor causing oncogenic osteomalacia," *Clinical Nuclear Medicine*, vol. 40, no. 1, pp. e6–e10, 2015.

[43] D. Wild, H. R. Mäcke, B. Waser et al., "68Ga-DOTANOC: a first compound for PET imaging with high affinity for somatostatin receptor subtypes 2 and 5," *European Journal of Nuclear Medicine and Molecular Imaging*, vol. 32, no. 6, p. 724, 2005.

[44] S. Breer, T. Brunkhorst, F. T. Beil et al., "68Ga DOTA-TATE PET/CT allows tumor localization in patients with tumor-induced osteomalacia but negative 111In-octreotide SPECT/CT," *Bone*, vol. 64, pp. 222–227, 2014.

[45] A. M. Dissanayake, J. L. Wilson, I. M. Holdaway, and I. R. Reid, "Oncogenic osteomalacia: culprit tumour detection whole body magnetic resonance imaging," *Internal Medicine Journal*, vol. 33, no. 12, pp. 615-616, 2003.

[46] P. Andreopoulou, C. E. Dumitrescu, M. H. Kelly et al., "Selective venous catheterization for the localization of phosphaturic mesenchymal tumors," *Journal of Bone and Mineral Research*, vol. 26, no. 6, pp. 1295–1302, 2011.

[47] D. M. Sciubba, R. J. Petteys, S. F. Shakur et al., "En bloc spondylectomy for treatment of tumor-induced osteomalacia: case report," *Journal of Neurosurgery: Spine*, vol. 11, no. 5, pp. 600–604, 2009.

[48] A. Bahrami, S. W. Weiss, E. Montgomery et al., "RT-PCR analysis for FGF23 using paraffin sections in the diagnosis of phosphaturic mesenchymal tumors with and without known tumor induced osteomalacia," *American Journal of Surgical Pathology*, vol. 33, no. 9, pp. 1348–1354, 2009.

[49] S. Krishnamurthy, C. Y. Inwards, A. M. Oliveira, and A. L. Folpe, "Frequent expression of fibroblast growth factor-23 (FGF-23) mRNA in aneurysmal bone cyst (ABC)," in *Laboratory Investigation*, Nature Publishing Group, New York, NY, USA, 2011.

[50] A. Khosravi, C. M. Cutler, M. H. Kelly et al., "Determination of the elimination half-life of fibroblast growth factor-23," *Journal of Clinical Endocrinology & Metabolism*, vol. 92, no. 6, pp. 2374–2377, 2007.

[51] E. Hesse, H. Rosenthal, and L. Bastian, "Radiofrequency ablation of a tumor causing oncogenic osteomalacia," *New England Journal of Medicine*, vol. 357, no. 4, pp. 422–424, 2007.

[52] F. Paglia, S. Dionisi, and S. Minisola, "Octreotide for tumor-induced osteomalacia," *New England Journal of Medicine*, vol. 346, no. 22, pp. 1748-1749, 2002.

[53] T. O. Carpenter, E. A. Imel, M. D. Ruppe et al., "Randomized trial of the anti-FGF23 antibody KRN23 in X-linked hypophosphatemia," *Journal of Clinical Investigation*, vol. 124, no. 4, pp. 1587–1597, 2014.

44

Undiagnosed Sjögren's Syndrome Presenting as Mesenteric Panniculitis

Rebecca L. Burns[1] and Sharukh J. Bhavnagri[2]

[1]*Division of Rheumatology, University of Michigan Health System, Suite 7C27, North Ingalls Building,
300 North Ingalls Street, SPC 5422, Ann Arbor, MI 48109-5422, USA*
[2]*Department of Diagnostic Radiology and Molecular Imaging, Oakland University William Beaumont
School of Medicine, 3601 West 13 Mile Road, Royal Oak, MI 48073, USA*

Correspondence should be addressed to Rebecca L. Burns; rburns24@gmail.com

Academic Editor: Mario Salazar-Paramo

Mesenteric panniculitis is a rare inflammatory and fibrotic process that affects the small intestine mesentery. It may occur following abdominal surgery or in association with a variety of conditions, including malignancy, infection, and certain autoimmune and inflammatory conditions. Herein, an unusual case of mesenteric panniculitis in a patient with primary Sjögren's syndrome will be presented. The patient presented with abdominal pain, weight loss, sicca symptoms, fatigue, and arthralgia. An abdominal CT revealed mesenteric fat stranding and prominent lymph nodes of the small intestine mesentery. She was found on laboratory workup to have positive antinuclear and anti-SSa antibodies. Minor salivary gland lip biopsy revealed focal lymphocytic sialadenitis. The patient's symptoms and CT findings improved with corticosteroids. This case suggests that Sjögren's syndrome should be considered as an underlying disease process in the evaluation of patients with mesenteric panniculitis.

1. Introduction

Mesenteric panniculitis is an acute and chronic inflammatory and fibrotic process that affects the small intestine mesentery [1, 2]. It may be associated with a variety of conditions, including malignancy, prior abdominal surgery, infection, and certain autoimmune and inflammatory conditions [3]. Presenting symptoms include abdominal pain, bloating, weight loss, and intestinal obstruction [4]. Evaluation by CT may reveal soft tissue masses, prominent lymph nodes, and fibrosis or inflammation of the small bowel mesentery. Primary Sjögren's syndrome (pSS) is a chronic autoimmune disorder characterized by lymphocytic infiltration of salivary and lacrimal glands, resulting in severe sicca symptoms. pSS patients may also present with extraglandular features. A rare case of mesenteric panniculitis in a patient with pSS will be presented here.

2. Case Presentation

A 44-year-old female presented to rheumatology clinic with complaints of progressively worsening epigastric abdominal pain and distention over 7 months. She had previously been diagnosed with mesenteric panniculitis and was referred for further management. The abdominal pain began following a laparoscopic hysterectomy. At the time of rheumatologic consultation, she had lost 40 lbs. She complained of severe constipation and ability to have bowel movements only with heavy use of laxatives. She had a small amount of bright red blood in her stool intermittently, which had been attributed to hemorrhoids. Review of systems was negative for fevers, rashes, photosensitivity, oral or nasal ulcers, hair loss, or pleurisy. She admitted to having severe dryness of her eyes and mouth, diffuse arthralgia, fatigue, and chills. She had no history of renal failure, thrombosis, or miscarriage. EGD and colonoscopy performed previously were significant only for

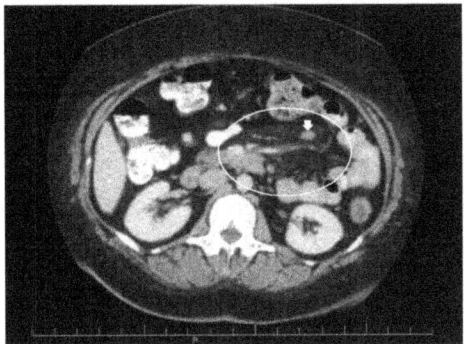

FIGURE 1: Axial CT image demonstrating mesenteric fat stranding (oval) with enlarged mesenteric lymph nodes (arrow) indicative of mesenteric panniculitis.

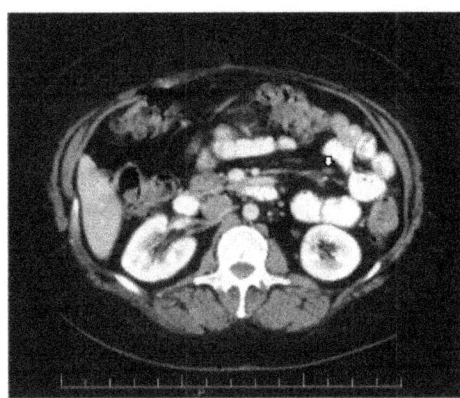

FIGURE 2: Axial CT image after therapeutic intervention reveals response to therapy with a decrease in the size of the mesenteric lymph node (arrow) and resolution of mesenteric fat stranding.

mild gastritis. A CT scan performed 5 months after the pain had begun revealed mesenteric fat stranding and prominent mesenteric lymph nodes concerning for mesenteric panniculitis (Figure 1).

Past medical history was significant for knee osteoarthritis, gastroesophageal reflux disease, and peptic ulcer with *H. pylori* infection. Prior surgeries preceding the laparoscopic hysterectomy included cholecystectomy, cesarean section, and partial hysterectomy. Family history was negative for rheumatic disease. Home medications included acetaminophen, lansoprazole, and laxative agents.

On physical exam, she was afebrile with normal vital signs. Mucous membranes were noted to be dry. Her abdomen was soft and nondistended, with moderate tenderness and guarding upon palpation over her epigastric region. Cardiac, pulmonary, neurologic, and joint exams were entirely unremarkable.

Laboratory workup revealed normal CBC, renal panel, and liver function panel. ESR was elevated at 54 mm. She had unremarkable urinalysis and urine protein-to-creatinine ratio. Antinuclear antibody (ANA) by immunofluorescence was positive with a titer of 1 : 640 in a speckled pattern. Anti-SSa antibody was positive. Anti-double stranded DNA (dsDNA), SSb, chromatin, Sm, RNP, scl-70, and centromere antibodies were all negative. Serum complements were normal, and serum protein electrophoresis revealed a polyclonal increase in gamma globulins, with no monoclonal protein present. Serum IgG4 level was 33.5 (normal range 8–150 mg/dL). A minor salivary gland biopsy revealed focal lymphocytic sialadenitis with a focus score of 1. A diagnosis of primary Sjögren's syndrome was made based on her presentation and laboratory findings.

The patient was started on oral prednisone 60 mg daily. She had near-complete resolution of her abdominal symptoms and joint pain within weeks, and the steroid was tapered over 3 months. She was transitioned to colchicine. Hydroxychloroquine was initiated for pSS-related arthralgia and fatigue. Repeat CT scan showed improvement of the previously noted changes of mesenteric panniculitis, with decrease in size of the enlarged mesenteric lymph nodes and mesenteric fat stranding (Figure 2). She remains stable on colchicine and hydroxychloroquine.

3. Discussion

Mesenteric panniculitis is a rare inflammatory and fibrotic process that affects the small intestine mesentery [1, 2]. It may be associated with a variety of conditions, including malignancy, liver cirrhosis, infection, and certain autoimmune and inflammatory conditions [3]. It may also be associated with a prior history of abdominal surgery [4]. A variety of systemic and gastrointestinal symptoms may arise from the disease process, including abdominal pain, bloating, weight loss, nausea and vomiting, diarrhea, constipation, fever, and intestinal obstruction. A palpable abdominal mass or chylous ascites may also be present. The disorder usually occurs in middle or late adulthood with a slight male predominance [5]; however, one large study of 7620 abdominal CT scans showed a female predominance [3].

Various terms have been used in the description of mesenteric panniculitis, including retractile mesenteritis, mesenteric lipodystrophy, and sclerosing mesenteritis [5–8]. The different terms are likely more appropriate to describe different points in the progression of the disease; it begins as adipocyte necrosis (mesenteric lipodystrophy), followed by a chronic inflammatory state (mesenteric panniculitis), and finally progressing to fibrosis (sclerosing or retractile mesenteritis).

An abdominal CT is often used for diagnosis. CT findings may include a single or multiple soft tissue masses in the root of the mesentery, often with calcification [3, 4]. Rarely, infiltration of the pancreas or porta hepatis may occur [9]. There may be increased density of the mesenteric fat without a discrete mass, suggesting fibrosis or inflammation, as well as prominence of retroperitoneal and mesenteric lymph nodes. A hypodense fatty halo may be found surrounding vessels and nodules [3]. If there is significant involvement of the mesenteric vessels, bowel ischemia may result [9].

When biopsy is obtained, histopathologic features may include fibrosis, inflammation, and fat necrosis [4]. Lipid-laden foamy macrophages may be found infiltrating the mesenteric fat.

Mesenteric panniculitis may be associated with many autoimmune conditions, including primary sclerosing cholangitis, systemic lupus erythematosus (SLE), retroperitoneal fibrosis, and Riedel thyroiditis [9,10]. Additionally, it has been suggested that the disease process may be associated with sclerosing pancreatitis and IgG4-related disease [4, 11].

The case presented here is an unusual one. Review of the literature revealed only 3 other case reports of mesenteric panniculitis associated with SS [12–14]. In addition, 2 patients with sclerosing mesenteritis from the study by Akram et al. had SS [4]. In the case presented by Batten and Ng, a 64-year-old male diagnosed with SS based on sicca symptoms and salivary gland biopsy underwent CT evaluation for abdominal pain and night sweats [13]. CT revealed edema of the mesenteric fat and lymph nodes in the jejunal mesentery. The patient improved symptomatically with a steroid taper; however, there was minimal improvement in the CT findings of mesenteric panniculitis. Sugihara et al. presented a case of a female with SS who developed abdominal pain, fever, and skin rash [12]. She was found to have systemic panniculitis involving the mesenteric adipose tissue as well as the skin. She also improved with corticosteroids alone. Osato et al. described a case of mesenteric panniculitis in a Human T-cell Lymphotropic Virus Type-I (HTLV-1) carrier with renal failure, pancytopenia, subcutaneous panniculitis, and uveitis [14]. The patient had a sicca syndrome thought to be HTLV-I associated SS. She had positive ANA with negative anti-SSa and anti-SSb antibodies. She underwent laparotomy for acute abdominal pain and was found to have mesenteric panniculitis with appendicitis. She later died from a mechanical ileus which developed at the surgical site.

It is important to exclude underlying malignancy in patients found to have mesenteric panniculitis. In the study by Daskalogiannaki et al., 69.4% of patients with mesenteric panniculitis were found to have a coexistent malignancy [3]. These included non-Hodgkin's lymphoma, breast and lung carcinomas, and various GI and gynecologic malignancies. Several patients had coexisting benign diseases, including SLE. Our patient was referred to general surgery for consideration of mesenteric biopsy to exclude lymphoproliferative process; however, she experienced such a dramatic improvement in symptoms and CT findings that a tissue diagnosis was thought to be unnecessary. She has undergone other age-appropriate cancer screenings without evidence for malignancy. She has had no other signs of symptoms to warrant further testing.

There is no standard treatment protocol for mesenteric panniculitis. Various treatment regimens have been proposed in small case series, including corticosteroids, tamoxifen, colchicine, azathioprine, thalidomide, and cyclophosphamide [4, 15–18]. Corticosteroids and other immunosuppressive agents appear to be the most promising due to their anti-inflammatory effects. While colchicine does not have a direct indication for the treatment of pSS, its efficacy in the management of mesenteric panniculitis, when combined with corticosteroids, has been demonstrated by Généreau et al. [15]. Fortunately, our patient improved with corticosteroids and was transitioned successfully to colchicine.

This case demonstrates the importance of considering Sjögren's syndrome as an underlying disease process in the evaluation of patients with mesenteric panniculitis.

Competing Interests

The authors declare that there are no competing interests regarding publication of this paper.

References

[1] Y. Gunduz, L. Tatli, and R. O. Kara, "Mesenteric panniculitis: a case report and review of the literature," *Maedica*, vol. 7, pp. 344–347, 2012.

[2] I. Issa and H. Baydoun, "Mesenteric panniculitis: various presentations and treatment regimens," *World Journal of Gastroenterology*, vol. 15, no. 30, pp. 3827–3830, 2009.

[3] M. Daskalogiannaki, A. Voloudaki, P. Prassopoulos et al., "CT evaluation of mesenteric panniculitis: prevalence and associated diseases," *American Journal of Roentgenology*, vol. 174, no. 2, pp. 427–431, 2000.

[4] S. Akram, D. S. Pardi, J. A. Schaffner, and T. C. Smyrk, "Sclerosing mesenteritis: clinical features, treatment, and outcome in ninety-two patients," *Clinical Gastroenterology and Hepatology*, vol. 5, no. 5, pp. 589–596, 2007.

[5] A. L. Durst, H. Freund, E. Rosenmann, and D. Birnbaum, "Mesenteric panniculitis: review of the literature and presentation of cases," *Surgery*, vol. 81, no. 2, pp. 203–211, 1977.

[6] R. E. Kipfer, C. G. Moertel, and D. C. Dahlin, "Mesenteric lipodystrophy," *Annals of Internal Medicine*, vol. 80, no. 5, pp. 582–588, 1974.

[7] W. W. Ogden II, D. M. Bradburn, and J. D. Rives, "Mesenteric panniculitis: review of 27 cases," *Annals of Surgery*, vol. 161, pp. 864–875, 1965.

[8] J. K. Kelly and W.-S. Hwang, "Idiopathic retractile (sclerosing) mesenteritis and its differential diagnosis," *American Journal of Surgical Pathology*, vol. 13, no. 6, pp. 513–521, 1989.

[9] K. M. Horton, L. P. Lawler, and E. K. Fishman, "CT findings in sclerosing mesenteritis (panniculitis): spectrum of disease," *RadioGraphics*, vol. 23, no. 6, pp. 1561–1567, 2003.

[10] A. M. Dor, J. L. Kohler, and P. Aubrespy, "Mesenteric panniculitis, an unusual initial stage of acute lupus erythromatosus in a ten-year old girl," *Archives d'Anatomie et de Cytologie Pathologiques*, vol. 30, no. 2, pp. 121–124, 1982.

[11] J. H. Kim, J. H. Byun, S. S. Lee, H. J. Kim, and M.-G. Lee, "Atypical manifestations of IgG4-related sclerosing disease in the abdomen: imaging findings and pathologic correlations," *American Journal of Roentgenology*, vol. 200, no. 1, pp. 102–112, 2013.

[12] T. Sugihara, R. Koike, Y. Nosaka et al., "Case of subcutaneous and mesenteric acute panniculitis with Sjögren's syndrome," *Japanese Journal of Clinical Immunology*, vol. 25, no. 3, pp. 277–284, 2002.

[13] R. L. Batten and W. F. Ng, "A case report of mesenteric panniculitis and primary Sjögren's syndrome," *Open Journal of Rheumatology and Autoimmune Diseases*, vol. 3, pp. 227–230, 2013.

[14] M. Osato, K. Yamaguchi, S. Tamiya et al., "A human T-cell lymphotropic virus type-I carrier with chronic renal failure, aplastic anemia, myelopathy, uveitis, Sjögren's syndrome and panniculitis," *Internal Medicine*, vol. 35, no. 9, pp. 742–745, 1996.

[15] T. Généreau, M.-F. Bellin, B. Wechsler et al., "Demonstration of efficacy of combining corticosteroids and colchicine in two patients with idiopathic sclerosing mesenteritis," *Digestive Diseases and Sciences*, vol. 41, no. 4, pp. 684–688, 1996.

[16] P. M. Ginsburg and E. D. Ehrenpreis, "A pilot study of thalidomide for patients with symptomatic mesenteric panniculitis," *Alimentary Pharmacology and Therapeutics*, vol. 16, no. 12, pp. 2115–2122, 2002.

[17] A. Bala, S. P. Coderre, D. R. E. Johnson, and V. Nayak, "Treatment of sclerosing mesenteritis with corticosteroids and azathioprine," *Canadian Journal of Gastroenterology*, vol. 15, no. 8, pp. 533–535, 2001.

[18] R. W. Bush, S. P. Hammar, and R. H. Rudolph, "Sclerosing mesenteritis. Response to cyclophosphamide," *Archives of Internal Medicine*, vol. 146, no. 3, pp. 503–505, 1986.

45

NXP-2 Positive Dermatomyositis: A Unique Clinical Presentation

Zeeshan Butt,[1] **Leeza Patel,**[2] **Manash K. Das,**[1] **Christopher A. Mecoli,**[3] and **Alim Ramji**[3]

[1]*Internal Medicine Residency Program, Prince George's Hospital Center, 3001 Hospital Dr, Cheverly, MD 20785, USA*
[2]*Department of Rheumatology, University of Arkansas for Medical Sciences, Little Rock, AR, USA*
[3]*Division of Rheumatology, John Hopkins University School of Medicine, 733 N Broadway, Baltimore, MD 21205, USA*

Correspondence should be addressed to Zeeshan Butt; zeeshantufail@gmail.com

Academic Editor: Remzi Cevik

Dermatomyositis (DM), a myopathy associated with inflammation and muscle weakness, has historically been difficult to diagnose. Recently, nuclear matrix protein (NXP-2) antibodies have been described as a myositis-specific antibody that may aid in the diagnostic evaluation. We present the case of a 21-year-old, previously healthy, African American male with DM. He presented to our outpatient clinic with periorbital swelling and a rash, for which he was started on prednisone by an ophthalmologist. Towards the end of the prednisone taper, he began to experience muscle weakness, a worsening rash, and dysphagia to solids with a resultant loss of 60 pounds within a month. He was transferred to a tertiary care hospital where he was further evaluated and ultimately diagnosed with dermatomyositis, supported by skin and muscle biopsies, and was found to be positive for NXP-2. He was given intravenous immunoglobulin (IVIG) and high-dose steroids with improvement.

1. Introduction

Dermatomyositis (DM) is a systemic disease characterized by chronic inflammation of the skin and muscle [1, 2]. There is significant clinical heterogeneity with respect to lung, muscle, joint, and cutaneous involvement, as well as variability in its association with malignancy and response to therapy [2–5]. Many patients with DM have circulating antibodies which are often associated with distinct clinical phenotypes [6, 7].

Recent studies identified new autoantibody specificities that include melanoma differentiation-associated protein 5 (MDA-5), transcription intermediary factor 1γ (TIF-1γ), and nuclear matrix protein (NXP-2) [8]. NXP-2 (also known as anti-MJ), a myositis-specific antibody, has been previously identified in 25% of juvenile dermatomyositis patients, and studies have shown its association with calcinosis and severe muscle weakness as well as potential gastrointestinal involvement [4, 7].

Here we present a case of adult NXP-2 positive DM.

2. Case Presentation

A 21-year-old African American male with no past medical history was in his usual state of health until January 2014, when he developed unusual periorbital swelling and a rash. He was evaluated at an outpatient ophthalmology clinic and was started on 60 mg prednisone daily. His periorbital swelling improved with this therapy, but as the prednisone was tapered he began experiencing symmetric bilateral proximal muscle weakness and soreness of the upper and lower extremities. This was accompanied by a hyperpigmented rash on the trunk, extensor surface of the arms, and upper thighs with associated soft tissue swelling. Two weeks after the completion of the prednisone taper, he began experiencing dysphagia to solids more than to liquids and suffered several choking episodes. This forced a change in his diet to thick liquids; as a result, by the end of the month he had lost 60 pounds. Given his worsening symptoms, he presented to our outpatient clinic in July 2014. Blood work for autoantibodies

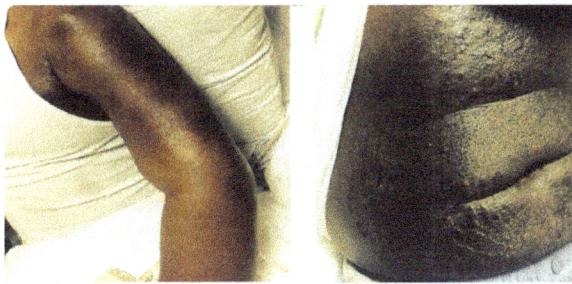

FIGURE 1: On physical exam, the patient was found to have a patchy, raised, nonulcerative healing rash with hypopigmentation on bilateral arms and forearms and anterior and lateral thighs, a patch of hyperpigmented rash on chest, and a diffuse rash over abdomen.

including ANA and dsDNA was negative. He was found to have an elevated total CK (1274 IU/L). ESR and CRP were normal. An upper endoscopy did not reveal any structural abnormalities.

In August 2014 during a follow-up visit at our clinic he was found to be very weak, barely able to climb stairs or stand up from a seated position. On examination, hyperpigmented pruritic frank macules were noted on the extensor surface of his arms, trunk, and upper thighs in multiple phases of healing (Figure 1). His hands and lips were swollen. Hand grip strength was reduced bilaterally. He had 3/5 strength in the left upper extremity and 4/5 on the right upper extremity. He was not able to raise his arm above his head; muscle bulk was decreased in the upper arm compared to the lower extremity. Hip flexors were 3/5 bilaterally, but quadriceps and hamstrings were 4/5 (Table 1). In this setting he was immediately transferred to a tertiary care facility.

Initial lab work there revealed elevated enzymes with AST of 75 U/L, creatinine kinase level of 1017 IU/L, myoglobin level of 233 ng/mL, LDH level of 386 U/L, ferritin 3151 ng/mL and ESR 33 mm/hr, uric acid 6.8 mg/dL, and being HIV negative (Table 1). Based on the clinical presentation and history, inflammatory myositis was suspected and rheumatology and dermatology were consulted. Blood works including an ANA, anti-Jo-1, anti-Ro, anti-La, anti-RNP/Smith, serum myoglobin, aldolase, CMV/EBV titers, and anti-histone antibodies were all negative.

He underwent CT scan and MRI of his chest, abdomen, and pelvis. Edema found in the bowel wall on CT (Figure 2(a)) prompted a colonoscopy with biopsy but results were nonspecific. MRI revealed intramuscular and subcutaneous edema (Figure 2(b)), but no occult malignancy. Skin biopsies were obtained from his right extensor arm and anterior chest which revealed a vacuolar interface dermatitis with dermal mucin deposition. A muscle biopsy of his left biceps demonstrated perifascicular atrophy and inflammation consistent with dermatomyositis. For his dysphagia, he was evaluated by a speech-language pathologist and underwent a cine esophagram which showed severe swallowing weakness with aspiration; a PEG tube was subsequently placed. He then began therapy with IVIG and pulse-dose pulse steroids with an eventual taper to 60 mg prednisone. Following IVIG treatment his hemoglobin dropped to 6.9 mg/dL with an

increased total bilirubin and LDH suggestive of intravascular hemolysis. Fecal occult blood test was negative and upper-GI bleed was not suspected leading to a glucose-6-phosphate dehydrogenase (G6PD) assay that confirmed very low activity of the enzyme. Thus he was diagnosed with G6PD deficiency and appropriate medication adjustments were made. Hemolysis was thought to be the result of stress from hospitalization. After 1 unit PRBC transfusion his hemoglobin remained stable for the course of the admission and he did not require any more transfusions. He demonstrated clinical improvement over the ensuing days, at which time his antibody testing for NXP-2 antibodies came back positive. NXP-2 antibodies were detected by the Oklahoma Myositis Research Foundation Panel.

3. Discussion

Dermatomyositis is a systemic disease that can be difficult to diagnose in its early stages [5]. The presence of myositis-specific autoantibodies allows for a more confident diagnosis,

TABLE 1: A summary of the significant lab results, immunologic test results, and results from the detailed motor strength test.

Lab results	
AST	75 U/L (0–35 U/L)
CK	1017 IU/L (30–170 U/L)
Myoglobin, serum	233 ng/mL (0–85 ng/mL)
LDH	386 U/L (60–100 U/L)
Ferritin	3151 ng/mL (15–200 ng/mL)
ESR	33 mm/hr (0–15 mm/hr)
Uric acid	6.8 mg/dL (3.7–8.0 mg/dL)
HIV	−ve
Immunologic tests	
ANA	−ve
Anti-Jo	−ve
Anti-Ro	−ve
Anti-LA	−ve
Anti-RNP	−ve
Anti-Smith	−ve
Anti-histone	−ve
CMV/EBV	−ve
Motor strength	
Neck flexion	2/5
Deltoids	3/5 bilaterally
Biceps	4/5 bilaterally
Triceps	4+/5 bilaterally
Wrist flexion	4+/5 on L, 4/5 on R
Wrist extension	4+/5 on L, 4/5 on R
Hand grip	4+/5 bilaterally
Hip extension and flexion	4/5 bilaterally
Knee extension and flexion	4+/5 bilaterally
Ankle flexion and dorsiflexion	5/5 bilaterally

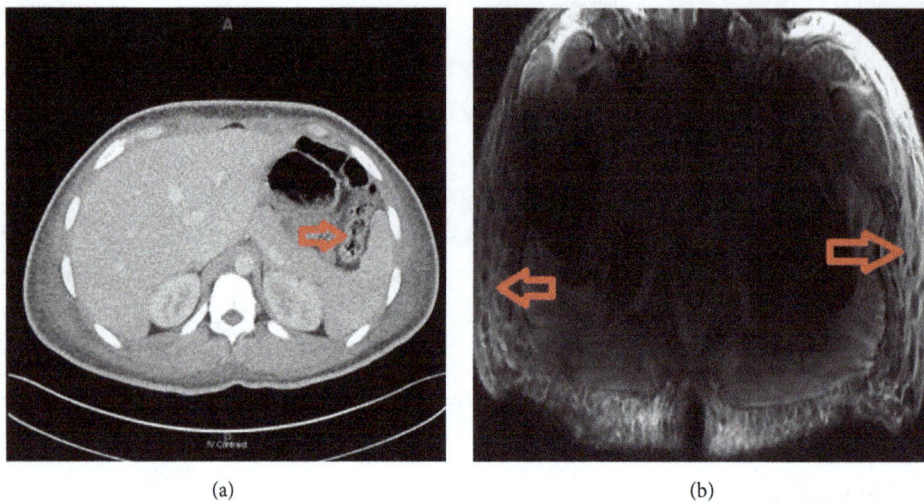

(a)   (b)

FIGURE 2: (a) CT of the abdomen showing thickening of the bowel wall (red arrow). (b) MRI showing edema of the soft tissue (red arrows).

better phenotype classification, and potentially more targeted treatments. Herein we present a patient with NXP-2 positive DM with dysphagia, unusual bowel wall edema, and diffuse soft tissue and muscle inflammation responsive to IVIG and corticosteroids.

Anti-NXP-2 antibodies were originally described in a subset of patients with juvenile DM and were associated with severe muscle weakness, polyarthritis, joint contractures, and intestinal vasculitis [7]. Anti-NXP-2 is also strongly associated with malignancy [8]. Until recently, there has been limited literature regarding its association in adult DM.

A recent study showed 1.6% of adult Japanese patients with inflammatory myopathy had anti-NXP-2 antibodies [9]. Anti-NXP-2 antibodies were found to be the most prevalent specificity in an Italian cohort followed by other known MSAs, such as anti-Jo-1 and Mi-2, and it was found to be similar to two juvenile DM studies performed in Argentina, the United Kingdom, and Ireland [7].

Two recently published studies have demonstrated that NXP-2 autoantibodies are associated with dysphagia and soft tissue/peripheral edema. Rogers et al. observed that in 20 patients with antibodies to NXP-2 dysphagia and peripheral edema were present in 74% and 35%, respectively [10]. In another study by Albayda et al., dysphagia and subcutaneous edema were present in 62% and 36% of anti-NXP-2 positive adult dermatomyositis patients [11]. In both studies, patients negative for NXP-2 autoantibodies had significantly less dysphagia and peripheral edema.

We describe a case of NXP-2 positive DM in a 21-year-old African American man with gastrointestinal involvement and soft tissue edema. This adds to the growing body of evidence that NXP-2 antibodies may reflect a unique phenotype of DM.

Acknowledgments

The authors would like to acknowledge the contributions of Devendra Patel, M.D., an Internal Medicine Resident at Prince George's Hospital Center in Cheverly, MD.

References

[1] J. P. Callen, "Dermatomyositis," *Lancet*, vol. 355, no. 9197, pp. 53–57, 2000.

[2] J. P. Callen and R. L. Wortmann, "Dermatomyositis," *Clinics in Dermatology*, vol. 24, no. 5, pp. 363–373, 2006.

[3] J. M. Olazagasti, P. J. Baez, D. A. Wetter, and F. C. Ernste, "Cancer Risk in Dermatomyositis: A Meta-Analysis of Cohort Studies," *American Journal of Clinical Dermatology*, vol. 16, no. 2, pp. 89–98, 2015.

[4] A. Bohan and J. B. Peter, "Polymyositis and dermatomyositis II," *The New England Journal of Medicine*, vol. 292, no. 8, pp. 403–407, 1975.

[5] A. Bohan and J. B. Peter, "Polymyositis and dermatomyositis," *The New England Journal of Medicine*, vol. 292, no. 7, pp. 344–347, 1975.

[6] M. Zong and I. E. Lundberg, "Pathogenesis, classification and treatment of inflammatory myopathies," *Nature Reviews Rheumatology*, vol. 7, no. 5, pp. 297–306, 2011.

[7] A. Ceribelli, M. Fredi, M. Taraborelli et al., "Anti-MJ/NXP-2 autoantibody specificity in a cohort of adult Italian patients with polymyositis/dermatomyositis," *Arthritis Research and Therapy*, vol. 14, no. 2, article no. R97, 2012.

[8] D. F. Fiorentino, L. S. Chung, L. Christopher-Stine et al., "Most patients with cancer-associated dermatomyositis have antibodies to nuclear matrix protein NXP-2 or transcription intermediary factor 1γ," *Arthritis and Rheumatism*, vol. 65, no. 11, pp. 2954–2962, 2013.

[9] Y. Ichimura, T. Matsushita, Y. Hamaguchi et al., "Anti-NXP2 autoantibodies in adult patients with idiopathic inflammatory myopathies: Possible association with malignancy," *Annals of the Rheumatic Diseases*, vol. 71, no. 5, pp. 710–713, 2012.

[10] A. Rogers, L. Chung, S. Li, L. Casciola-Rosen, and D. F. Fiorentino, "The cutaneous and systemic findings associated with nuclear matrix protein-2 antibodies in adult dermatomyositis patients," *Arthritis Care & Research*, 2017.

[11] J. Albayda, I. Pinal-Fernandez, W. Huang et al., "Dermatomyositis patients with anti-nuclear matrix protein-2 autoantibodies have more edema, more severe muscle disease, and increased malignancy risk," *Arthritis care & research*, 2017, doi: 10.1002/acr.23188. [Epub ahead of print].

46

Poncet's Disease in the Preclinical Phase of Rheumatoid Arthritis

Myat Tun Lin Nyo,[1] **Mahmood M. T. M. Ally**(ID),[2] **Elsa Magreta Van Duuren,**[3] **and Regan Arendse**(ID)[4]

[1]Department of Medicine, Division of Rheumatology, Sefako Makgatho Health Sciences University, Pretoria, South Africa
[2]Department of Internal Medicine, Division of Rheumatology, University of Pretoria, Pretoria, South Africa
[3]Department of Medicine, Division of Rheumatology, Sefako Makgatho Health Sciences University, Pretoria, South Africa
[4]Division of Rheumatology, Community Rheumatology Care, University of Saskatchewan, 301-39 23rd St. East, Saskatoon, SK, Canada S7K 0H6

Correspondence should be addressed to Regan Arendse; regan@arendse.biz

Academic Editor: Tsai-Ching Hsu

We report on a patient with seropositive polyarthritis retrospectively diagnosed as Poncet's disease in the preclinical phase of seropositive rheumatoid arthritis. Our patient developed rheumatoid arthritis more than 2 years after being successfully treated for pulmonary tuberculosis and an initial inflammatory polyarthritis consistent with the diagnosis of Poncet's disease. This case illustrates the importance of recognizing Poncet's disease in a patient presenting with polyarthritis in order to avoid inappropriate long-term disease modifying antirheumatic treatment. It also illustrates the need for adequate follow-up of patients with Poncet's disease after treatment with antituberculosis treatment so that progression to a primary inflammatory arthritis such as rheumatoid arthritis may be identified timeously. Although seropositivity for rheumatoid arthritis has been reported in Poncet's disease as well as in tuberculosis, it is rather uncommon, and long-term follow-up of patients with Poncet's disease is essential particularly if they have positive serological tests for rheumatoid arthritis. In this case report, we describe the first reported case of Poncet's disease in the preclinical phase of rheumatoid arthritis and review the literature related to this rare disease presentation.

1. Introduction

Poncet's disease (PD), also known as tuberculosis-associated arthritis, is a nonerosive inflammatory arthritis that may follow a tuberculosis infection without direct mycobacterial presence in the involved joints. PD can mimic rheumatoid arthritis (RA) both clinically and serologically. Serological tests such as rheumatoid factor (RF) and anticitrullinated peptide antibody (ACPA) may be positive in patients with TB without documented clinical evidence of rheumatoid arthritis. In patients with TB without RA, positive ACPA is reported in up to 37% and positive IgM RF in up to 62%. While it is important to recognize PD in a patient presenting with polyarthritis in order to avoid inappropriate long-term disease-modifying antirheumatic treatment, it is also equally important to adequately follow up a patient with PD so that the evolution to a primary inflammatory arthritis such as RA does not go undetected.

2. Case Report

In December 2013, a 64-year-old African female was referred to the rheumatology clinic at our hospital with suspected RA. She reported painful hands and knees associated with early morning stiffness of two to three hours for the duration of one year. On further questioning, she reported that she had been diagnosed with pulmonary tuberculosis (TB) on the basis of positive sputum testing eight months prior to the time. The Gene Xpert test on her sputum had detected Mycobacterium tuberculosis complex, which was sensitive to rifampicin. She had subsequently been started on anti-tuberculosis (TB) chemotherapy, which included rifampicin, isoniazid, ethambutol, and pyrazinamide. However, she had taken the treatment for only three months reportedly due to intolerance of the chemotherapy.

Rheumatological examination at that visit revealed a clinical picture suggestive of RA. She had seven swollen joints all of which were metacarpophalangeal joints and seven tender joints including the wrists, knees, and meta-carpophalangeal joints. Her patient global assessment was seven, and physician global assessment was four. This indicated high disease activity with a calculated clinical disease activity index (CDAI) of 25. Her chest radiograph showed features suggestive of active tuberculosis in the right upper lobe. Periarticular osteoporosis suggestive of an early inflammatory arthritis was identified on plain radiographs of hands and feet. There were no erosions or joint space narrowing identified on the latter. Blood investigations revealed positive serological tests for RA, with a rheumatoid factor (RF) of 69 international units per millilitre (normal value < 15) and an anti-citrullinated peptide antibody (ACPA) of 53 units per millilitre (normal value < 20). Inflammatory markers were also elevated which could be either due to active arthritis or as a result of active pulmonary tuberculosis.

On the basis of chronic symmetrical polyarthritis involving predominantly small joints, plain radiographs suggestive of an early inflammatory arthritis, and supportive serological features, we diagnosed her arthritic condition as RA. Recognizing that she had not completed her anti-TB chemotherapy and she still had clinicoradiological features suggestive of active pulmonary TB, the original anti-TB chemotherapy was restarted and she was referred to the local clinic to continue the treatment for six months. As for RA, we decided not to initiate methotrexate until anti-TB chemotherapy was completed. We opted instead for a combination therapy of chloroquine and low-dose prednisone for the arthritis. In the follow-up clinic, a month later, we added sulfasalazine as her disease activity was persistently high. She subsequently defaulted the RA treatment. She however continued going to the local TB clinic to complete anti-TB chemotherapy.

When she finally returned to the rheumatology clinic after completion of six months of anti-TB therapy, we found that she had no residual symptoms and signs of RA without any specific therapy for at least 4 months. We felt that a complete resolution of arthritis would be very unlikely under anti-TB chemotherapy without adequate DMARD therapy if the patient had rheumatoid arthritis. This led to a retrospective diagnosis of PD, which is a condition known to completely resolve without joint damage on anti-TB chemotherapy.

In the subsequent 2-year follow-up without any form of pharmacological treatment, there was no relapse of the arthritis despite the serological tests for RA remaining positive, and she was discharged from the clinic. However, she presented again in January 2017 with a painful right foot, and she had been limping for a few months due to the pain. Clinical examination revealed swelling of the second and third metatarsophalangeal joints and tenderness of all of the right metatarsophalangeal joints. Repeated plain radiographs of the hands and feet revealed periarticular osteoporosis without erosions or joint space narrowing. Musculoskeletal ultrasound revealed active synovitis with increased Doppler signal in the right second and third metatarsophalangeal joints (Figure 1). No erosions were detected in the hand joints on ultrasound examination either. Serum RF was 166 international unit per millilitre, and serum ACPA was 100 units per millilitre. Serum C-reactive protein was mildly elevated at 17 milligrams per litre. She had no features to suggest reactivation of TB or reinfection with TB at this time. RA was diagnosed, and she was then started on oral methotrexate, folate, and low-dose prednisone leading to improvement of her symptoms. Written informed consent was obtained from the patient to allow publication of her clinical diagnosis and management.

3. Discussion

PD is a nondestructive (nonerosive) inflammatory arthritis that may follow mycobacterial infection elsewhere with no direct infective agent identified in the involved joints. Antonin Poncet first described it in 1897 [1]. The definition of the disease was modified and improved to a more precise one by Bloxham and Addy in 1987 [2]. Multiple case reports of PD have been published globally since the original description of the disease. In 2013, Rueda et al. [3] systemically reviewed 198 case reports and studies concerning PD published to that date. The clinical characteristics of PD were synthesized from this analysis and a case from their academic centre. Based on the analysis of these 198 cases and a case of their own, PD was hypothesized to be an immunologically mediated disease caused by molecular mimicry between TB antigens and host cartilage in genetically predisposed individuals. The joint involvement improved spontaneously weeks after anti-TB therapy was completed without sequelae. Pulmonary TB was found to be the commonest site of TB infection (43.2%). The sites of extrapulmonary TB infection included lymphatic, renal, bone, skin, and other less common sites. Oligoarthritis was the most common rheumatological presentation (40%) followed by polyarthritis (27.6%) and monoarthritis (24.6%). The most frequently involved joints were the ankles (63%) and knees (59%). The wrists, elbows, interphalangeal joints, metacarpophalangeal joints, shoulders, and metatarsophalangeal joints were affected less frequently. Axial involvement has not yet been reported to date. More recently, Sharma et al. [4] reported a case series of 23 patients with PD. Oligoarthritis was found in 13 patients and polyarthritis in the remaining ten with the ankles being the most frequently involved joints. All patients in the series had nonerosive and nondeforming arthritis.

The RF status of PD has frequently been documented in the previously published case reports and series. The majority of reports that have published the RF status of patients with PD have reported this status to be negative [5]. In contrast, the ACPA status is less often reported and was negative in a few case reports that documented its status. There is, however, a single case of PD that has reported high titres of RF and ACPA, which mimicked rheumatoid

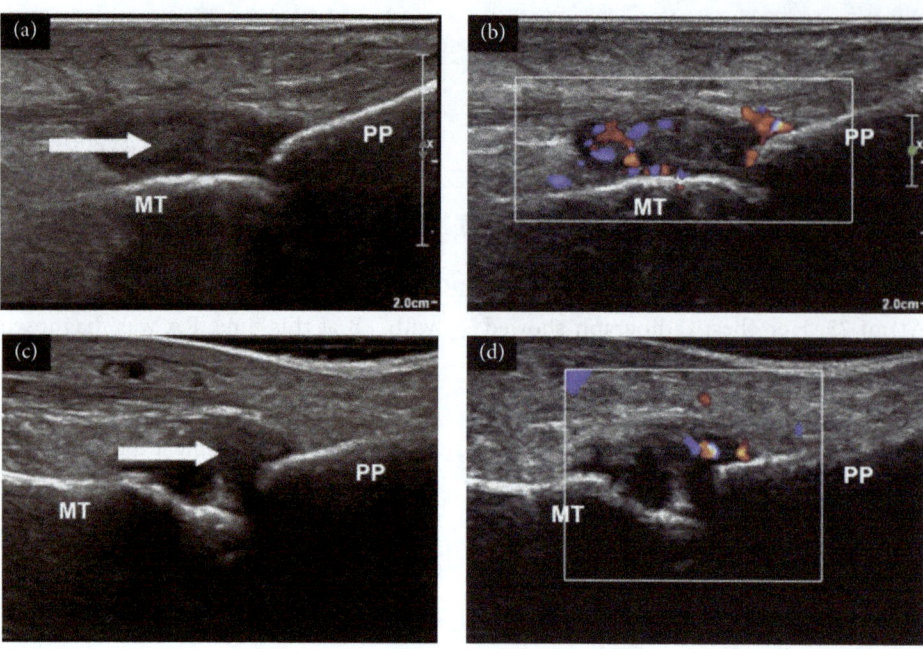

FIGURE 1: Musculoskeletal ultrasound images showing synovitis of right second and third metatarsophalangeal (MTP) joints. (a) Synovial hypertrophy of right second MTP joint (arrow); (b) increased Doppler signal indicating active inflammation; (c) synovial hypertrophy of right third MTP joint (arrow); (d) increased Doppler signal indicating active inflammation. MT: metatarsal; PP: proximal phalange.

arthritis [6]. This case did not report the duration of follow-up after resolution of arthritis or whether there was progression to rheumatoid arthritis. In addition, there are reports that the RF and ACPA tests may be positive in patients with TB without documented clinical evidence of rheumatoid arthritis. In patients with TB without RA, positive ACPA is reported in up to 37% and positive IgM RF in up to 62%. However, it is also not transparent in the latter reports that the patients were followed up for a defined period after treatment of the TB to exclude the progression to rheumatoid arthritis [7–12]. Our case is therefore unique in the literature in that once our patient completed TB therapy with resolution of the PD, the patient subsequently progressed over two years from an ACPA and RF positive status to the extent that she fulfilled the 2010 American College of Rheumatology/European League against Rheumatism (ACR/EULAR) classification criteria for rheumatoid arthritis [13, 14].

The preclinical or seropositive arthralgia phase of RA in which serological tests such as RF and ACPA are positive prior to the onset of clinical phenotype is well described. It is generally recognized that a positive ACPA status is a stronger predictor of progression to rheumatoid arthritis than a positive RF status. The predictors for progression from a seropositive RF and ACPA status to clinically evident rheumatoid arthritis include the demonstration of HLA alleles, *HLA-DRB1 ∗ 0401* and *HLA-DRB1 ∗ 0404*, the presence of raised inflammatory markers, the strength of the ACPA titre, and the presence of subclinical synovitis detected by either ultrasound or MRI examination [15]. Furthermore, it has been postulated that 100% of patients will progress to rheumatoid arthritis within five years if they are both ACPA and RF positive regardless of the background

incidence of rheumatoid arthritis in the population from which the patient originates [15]. There is also tentative evidence that preemptive treatment of the arthralgia in a patient with positive ACPA status with anti-CD20 therapy rituximab may delay the onset and the severity of RA [16].

Periarticular osteoporosis is a well-described radiologic observation in both Poncet's disease [17] and early rheumatoid arthritis [18]. Periarticular osteoporosis is defined as "*a decrease in radiographic density in the osseous structure surrounding the joints*" and is frequently described at the proximal phalanges and metacarpals in early rheumatoid arthritis [18]. However, interobserver agreement in controlled studies evaluating the radiographic diagnosis of periarticular osteoporosis is moderate at best [18]. As a consequence of the high observational variation in reporting periarticular osteoporosis in patients with early rheumatoid arthritis, this radiographic feature has not been included in the 2010 ACR classification criteria [18]. The observation of the presence of periarticular osteoporosis in our patient's first radiographs did not allow us to distinguish between rheumatoid arthritis and Poncet's disease. We are confident therefore that our patient's initial clinical course was consistent with a diagnosis of Poncet's disease and that there was the subsequent development of rheumatoid arthritis.

Palindromic rheumatism is a condition in which a person with positive RF and ACPA serology may report self-limiting, intermittent joint pain, and swelling [19]. The episodes of joint pain and swelling may be present for days to weeks. The joint inflammation is described to resolve spontaneously or in response to symptomatic treatment. The episodes of joint inflammation may be interspersed with symptom-free periods that may range from weeks to years [20]. Palindromic rheumatism is distinct from early RA in that it does not have the persistent joint symptoms of pain and swelling for more than 6 weeks, which are required to fulfill the 2010 ACR/EULAR classification criteria for RA. We considered palindromic rheumatism in the differential diagnosis of our patients' condition, as there was a two-year interval of spontaneous improvement not attributed to the use of conventional DMARDs but to the treatment of the pulmonary tuberculosis. However, the initial and January 2017 presentations of small joint pain and swelling for periods of more than one year and more than a few months, respectively, are inconsistent with the definition of palindromic rheumatism which requires that the swelling be present for less than six weeks. For this reason, we do not believe that palindromic rheumatism may account for the two distinct periods of the inflammatory arthritis interspersed by the two-year period of improvement in joint symptoms. Rather the initial and January 2017 periods of joint swelling may be attributed to successive diagnoses of Poncet's disease and rheumatoid arthritis, respectively.

We hypothesize that our patient initially developed PD in response to the untreated tuberculosis infection. We base this hypothesis on the temporal association between the presentation of the polyarthritis and the presence of tuberculosis and the subsequent resolution once the tuberculosis infection had been treated. We think it is unlikely but not impossible that the PD may have been a form of early RA transiently unmasked by TB. Rather, we hypothesize that elimination of the mycobacterial antigen with antituberculosis therapy may have reduced the antigen load and minimized subsequent molecular mimicry with resolution of the PD. We have not found evidence that the antituberculosis therapy may have a beneficial effect on the activity of RA if the initial PD was in fact an early flare of RA. Neither do we think that the initial presentation of PD was a form of palindromic rheumatism. The absence of prior episodes and subsequent absence of similar episodes within the two-year follow-up after completing the TB treatment suggest that the diagnosis of PD is distinct from palindromic rheumatism.

We further hypothesize that our patient subsequently evolved to rheumatoid arthritis as a result of the predictive features of elevated inflammatory markers and strongly positive serology. While we place emphasis on the presence of the predictive features, we acknowledge that it is also possible that the mycobacterial infection may have been contributory to the progression to RA. In this regard, there has been interest in the role of mycobacterial 65-kd heat-shock protein (BHSP65) in the pathogenesis of adjuvant-induced arthritis in rodents and RA in humans [21–24]. Despite the convincing data for the relationship between BHSP65 and experimental arthritis in rodents, the causative role of BHSP65 in human RA remains unproven. We suspect that the case reported by Sasaki et al. [6] of PD with positive RF and ACPA serology may have also eventually progressed to RA if monitored for a similar or longer period of time. The absence of TB infection and the absence of predictive features may have limited the progression to RA within the period reported by Sasaki et al. [6].

4. Conclusion

We report a unique case of a patient with seropositive polyarthritis retrospectively diagnosed as PD in the preclinical phase of seropositive RA. She developed RA more than 2 years after being successfully treated for pulmonary TB and an initial inflammatory polyarthritis consistent with the diagnosis of PD. While this case illustrates the importance of recognizing PD in a patient presenting with polyarthritis in order to avoid unnecessary long-term disease-modifying antirheumatic treatment, it also illustrates the need for adequate follow-up in patients with PD so that the possibility of RA is not overlooked. The existence of a preclinical phase of RA in which serological tests such as RF and ACPA can be positive for years before the onset of clinical phenotype is well recognized in the literature. Although seropositivity for RA has been reported in PD as well as in TB, it is rather uncommon and long-term follow-up of patients with PD is essential particularly if they have positive serological tests for RA. This is the first description of PD in the preclinical phase of RA.

References

[1] A. Poncet, "De la polyarthrite tuberculeuse deformante ou pseudo- rheumatisme chronique tuberculeux," *Congres Francaise de Chirurgie*, vol. 1, pp. 732–739, 1897.

[2] C. A. Bloxham and D. P. Addy, "Poncet's disease: para-infective tuberculous polyarthropathy," *British Medical Journal*, vol. 1, no. 6127, p. 1590, 1978.

[3] J. C. Rueda, M. F. Crepy, and R. D. Mantilla, "Clinical features of Poncet's disease. From the description of 198 cases found in the literature," *Clinical Rheumatology*, vol. 32, no. 7, pp. 929–935, 2013.

[4] A. Sharma, B. Pinto, S. Dogra et al., "A case series and review of Poncet's disease, and the utility of current diagnostic criteria," *International Journal of Rheumatic Diseases*, vol. 19, no. 10, pp. 1010–1017, 2016.

[5] E. Erkol Inal, D. Keskin, and H. Bodur, "A case of Poncet's disease: tuberculous rheumatism," *Türkiye Fiziksel Tip ve Rehabilitasyon Dergisi*, vol. 61, no. 1, pp. 77–79, 2015.

[6] H. Sasaki, M. Inagaki, M. Shioda, and K. Nagasaka, "Poncet's disease with high titers of rheumatoid factor and anti-citrullinated peptide antibodies mimicking rheumatoid arthritis," *Journal of Infection and Chemotherapy*, vol. 21, no. 1, pp. 65–69, 2015.

[7] I. Lima, R. C. Oliveira, A. Atta et al., "Antibodies to citrullinated peptides in tuberculosis," *Clinical Rheumatology*, vol. 32, no. 5, pp. 685–687, 2013.

[8] I. Lima and M. Santiago, "Antibodies against cyclic citrullinated peptides in infectious diseases–a systematic review," *Clinical Rheumatology*, vol. 29, no. 12, pp. 1345–1351, 2010.

[9] M. Karkucak, E. Çapkin, Ö. F. Barçak, H. Çakirbay, M. Tosun, and F. Gökmen, "Anti-CCP antibody and rheumatoid factor positivity in a case of tuberculosis arthritis," *Turkish Journal of Rheumatology*, vol. 25, no. 2, pp. 95–98, 2010.

[10] P. Kakumanu, H. Yamagata, E. S. Sobel, W. H. Reeves, E. K. Chan, and M. Satoh, "Patients with pulmonary tuberculosis are frequently positive for anti-cyclic citrullinated

peptide antibodies, but their sera also react with unmodified arginine-containing peptide," *Arthritis and Rheumatism*, vol. 58, no. 6, pp. 1576–1581, 2008.

[11] O. Elkayam, R. Segal, M. Lidgi, and D. Caspi, "Positive anti-cyclic citrullinated proteins and rheumatoid factor during active lung tuberculosis," *Annals of the Rheumatic Diseases*, vol. 65, no. 8, pp. 1110–1112, 2006.

[12] S. Mori, H. Naito, S. Ohtani, T. Yamanaka, and M. Sugimoto, "Diagnostic utility of anti-cyclic citrullinated peptide antibodies for rheumatoid arthritis in patients with active lung tuberculosis," *Clinical Rheumatology*, vol. 28, no. 3, pp. 277–283, 2009.

[13] F. C. Arnett, S. M. Edworthy, D. A. Bloch et al., "The American Rheumatism Association 1987 revised criteria for the classification of rheumatoid arthritis," *Arthritis and Rheumatism*, vol. 31, no. 3, pp. 315–324, 1988.

[14] D. Aletaha, T. Neogi, A. J. Silman et al., "2010 rheumatoid arthritis classification criteria: an American College of Rheumatology/European League Against Rheumatism collaborative initiative," *Annals of the Rheumatic Diseases*, vol. 69, no. 9, pp. 1580–1588, 2010.

[15] K. D. Deane, J. M. Norris, and V. M. Holers, "Pre-clinical rheumatoid arthritis: identification, evaluation and future directions for investigation," *Rheumatic Disease Clinics of North America*, vol. 36, no. 2, pp. 213–241, 2010.

[16] D. M. Gerlag, J. M. Norris, and P. P. Tak, "Towards prevention of autoantibody-positive rheumatoid arthritis: from lifestyle modification to preventive treatment," *Rheumatology*, vol. 55, no. 4, pp. 607–614, 2016.

[17] C. Hugosson, R. S. Nyman, J. Brismar, S. G. Larsson, S. Lindahl, and C. Lundstedt, "Imaging of tuberculosis," *Acta Radiologica*, vol. 37, no. 4, pp. 512–516, 1996.

[18] S. J. Moon, I. E. Ahn, S. K. Kwok et al., "Periarticular osteoporosis is a prominent feature in early rheumatoid arthritis: estimation using shaft to periarticular bone mineral density ratio," *Journal of Korean Medical Science*, vol. 28, no. 2, pp. 287–294, 2013.

[19] S. Cabrera-Villalba and R. Raimon Sanmartí, "Palindromic rheumatism: a reappraisal," *International Journal of Clinical Rheumatology*, vol. 8, no. 5, pp. 569–577, 2013.

[20] A. Powell, P. Davis, N. Jones, and A. S. Russell, "Palindromic rheumatism is a common disease: comparison of new-onset palindromic rheumatism compared to new-onset rheumatoid arthritis in a 2-year cohort of patients," *Journal of Rheumatology*, vol. 35, no. 6, pp. 992–994, 2008.

[21] W. van Eden, E. J. Hogervorst, R. van der Zee, J. D. van Embden, E. J. Hensen, and I. R. Cohen, "The mycobacterial 65 kD heat-shock protein and autoimmune arthritis," *Rheumatology International*, vol. 9, no. 3–5, pp. 187–191, 1989.

[22] P. Res, J. Thole, and R. de Vries, "Heat-shock proteins and autoimmunity in humans," *Springer Seminars in Immunopathology*, vol. 13, no. 1, pp. 81–98, 1991.

[23] G. Rook, P. Lydyard, and J. Stanford, "Mycobacteria and rheumatoid arthritis," *Arthritis and Rheumatism*, vol. 33, no. 3, pp. 431–435, 1990.

[24] M. N. Huang, H. Yu, and K. D. Moudgil, "The involvement of heat-shock proteins in the pathogenesis of autoimmune arthritis: a critical appraisal," *Seminars in Arthritis and Rheumatism*, vol. 40, no. 2, pp. 164–175, 2010.

47

Granulomatosis with Polyangiitis Presenting as Pyrexia of Unknown Origin, Leukocytosis, and Microangiopathic Haemolytic Anemia

Sima Terebelo and Iona Chen

Maimonides Medical Center, Brooklyn, NY, USA

Correspondence should be addressed to Sima Terebelo; sima.terebelo@gmail.com

Academic Editor: George S. Habib

A 66-year-old woman presented to the Emergency Department with a florid sepsis-like picture, a two-week history of fever, relative hypotension with end organ ischemia (unexplained liver enzyme and troponin elevations), and nonspecific constitutional symptoms. She was initially found to have a urinary tract infection but, despite appropriate treatment, her fever persisted and her white blood cell count continued to rise. During her hospitalization the patient manifested leukocytosis to 47,000 WBC/μL, ESR 67 mm/hr (normal range 0–42 mm/hr), CRP 17.5 mg/dL (normal range 0.02–1.20 mg/dL), and microangiopathic haemolytic anemia, with declining haemoglobin and haematocrit. An infectious aetiology was not found despite extensive bacteriologic studies and radiographic imaging. The patient progressed to acute kidney injury with "active" urinary sediment and proteinuria. Kidney biopsy results and serological titres of myeloperoxidase positive perinuclear-antineutrophil cytoplasmic antibodies (MPO+ p-ANCA) led to a diagnosis of granulomatosis with polyangiitis. Immunosuppressive treatment with high dose methylprednisolone and rituximab led to resolution of the leukocytosis and return of the haemoglobin and haematocrit values toward normal without further signs of hemolysis.

1. Introduction

Granulomatosis with polyangiitis (GPA) is an uncommon autoimmune disease characterized by a pauci-immune necrotizing vasculitis of small and medium sized vessels. It most commonly occurs in Caucasian patients between 45 and 65 years, without gender predilection, and characteristically affects the upper and lower respiratory tract and kidneys. We report a 66-year-old Afro-Caribbean woman whose presenting symptoms and findings suggested sepsis syndrome and included fever, hypotension with end organ ischemia, leukocytosis to 47,000 WBC/μL, and microangiopathic haemolytic anemia (MAHA). An extensive workup failed to show any infectious or neoplastic aetiology. The patient was ultimately diagnosed with GPA based on kidney biopsy results and MPO+ p-ANCA. To our knowledge, leukocytosis to this extent has not been previously described with GPA. Additionally, MAHA rarely accompanies GPA.

2. Description of Patient

A 66-year-old Afro-Caribbean woman presented to the Emergency Department with complaints of weakness, fever, fatigue, myalgia, hypotension × 2 weeks, and increased urinary frequency. The patient has a past medical history of hypertension, hypothyroidism, hearing loss, tinnitus, and "benign pulmonary nodules." Two weeks prior to presentation, the patient began experiencing daily fevers of 102 degrees Fahrenheit (38.9 degrees Celsius), severe body aches, nonproductive cough with pleuritic chest pain, and low blood pressure (90–100 mmHg systolic) without ingestion of antihypertensive medications. She visited her primary care physician three days prior to presentation and was given amoxicillin for presumed upper respiratory infection; however her symptoms continued to worsen.

The patient disclosed a two-year history of intermittent episodes of bronchitis and haemoptysis, which were treated with multiple courses of oral antibiotics. She had presented to our institution twice for evaluation of haemoptysis. On the first occasion, 1 year ago, she had minimal bloody expectorant and was treated for bronchitis. On her second presentation, three months ago, frank haemoptysis was present and the patient was admitted. Sputum samples were negative for acid fast bacilli and cultures were negative for tuberculosis. The patient was ultimately treated for community acquired pneumonia. Pulmonary nodules noted on radiographic imaging had been evaluated in an outpatient setting, and the patient indicated that she had been informed that these were "benign."

The patient was a nonsmoker and did not consume alcohol. She worked as a patient care technician in a hospital and had a history of positive purified protein derivative skin test for tuberculosis (PPD+). She recently traveled to Haiti.

In the Emergency Department, the patient was afebrile (had just taken paracetamol), with respiratory rate = 23, blood pressure 114/67, white blood cell count (WBC) 24,000/μL, 87% neutrophils, 4% lymphocytes, 7% monocytes, haemoglobin 9.1 g/dL with +anisocytosis and target cells, platelets 513,000/μL, troponin 0.11 ng/mL (normal 0.00–0.04 ng/mL), AST 399 IU/L (normal 8–26 IU/L), ALT 368 IU/L (normal 6–51 IU/L), alkaline phosphatase 131 IU/L (normal 33–92 IU/L), total bilirubin 0.4 mg/dL (normal 0.4–1.1 mg/dL), 0.1 mg/dL direct bilirubin (normal 0.1–0.2 mg/dL), and albumin 2.5 g/dL (normal 3.6–4.6 g/dL).

Physical exam was notable for decreased breath sounds over the right lower lobe and minimal lower extremity oedema bilaterally. There were no rashes, swollen joints, digital ulcers, or loss of digit pulp.

2.1. Clinical Course and Diagnostic Assessment.

Initial workup was significant for a urinary tract infection. Despite appropriate antibiotic therapy the patient continued to be intermittently febrile accompanied by increasing leukocytosis, with neutrophil counts ranging from 80 to 86%. Repeat urine culture was negative. No source of infection was found despite extensive investigation. Multiple blood cultures were negative. CT chest demonstrated chronic scarring and architectural distortion of the right upper lobe, thought to be due to prior granulomatous disease, which was unchanged from a prior CT. A left lung nodule was noted, unchanged from the patient's previous CT on 10/2015. Sputum samples were negative for acid fast bacilli by fluorochrome methodology. Further diagnostic studies were initiated due to the persistence of fever. Echocardiogram was negative for valvular vegetation. CT scan of the abdomen and pelvis was negative for occult abscess or osteomyelitis. MRI of the abdomen and pelvis was negative for infectious processes and pelvic ultrasound did not reveal gynecologic pathology. A peripheral blood smear examined by a haematology/oncology consultant was interpreted as reactive, without signs of neoplasia, and therefore there was no indication for bone marrow biopsy.

WBC count continued to increase from the admission level of 24,000/μL to a peak of 47,000/μL. Haemoglobin and haematocrit values gradually declined from admission values of 9.1 g/dL and 29.9% to 6.6 g/dL and 20% (Figure 1); schistocytes and target cells were identified on peripheral smear. Coombs test was negative for direct and indirect antibodies.

LDH rose from 251 IU/L to 409 IU/L (normal 84–193 IU/L) and haptoglobin was <3 (normal 34–200 mg/dL), consistent with microangiopathic haemolytic anemia (MAHA). Other relevant laboratory findings included serum iron 14 mcg/dL (normal 64–196 mg/dL), transferrin 105 mg/dL (normal 192–321 mg/dL), TIBC 147 mcg/dL (normal 279–449 mcg/dL), ferritin 452 ng/mL (normal 4.8–94.4 ng/mL), and reticulocyte count 5.6%, with absolute reticulocytes 0.160, and corrected reticulocyte count 2.9%.

Liver enzymes and cardiac troponin levels decreased to normal. Serological testing was negative for acute or chronic viral hepatitis, Epstein Barr virus, or cytomegalovirus infections.

Creatinine gradually increased from baseline 0.9 mg/dL (normal 0.5–1.2 mg/dL) to peak of 3.4 mg/dL. Urine microscopy revealed 5–10 red cell casts/LPF and 2–5 coarse granular casts/LPF. Urine protein : creatinine ratio was 1.8-gram protein/gram creatinine (normal <0.16 g/g creatinine) and increased to 2.4-gram protein/gram creatinine. Markers of inflammation revealed ESR 67 mm/hr (normal 0–42 mm/hr) and CRP 17.5 mg/dL (normal 0.02–1.20 mg/dL). Inflammatory markers were only measured once during the patient's hospital course. ANA was weakly positive 1 : 80 (homogenous) and p-ANCA was positive, 1 : 160, with MPO 115.2 units (normal ≤ 20.0 units). Pertinent negative laboratory values included c-ANCA negative, PR3 negative, C3 113 mg/dL (normal 75–161 mg/dL), C4 22 mg/dL (normal 14–45 mg/dL), Rheumatoid Factor negative, antiglomerular basement membrane antibody negative (<0.02), and urine eosinophil smear negative.

Renal biopsy demonstrated pauci-immune necrotizing glomerulonephritis with crescents and vascular and interstitial necrosis. There was full thickness fibrinoid necrosis of the vessels with surrounding interstitial necrosis. There was 30% interstitial fibrosis associated with tubular atrophy and dense lymphocytic inflammatory infiltrate. Fibrinogen staining showed crescents and necrosis of an artery (Figures 2–4).

2.2. Treatment/Outcome.

The patient was treated with methylprednisolone 1000 mg IV × 5 days. Rituximab 375 mg/m^2 was started while being inpatient and was continued weekly for a total of 4 weeks. The patient had been manifesting frequent fevers within the range of 100.4–102.7 degrees Fahrenheit (38.0–39.3 degrees Celsius). The day following solumedrol infusion fevers ceased and patient's body temperature thereafter remained in the normal range. WBC count initially rose from 35,000/μL with 87% neutrophils to 47,000/μL with 82% neutrophils after methylprednisolone administration for two days and after the first dose of rituximab was administered. The following day WBC count declined to 31,500/μL with 83% neutrophils and continued to decline gradually. One week after beginning methylprednisolone and rituximab therapy WBC count was 25,700/μL with 81% neutrophils and declined to 20,100/μL with 86% neutrophils following the second dose of methylprednisolone. Creatinine slowly declined and haemoglobin and haematocrit levels slowly rose. Urine protein : creatinine ratio declined to 1.6-gram protein/gram creatinine. Corticosteroids were gradually

Granulomatosis with Polyangiitis Presenting as Pyrexia of Unknown Origin, Leukocytosis, and Microangiopathic...

221

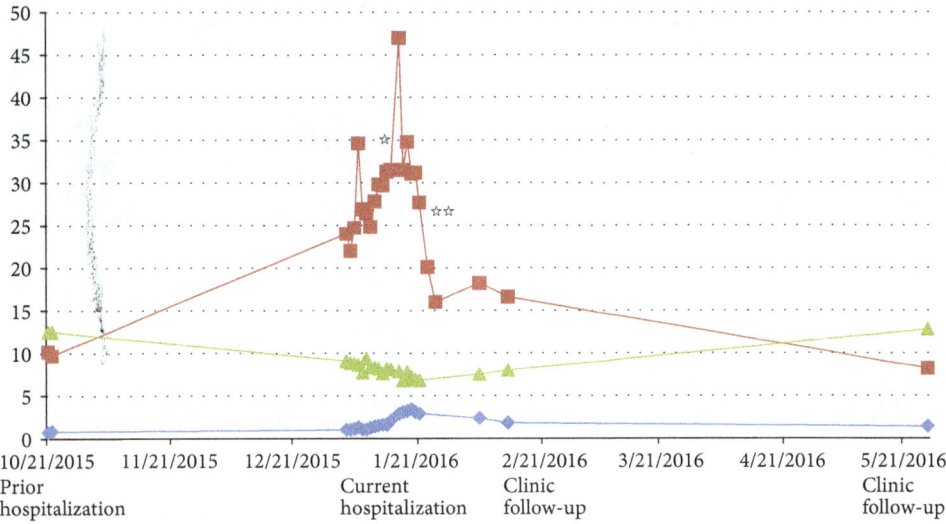

☆ Methylprednisolone and first dose of rituximab were given
☆☆ Second dose of rituximab was given
◆ Creatinine
■ WBC
▲ Haemoglobin

FIGURE 1: *Relationship between serum creatinine, WBC, and haemoglobin.* Upon initial presentation to our hospital several months earlier, patient had normal laboratory values. At this admission the patient had leukocytosis, anemia, and rising creatinine values. Administration of methylprednisolone and rituximab (star) was associated with an initial rise in WBC count. Within several days leukocyte counts began to decline, most notably after the second rituximab infusion (two stars). Haemoglobin and creatinine levels also responded appropriately. At the outpatient clinic follow-up the patient received another two doses of rituximab. Laboratory testing continued to show improved WBC count, haemoglobin, and creatinine levels.

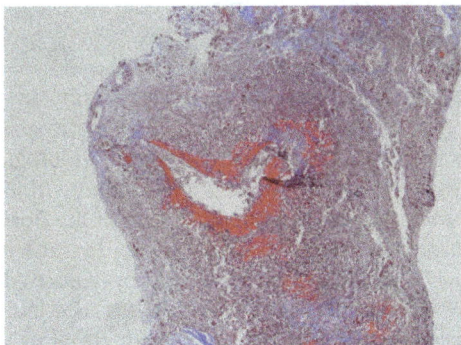

FIGURE 2: Full thickness fibrinoid necrosis of the vessels with surrounding interstitial necrosis.

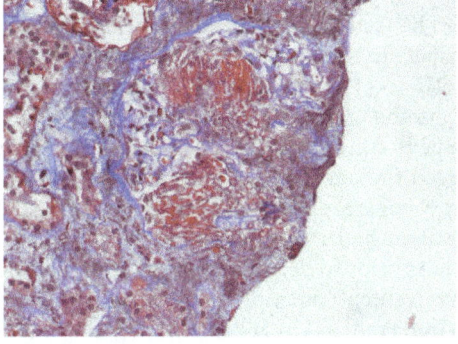

FIGURE 3: Tubular atrophy with dense lymphocytic inflammatory infiltrate and interstitial fibrosis.

tapered. The patient tolerated the treatment well and clinical symptomatology resolved. Lab values, 5 months after hospitalization, revealed WBC 8.2k/μL, haemoglobin 12.8 g/dL, haematocrit 39.2%, platelets 210k/UL, BUN 22 mg/dL and creatinine 1.4 mg/dL, AST 23 IU/L, and ALT 16 IU/L (Figure 1).

3. Discussion and Literature Review

Over a 2-year period, the patient experienced limited lung disease and developed hearing loss and tinnitus. She then abruptly developed a sepsis-like condition, which rapidly progressed to include persistent fever, increasing leukocytosis, MAHA, and acute necrotizing pauci-immune glomerulonephritis. The lack of response to antibiotic therapy prompted a search for occult infection or malignancy. Despite multiple blood and sputum cultures, extensive imaging studies (including a CT of the chest, abdomen, and pelvis, an MRI of the abdomen and pelvis, and a pelvic ultrasound), and peripheral blood smear evaluation by an oncologist, no source of abscess, infection, or neoplasm could be found to explain the patient's fevers and leukocytosis. The increase

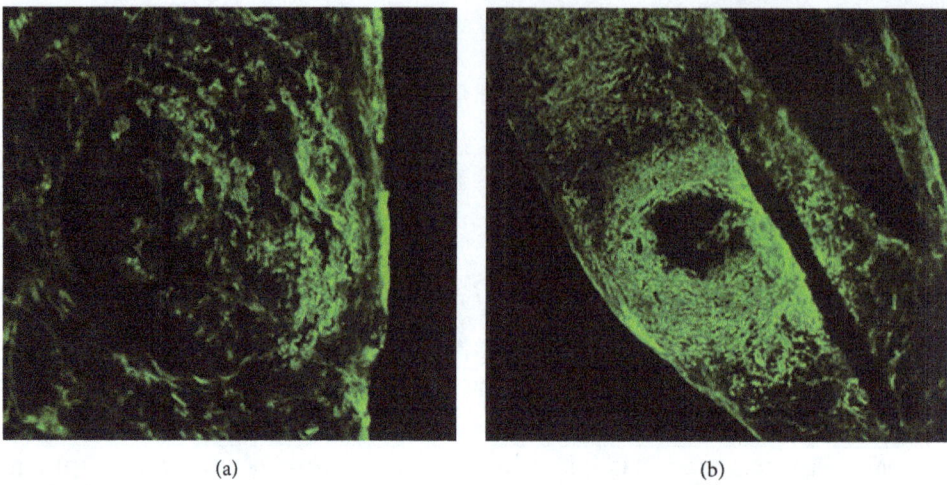

(a)   (b)

FIGURE 4: Fibrinogen staining shows cellular crescents (a) and necrosis of an artery (b).

in creatinine and onset of proteinuria with active urinary sediment led to renal biopsy, the histology of which supported the diagnosis of GPA in the setting of the past history of haemoptysis, hearing loss, tinnitus, and positive serological markers for p-ANCA and MPO.

GPA is an uncommon autoimmune disease most prevalent in Caucasian patients with disease onset usually between 45 and 65 y [1]. Notably, the prevalence of GPA is very low in non-Caucasians, and this patient is Afro-Caribbean. In a survey of 701 patients in North America, only 2% of patients diagnosed with GPA were not Caucasian [1]. The diagnosis of GPA can be challenging, as the entity commonly presents with nonspecific symptoms such as fatigue, joint pains, and sinusitis [1–3]. Organ systems involved at the time of diagnosis are the upper and lower airways, ears, lung, joints, and kidneys [1–3]. Most patients are diagnosed within 3–12 months from the onset of symptomatology, and on average two organ systems are involved at time of diagnosis [1].

Our patient had a two-year indolent phase with minor exacerbations prior to her acute presentation. Isolated organ system involvement, such as isolated lung nodules, is rare in GPA. The French Vasculitis Study Group identified 16 patients with isolated GPA occurring for as long as 58 months without progression to systemic disease [4]. However, such patients may progress if followed long enough. One case report described a patient with limited tracheobronchial disease which then suddenly flared twenty years after the initial presentation [5].

Unexplained fever and increasing leukocytosis were significant features of our patient's presentation and course. In one retrospective survey, fever was described as the first symptom in 33% of patients [1]. Fever suggestive of an infectious aetiology is not uncommon in GPA. Several case reports describe fever and pulmonary symptoms with abnormal chest imaging studies (often initially interpreted to be pneumonia), as in our patient's diagnosis from her prior admission [6–8]. Tuberculosis was suspected in our patient on both hospitalizations due to exposure risks in Haiti and in

her role as a healthcare worker, along with the presence of a positive tuberculin skin test.

Occasionally GPA can present with protracted fever without localizing signs, as in our patient, although this is uncommon. Pyrexia of unknown origin (PUO) is most commonly secondary to infectious disease. Fever secondary to occult collagen vascular disease is less common [9, 10]. In a retrospective cohort of 857 patients, 16% (137 patients) had fever due to collagen vascular disease. Only 3/137 (0.3% of the entire cohort) had fever secondary to GPA [11]. Our patient's fever resolved completely after the first dose of methylprednisolone.

Our patient's course was unusual in that her WBC count increased to 47,000. As such, there was significant concern for infectious or neoplastic source. We were unable to find an infectious source despite extensive microbiologic studies and imaging. The decision to begin treatment with high dose corticosteroids remained difficult in face of the florid leukocytosis, despite the negative sepsis workup. To our knowledge, leukocytosis at this level has not been previously described in the literature in association with GPA. The leukocytosis resolved completely after treatment with rituximab, further supporting its association with GPA.

Neutrophilic leukocytosis is commonly seen in association with an acute infectious process [12]. At times inflammatory processes or physiologic stressors can stimulate leukocytosis. For example, patients with rheumatoid arthritis, adult Still's disease, and noncystic fibrosis bronchiectasis have been found to develop leukocytosis with disease flare-ups [13–15]. Trauma patients have also been observed to have sterile neutrophilia with negative blood cultures [16]. In our patient, a possible mechanism for the observed leukocytosis could be as a response to extreme physiologic stress causing a profound inflammatory response and upregulating the immune system. Additionally, stimulation of bone marrow, such as that seen in haemolytic anemia, can rarely precipitate significant leukocytosis, possibly via overstimulation of the bone marrow in response to the anemia [17].

The patient's haemoglobin/haematocrit had declined in comparison to levels during the previous months. Her red blood cell levels continued to decline with schistocytes and target cells identified on peripheral smear. Laboratory evidence of MAHA included elevated LDH, undetectable haptoglobin, and negative Coombs test. MAHA is a rare complication of the immune activation in GPA and has been reported occasionally [18, 19]. In our patient the haemolytic anemia resolved completely after treatment with rituximab, further supporting the association.

Finally, c-ANCA with PR3 positive autoantibodies are diagnostic markers for GPA and are present in 70% to 90% of patients [20]. Our patient was p-ANCA MPO+, which is unusual in GPA, although it has been reported in 5% to 10% of cases [20]. In non-Caucasian populations, MPO+ p-ANCA may be more common. In a case series from China 60% of GPA patients were MPO+ p-ANCA. Those patients were more likely to have elevated serum creatinine at the onset of illness and less likely to have arthralgia, rash, and ophthalmic and ear involvement [20]. Our patient did not have arthralgia, rash, or ophthalmic involvement; however she did have tinnitus and a history of decreased hearing acuity.

4. Conclusion

GPA is a rare disorder with protean manifestations. It is important to consider the diagnosis of GPA early in order to begin immunosuppressive therapy. If not treated aggressively and promptly the patient can rapidly progress to renal failure. In this patient, the clinical picture of infection was misleading and made our decision to treat with corticosteroids and rituximab a very difficult one. We believe this is the first report of a patient with extreme leukocytosis in the setting of GPA and the absence of an infectious aetiology.

Acknowledgments

The authors thank Dr. Stephan Kamholz and Dr. Carl Schiff for their expert review of the manuscript and their insightful comments.

References

[1] N. I. Abdou, G. J. Kullman, G. S. Hoffman et al., "Wegener's granulomatosis: survey of 701 patients in North America. changes in outcome in the 1990s," *The Journal of Rheumatology*, vol. 29, no. 2, pp. 309–316, 2002.

[2] J. H. Takala, H. Kautiainen, H. Malmberg, and M. Leirisalo-Repo, "Wegener's granulomatosis in Finland in 1981-2000: clinical presentation and diagnostic delay," *Scandinavian Journal of Rheumatology*, vol. 37, no. 6, pp. 435–438, 2008.

[3] J. U. Holle, W. L. Gross, U. Latza et al., "Improved outcome in 445 patients with Wegener's granulomatosis in a German vasculitis center over four decades," *Arthritis and Rheumatism*, vol. 63, no. 1, pp. 257–266, 2011.

[4] C. Pagnoux, M. Stubbe, F. Lifermann et al., "Wegener's granulomatosis strictly and persistently localized to one organ is rare: Assessment of 16 patients from the French Vasculitis Study Group database," *Journal of Rheumatology*, vol. 38, no. 3, pp. 475–478, 2011.

[5] J. E. Peters, A. D. Salama, and P. W. Ind, "Wegener's granulomatosis presenting as acute systemic vasculitis following 20 years of limited tracheobronchial disease," *Journal of Laryngology and Otology*, vol. 123, no. 12, pp. 1375–1377, 2009.

[6] A. B. S. Zubairi, H. B. Liaquat, S. J. Jusain, and K. Fatima, "Wegeners granulomatosis: a diagnostic challenge," *Journal of Pakistani Medical Association*, vol. 59, no. 12, pp. 853–855, 2009.

[7] S. J. Spalding, M. Cambria, and T. Arkachaisri, "Distinguishing wegener's granulomatosis from necrotizing community acquired pneumonia: a case report and comparison of radiographic findings," *Pediatric Pulmonology*, vol. 44, no. 2, pp. 195–197, 2009.

[8] B. P. Paudyal, S. Pantha, N. Ranjitkar, A. Manandhar, and A. Arjyal, "A diagnosis missed for several years-Wegener's granulomatosis," *Kathmandu University Medical Journal*, vol. 35, no. 9, pp. 218–221, 2011.

[9] M. A. Islam, F. Bagheri, D. Bencomo et al., "Wegener's granulomatosis presenting as fever of unknown origin in an African-American male," *Proceedings of the Western Pharmacology Society*, vol. 50, pp. 136–139, 2007.

[10] E. Bayrak, Ö. Dönderici, R. Serter, and F. K. Efe, "A case with fever of unknown origin diagnosed as wegener granulomatosis," *Turkish Journal of Rheumatology*, vol. 25, no. 3, pp. 159–161, 2010.

[11] O. R. Sipahi, S. Senol, G. Arsu et al., "Pooled analysis of 857 published adult fever of unknown origin cases in Turkey between 1990-2006," *Medical Science Monitor*, vol. 13, no. 7, pp. CR318–CR322, 2007.

[12] Y. R. Lawrence, D. Raveh, B. Rudensky, and G. Munter, "Extreme leukocytosis in the emergency department," *QJM*, vol. 100, no. 4, pp. 217–223, 2007.

[13] K. M. Syed and R. S. Pinals, "Leukocytosis in rheumatoid arthritis," *Journal of Clinical Rheumatology*, vol. 2, no. 4, pp. 197–202, 1996.

[14] J. Pouchot, J. S. Sampalis, F. Beaudet et al., "Adult Stills disease: manifestations, disease course and outcomes in 62 patients," *Medicine*, vol. 70, no. 2, pp. 118–136, 1991.

[15] C. B. Wilson, P. W. Jones, C. J. O'Leary et al., "Systemic markers of inflammation in stable bronchiectasis," *European Respiratory Journal*, vol. 12, no. 4, pp. 820–824, 1998.

[16] J. A. Claridge, J. F. Golob Jf, A. M. Fadlalla, M. A. Malangoni, J. Blatnick, and C. J. Yowler, "Fever and leukocytosis in critically ill traua patients: it is not the blood," *Am Surg*, vol. 75, no. 5, pp. 405–410, 2009.

[17] S. J. Jea, S. Y. Kim, B. M. Choi, J. H. Lee, K. C. Lee, and C. W. Woo, "A pediatric case of autoimmune hemolytic anemia followed by excessive thrombocytosis and leukocytosis," *Korean J Hematol*, vol. 42, no. 3, pp. 288–291, 2007.

[18] C. N. Ross, H. Reuter, D. Scott, and D. V. Hamilton, "Microangiopathic haemolytic anaemia and systemic vasculitis," *British Journal of Rheumatology*, vol. 35, no. 4, pp. 377–379, 1996.

[19] J. Jordan, M. Manning, and N. B. Allen, "Multiple unusual man-
      ifestatiosn of Wegeners granulomatosis: breast mass, micran-
      giopathic haemolytic anemia, consumptive coagulopathy, and
      low erythrocyte sedimentation rate," *Arthritis Rheumatism*, vol.
      29, no. 12, pp. 1527–1531, 1986.

[20] M. Chen, F. Yu, Y. Zhang, W.-Z. Zou, M.-H. Zhao, and H.-
      Y. Wang, "Characteristics of Chinese patients with Wegener's
      granulomatosis with anti-myeloperoxidase autoantibodies,"
      Kidney International, vol. 68, no. 5, pp. 2225–2229, 2005.

48

Erosive Arthritis, Fibromatosis, and Keloids: A Rare Dermatoarthropathy

Fawad Aslam[ID],[1] Jonathan A. Flug,[2] Yousif Yonan,[3] and Shelley S. Noland[4,5]

[1]Division of Rheumatology, Department of Internal Medicine, Mayo Clinic, Scottsdale, AZ, USA
[2]Department of Radiology, Mayo Clinic, Scottsdale, AZ, USA
[3]Department of Dermatology, Mayo Clinic, Scottsdale, AZ, USA
[4]Division of Plastic Surgery, Department of Surgery, Mayo Clinic Hospital, Phoenix, AZ, USA
[5]Department of Orthopedic Surgery, Mayo Clinic Hospital, Phoenix, AZ, USA

Correspondence should be addressed to Fawad Aslam; fawadaslam2@gmail.com

Academic Editor: Tsai-Ching Hsu

Polyfibromatosis is a rare disease characterized by fibrosis manifesting in different locations. It is commonly characterized by palmar fibromatosis (Dupuytren's contracture) in variable combinations with plantar fibromatosis (Ledderhose's disease), penile fibromatosis (Peyronie's disease), knuckle pads, and keloids. There are only three reported cases of polyfibromatosis and keloids with erosive arthritis. We report one such case and review the existing literature on this rare syndrome.

1. Introduction

Polyfibromatosis is a rare disease characterized by fibrosis manifesting in different locations. It is commonly characterized by palmar fibromatosis (Dupuytren's contracture) in variable combinations with plantar fibromatosis (Ledderhose's disease), penile fibromatosis (Peyronie's disease), knuckle pads, and keloids [1]. The aforementioned are all categories of superficial fibromatoses. Coexistence of fibromatosis and keloid formation is also very rare [2, 3], and it is not entirely clear if keloids are formally part of the polyfibromatosis syndrome. Nevertheless, this association is rare. To identify previous reports, a nonrestricted PubMed search was carried out using the key words Dupuytren's contracture, keloid, fibrosis, arthritis, osteolysis, erosive arthritis, and their varying combinations. Bibliographies of identified relevant studies were also reviewed for further pertinent cases. A few case reports have described presence of erosive and/or osteolytic disease in patients with polyfibromatosis [4–6]. There are only three reported cases of simultaneous occurrence of fibromatosis, keloids, and erosive arthritis, all in males [7–9]. Interestingly, the keloid formation is also spontaneous in these cases. We report a fourth such case and review the existing literature.

2. Case Presentation

A 23-year-old male presented to the primary care clinic to establish care after relocating to Arizona. His past medical history was significant for severe, mostly spontaneous, keloid formation since puberty. He complained of a right ring finger mass and a left ring finger deformity, bilateral foot pain, and worsening keloids and skin nodules.

Over the last four months, he had noticed a spontaneous, slowly enlarging mass on his right ring finger. It bothered him when directly pressed upon or during rock climbing. There were no associated neurological symptoms, redness, or erythema. He also reported a contracture in the left ring finger over the last six months. He had undergone a left small finger proximal interphalangeal joint arthrodesis for presumed camptodactyly at age 16. This surgery was complicated by fibromatosis and keloid scar formation, ultimately leading to amputation of the small finger. He now complained of excessive scar formation at that amputation site.

He gave a two-year history of bilateral forefoot pain. His right fourth toe was the most painful. He reported that this toe had become very stiff over this time. Other toes were involved as well, and prolonged standing exacerbated the symptoms. He did not report any redness, warmth, or swelling. He denied any acute joint pain episodes and hand or back pain.

With respect to his keloids and skin nodules, he had had them since puberty. He noted that some were related to sites of minor trauma, and others were spontaneous. He had multiple large keloids involving the chest, back, arms, and legs. Recently, some had involved the toes as well. He denied any genital involvement. Past treatments included intralesional steroid injections and radiation therapy with temporary improvements.

He was a lifelong nonsmoker and drank alcohol socially. He was an avid rock-climber. His family history was significant for keloid formation in his grandfather. A maternal cousin had rheumatoid arthritis. On review of systems, he denied any fatigue, morning stiffness, night sweats, weight loss, inflammatory eye disease, cough, shortness of breath, back pain, nephrolithiasis, Raynaud's phenomenon, or blood dyscrasias. He did not take any chronic medications.

On examination, he was afebrile with normal vital signs and appropriate weight. There was no glandular swelling or gingival hypertrophy. Hand examination showed severe left ring finger proximal interphalangeal (PIP) joint contracture of 80°, with palmar fibromatosis and keloid scar formation (Figures 1 and 2). There was no intrinsic degeneration of the PIP joint on X-ray or MRI. The right ring finger demonstrated a firm and immobile mass extending for the length of the middle phalanx on the ulnar aspect. Ring finger movement was intact. At the distal aspect of his prior amputation, he had a thickened scar. Mild tenderness to flexion and extension of his bilateral fourth and fifth digits was present. He had prominent fifth metatarsal heads bilaterally which were tender to palpation. Ankle and subtalar joint exam was normal. Ambulation was unrestricted. Multiple large areas of hypertrophic scarring and keloid formation involving the central chest (Figure 3), arms, and legs as well as some discrete nodules on the upper back were present.

Laboratory testing was unremarkable. He tested negative for rheumatoid factor, anticyclic citrullinated peptide, C-reactive protein, erythrocyte sedimentation rate, antinuclear antibody, HLA-B27 gene, and hepatitis serology. Routine laboratory markers including complete blood count, renal function, liver function, thyroid and parathyroid gland function, and uric acid and urinalysis were normal. A chest radiograph was unremarkable. A right hand X-ray film showed nonspecific soft tissue swelling of the right ring finger. The left hand film showed amputation of the small finger at the level of the proximal to mid fifth metacarpal and a flexion deformity of the ring finger at the PIP joint. Sacroiliac joints showed minimal degenerative changes on X-rays. Feet radiographs showed multiple erosions. Axial (Figure 4) and coronal (Figure 5) magnetic resonance imaging (MRI) of the feet obtained with gadolinium contrast administration demonstrated marginal

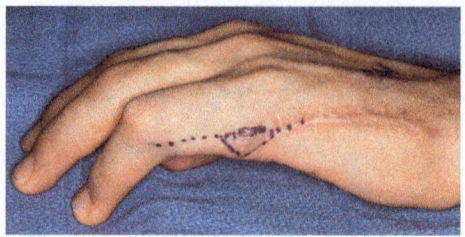

FIGURE 1: Severe left ring finger contracture with palmar fibromatosis and keloid scar formation.

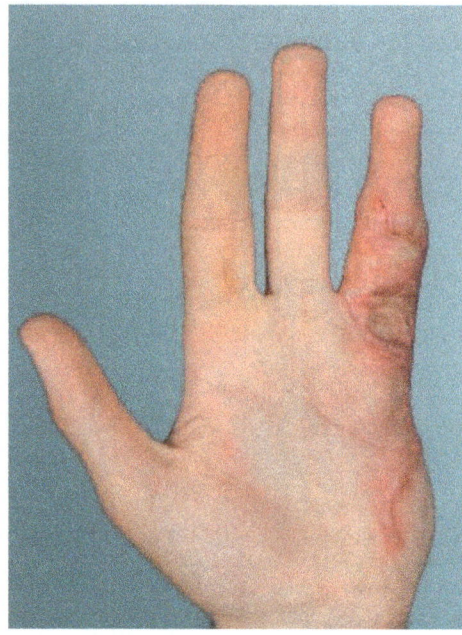

FIGURE 2: Severe left ring finger contracture with palmar fibromatosis and keloid scar formation.

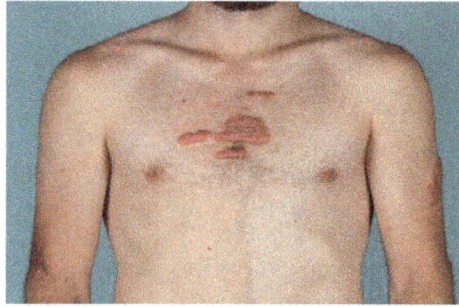

FIGURE 3: Keloids and hypertrophic scars on the chest and arms.

erosions, synovitis, and bone marrow enhancement. Enhancing inflammatory changes in the plantar soft tissues and heterogeneous enhancement of keloids was also seen.

To treat the contracture, the patient underwent a left ring finger palmar fasciectomy. Operative findings included severe fibromatosis of the left middle and ring finger and keloid formation that was confirmed by histopathology. After excision of diseased palmar fascia, the finger was able to be fully extended. A residual skin deficit required skin

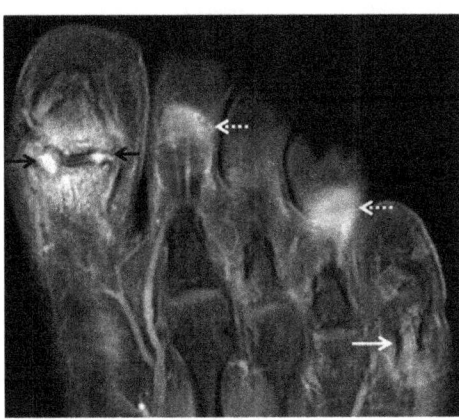

FIGURE 4: Axial T1 fat-saturated magnetic resonance imaging (MRI) of the foot obtained with gadolinium contrast administration demonstrated marginal erosions at the great toe interphalangeal joint, associated synovitis, and bone marrow enhancement (black arrows). Erosive changes involving the fifth metatarsophalangeal joint were present with bone marrow enhancement in the proximal phalanx (solid white arrow). Enhancing inflammatory changes in the second and fourth toe plantar soft tissues were present (dashed white arrows).

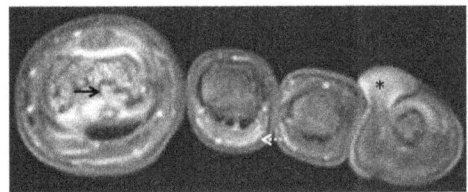

FIGURE 5: Coronal T1 fat-saturated magnetic resonance imaging (MRI) of the foot obtained with gadolinium contrast administration demonstrated marginal erosions at the great toe interphalangeal joint, associated synovitis, and bone marrow enhancement (black arrows). Enhancing inflammatory changes in the second and fourth toe plantar soft tissues were present (dashed white arrows). One of the several keloids is seen along the medial margin of the fourth toe at the level of the nail with moderate heterogeneous enhancement (asterisk).

grafting for closure. The entire palmar surface of the proximal phalanx was resurfaced with a full thickness skin graft. His nonoperative skin lesions were treated with a combination of intralesional methylprednisolone, 5-fluorouracil, and pulsed dye laser treatments. He was initiated on 15 mg of oral methotrexate for his erosive disease.

Aggressive occupational therapy was pursued after the surgery. At six-month follow-up, he reported improvement in his joint pain as well as keloids. The ring finger PIP joint flexion contracture had improved from 80° to 35°. However, continued keloid formation persisted over the surgical scars. His skin graft healed completely. Due to the scarring and keloids, no further surgery was recommended.

3. Discussion

Palmar fibromatosis is relatively uncommon as compared with keloids. It tends to predominantly occur in males after the age of 40. It has been associated with diabetes, alcohol use, smoking, liver disease, and those using vibratory hand tools [1, 3]. Keloid formation is more common, tends to favor the young, has no gender preference, and spares the hands and the feet. Both diseases can be familial [1, 3].

Polyfibromatosis with arthritis is extremely rare and presents with varying degrees of fibrotic features. Cases of fibromatosis with keloids without arthritic features have also been reported [2, 3]. It is clear that this syndrome presents with variable features as no reported patient has had all syndromic manifestations. Table 1 summarizes the reported cases of polyfibromatosis with arthritis. Incidence is primarily sporadic. One case was related to phenytoin exposure [4]. Keloid or fibromatosis was the primary reason for clinical presentation. No case presented to a rheumatology department. This likely implies that the arthritic process is secondary, being driven by the fibrotic disease process or that cosmetic concerns are paramount. It is not known if routine radiographic screening of patients with polyfibromatosis would reveal more silent erosive disease than is currently reported. Long-term data are not available on all of these reported patients, but the erosive findings remained unchanged in one patient at 10-year follow-up [10]. In the reported cases, there was no evidence of a systemic rheumatic disease process. Our case had no features of multicentric reticulohistiocytosis or fibroblastic rheumatism. It is interesting to note the presence of synovitis and enhancement of keloids on MRI in our case. A long-term follow-up in our or similar cases may shed more light on the natural history.

The pathogenesis of polyfibromatosis is unclear. Both palmar fibromatosis and keloids have increased production of type III collagen, and anoxia is thought to play an important role. The ischemia produces free oxygen radicals which may promote fibroblastic growth [11]. However, it is thought that the fibroblasts are inherently unstable in keloids in contrast to palmar fibromatosis [10]. One study found increased incidence of carotid atherosclerotic plaque in keloid patients when compared to those with palmar fibromatosis [12]. They speculated that the myofibroblasts in these diseases originated from different cellular precursors. Electron microscopy studies reveal that myofibroblasts are better organized in palmar fibromatosis as opposed to keloids [13]. The etiologic relationship between the musculoskeletal features and polyfibromatosis is unclear. A common triggering factor may be responsible [9]. Bone biopsy done in one case showed increased osteoclast activity [7]. Another common denominator in these conditions may be the matrix metalloproteinases [14–16]. Osteoclast and matrix metalloproteinases could be future therapeutic targets.

Immunosuppressive treatment is generally ineffective although one case responded to methotrexate [6]. Our patient has also had subjective improvement with methotrexate, but only a longer follow-up will reveal its success at prevention of new erosions or halting progression of the current ones. It is unknown if biological agents like tumor necrosis actor inhibitors (TNFi) are useful in this syndrome, but the presence of synovitis in our case and one

TABLE 1: Summary of polyfibromatosis cases with a musculoskeletal component.

Author/year/country	Age (years)/gender	Fibromatosis	Keloids	Musculoskeletal features	X-ray features	MRI features
Pierard and Lapiere 1979 [4], Belgium	20, male	Hand fibromatosis, knuckle pads, and "toughness" of skin	NA	Camptodactyly, tendon calcification, facial hypolasia, osteolysis, and scoliosis	Osteolysis of distal ulna, right ring finger proximal phalanx, and first metacarpal	NA
Fenton et al. 1986 [7], United Kingdom	48, male	Palmar fibromatosis, and Peyronie's disease	Keloids of arms, shoulders, and presternal area	Hand and foot stiffness	Erosions of shoulders, hands, and feet	NA
Chen et al. 2006 [5], Australia	65, male	Progressive fibrosis and contractures of wrist, elbows, knees, and ankles; linear fibrotic cords	None	Inflammatory pain of wrist, elbows, knees, and ankles	Erosions of left shoulder, elbows, wrists, hands, and feet	NA
Kim et al. 2009 [8], South Korea	44, male	Palmar and plantar nodules and fibromatosis	Multiple keloids of trunk and extremities	Asymptomatic	Erosions and osteolysis of hands	Multiple hand erosions
Cinotti et al. 2013 [9], Italy	53, male	Flexion contractures of wrists, fingers, ankles, and toes; gingival hyperplasia and conjunctival fibrosis	Multiple keloids	Severe hand and foot deformities and facial changes	Osteolysis of wrists, hands, and toes; ankylosis	NA
Albarran et al. 2015 [6], Spain	33, male	Palmar and plantar nodules, palmar fibromatosis, knee contractures and fibromatosis, and gingival hyperplasia	None	NA	Erosion in right foot	Synovitis and effusions in both knees
Present case 2018, USA	23, male	Finger flexion contractures	Multiple keloids of trunk and extremities	Mild foot pain	Erosions of feet; hands without erosions	Multiple erosions and synovitis of feet

another [6] indicates its potential usefulness. However, none of the cases had prominent inflammatory joint symptoms despite the aggressive radiological findings. Laboratory studies have shown the inhibitory effects of TNFi in Dupuytren's contracture by inhibiting myofibroblast activity and the contractile apparatus [17]. A phase II clinical trial will assess the role of intralesional adalimumab in early Dupuytren's contracture [18]. Thus, TNFi could possibly help address both the musculoskeletal and dermatological manifestations. Erosions could also possibly be repaired using an osteoclast development inhibitor like denosumab [19] but is untested in this dermatoarthropathy. Bisphosphonates have been used to treat musculoskeletal manifestation in some osteolytic disorders [20].

In conclusion, polyfibromatosis with arthritis is extremely rare with no established treatment. Our case will add to the limited repertoire of erosive polyfibromatosis cases with keloids and serve to increase awareness and thereby stimulate research and reporting of this rare syndrome.

References

[1] N. P. Burrows and C. R. Lovell, "Disorders of connective tissue," in *Rook's Textbook of Dermatology*, A. Rook and T. Burns, Eds., Wiley-Blackwell Hoboken, NJ, USA, 8th edition, 2010.

[2] R. Gonzalez-Martinez, S. Marin-Bertolin, and J. Amorrortu-Velayos, "Association between keloids and Dupuytren's disease: case report," *British Journal of Plastic Surgery*, vol. 48, no. 1, pp. 47-48, 1995.

[3] L. Ly and I. Winship, "X-linked recessive polyfibromatosis manifesting with spontaneous keloid scars and Dupuytren's contracture," *Australasian Journal of Dermatology*, vol. 53, no. 2, pp. 148–150, 2012.

[4] G. E. Pierard and C. M. Lapiere, "Phenytoin dependent fibrosis in polyfibromatosis syndrome," *British Journal of Dermatology*, vol. 100, no. 3, pp. 335–341, 1979.

[5] D. L. Chen, A. H. Chong, J. Green, D. Orchard, R. Williams, and L. Clemens, "A novel case of polyfibromatosis and interstitial granulomatous dermatitis with arthritis," *Journal of the American Academy of Dermatology*, vol. 55, no. 2, pp. S32–S37, 2006.

[6] C. Albarran Planelles, D. Jimenez Gallo, M. Linares Barrios, and J. M. Baez Baena, "Touraine's polyfibromatosis: a forgotten disease," *European Journal of Dermatology*, vol. 25, no. 4, pp. 357-358, 2015.

[7] D. A. Fenton, D. A. Yates, and M. M. Black, "Aggressive polyfibromatosis," *Journal of the Royal Society of Medicine*, vol. 79, no. 8, pp. 482-483, 1986.

[8] S. K. Kim, H. J. Kim, Y. H. Lee, K. J. Suh, S. H. Park, and J. Y. Choe, "Erosive arthropathy with osteolysis as a typical feature in polyfibromatosis syndrome: a case report and a review of the literature," *Journal of Korean Medical Science*, vol. 24, no. 2, pp. 326–329, 2009.

[9] E. Cinotti, G. Ferrero, F. Paparo et al., "Arthropathy, osteolysis, keloids, relapsing conjunctival pannus and gingival overgrowth: a variant of polyfibromatosis?," *American Journal of Medical Genetics Part A*, vol. 161, no. 6, pp. 1214–1220, 2013.

[10] Y. C. Lee, H. H. Chan, and M. M. Black, "Aggressive polyfibromatosis: a 10 year follow-up," *Australasian Journal of Dermatology*, vol. 37, no. 4, pp. 205–207, 1996.

[11] G. A. Murrell, M. J. Francis, and L. Bromley, "Free radicals and Dupuytren's contracture," *British Medical Journal*, vol. 295, no. 6610, pp. 1373–1375, 1987.

[12] S. Bhavsar, A. Nimigan, D. G. Hackam, D. B. O'Gorman, B. S. Gan, and J. D. Spence, "Keloid scarring, but not Dupuytren's contracture, is associated with unexplained carotid atherosclerosis," *Clinical and Investigative Medicine*, vol. 32, no. 2, pp. E95–E102, 2009.

[13] B. Eyden, "Electron microscopy in the study of myofibroblastic lesions," *Seminars in Diagnostic Pathology*, vol. 20, no. 1, pp. 13–24, 2003.

[14] D. E. Lee, R. M. Trowbridge, N. T. Ayoub, and D. K. Agrawal, "High-mobility group box protein-1, matrix metalloproteinases, and vitamin D in keloids and hypertrophic scars," *Plastic and Reconstructive Surgery–Global Open*, vol. 3, no. 6, p. e425, 2015.

[15] J. M. Wilkinson, R. K. Davidson, T. E. Swingler et al., "MMP-14 and MMP-2 are key metalloproteases in Dupuytren's disease fibroblast-mediated contraction," *Biochimica et Biophysica Acta*, vol. 1822, no. 6, pp. 897–905, 2012.

[16] J. A. Martignetti, A. A. Aqeel, W. A. Sewairi et al., "Mutation of the matrix metalloproteinase 2 gene (MMP2) causes a multicentric osteolysis and arthritis syndrome," *Nature Genetics*, vol. 28, no. 3, pp. 261–265, 2001.

[17] L. S. Verjee, J. S. Verhoekx, J. K. Chan et al., "Unraveling the signaling pathways promoting fibrosis in Dupuytren's disease reveals TNF as a therapeutic target," *Proceedings of the National Academy of Sciences*, vol. 110, no. 10, pp. E928–E937, 2013.

[18] J. Nanchahal, C. Ball, J. Swettenham et al., "Study protocol: a multi-centre, double blind, randomised, placebo-controlled, parallel group, phase II trial (RIDD) to determine the efficacy of intra-nodular injection of anti-TNF to control disease progression in early Dupuytren's disease, with an embedded dose response study," *Wellcome Open Research*, vol. 2, p. 37, 2017.

[19] J. Yue, J. F. Griffith, F. Xiao et al., "Repair of bone erosion in rheumatoid arthritis by denosumab: a high-resolution peripheral quantitative computed tomography study," *Arthritis Care & Research*, vol. 69, no. 8, pp. 1156–1163, 2017.

[20] K. Pichler, D. Karall, D. Kotzot et al., "Bisphosphonates in multicentric osteolysis, nodulosis and arthropathy (MONA) spectrum disorder–an alternative therapeutic approach," *Scientific Reports*, vol. 6, no. 1, p. 34017, 2016.

Permissions

All chapters in this book were first published in CRR, by Hindawi Publishing Corporation; hereby published with permission under the Creative Commons Attribution License or equivalent. Every chapter published in this book has been scrutinized by our experts. Their significance has been extensively debated. The topics covered herein carry significant findings which will fuel the growth of the discipline. They may even be implemented as practical applications or may be referred to as a beginning point for another development.

The contributors of this book come from diverse backgrounds, making this book a truly international effort. This book will bring forth new frontiers with its revolutionizing research information and detailed analysis of the nascent developments around the world.

We would like to thank all the contributing authors for lending their expertise to make the book truly unique. They have played a crucial role in the development of this book. Without their invaluable contributions this book wouldn't have been possible. They have made vital efforts to compile up to date information on the varied aspects of this subject to make this book a valuable addition to the collection of many professionals and students.

This book was conceptualized with the vision of imparting up-to-date information and advanced data in this field. To ensure the same, a matchless editorial board was set up. Every individual on the board went through rigorous rounds of assessment to prove their worth. After which they invested a large part of their time researching and compiling the most relevant data for our readers.

The editorial board has been involved in producing this book since its inception. They have spent rigorous hours researching and exploring the diverse topics which have resulted in the successful publishing of this book. They have passed on their knowledge of decades through this book. To expedite this challenging task, the publisher supported the team at every step. A small team of assistant editors was also appointed to further simplify the editing procedure and attain best results for the readers.

Apart from the editorial board, the designing team has also invested a significant amount of their time in understanding the subject and creating the most relevant covers. They scrutinized every image to scout for the most suitable representation of the subject and create an appropriate cover for the book.

The publishing team has been an ardent support to the editorial, designing and production team. Their endless efforts to recruit the best for this project, has resulted in the accomplishment of this book. They are a veteran in the field of academics and their pool of knowledge is as vast as their experience in printing. Their expertise and guidance has proved useful at every step. Their uncompromising quality standards have made this book an exceptional effort. Their encouragement from time to time has been an inspiration for everyone.

The publisher and the editorial board hope that this book will prove to be a valuable piece of knowledge for researchers, students, practitioners and scholars across the globe.

List of Contributors

Anupam Bansal
Atlantic University School of Medicine, Gros Islet Highway, Rodney Bay, Saint Lucia

Rupali Drewek
Phoenix Children's Hospital, 1919 E. Thomas Road, Phoenix, AZ 85016, USA

Elli-Sophia Tripodaki, Ioanna Skrapari, Giorgios Katsikas and Euaggelia Sioula
1st Department of Internal Medicine, Evangelismos General Hospital, Ypsilanti 45-47, 10676 Athens, Greece

Sotirios Kakavas
1st Department of Internal Medicine, Evangelismos General Hospital, Ypsilanti 45-47, 10676 Athens, Greece
9 Kosma Aitolou, Herakleio, 14121 Athens, Greece

Dimitrios Michas
Department of Neurology, Evangelismos General Hospital, Ypsilanti 45-47, 10676 Athens, Greece

Theodoros Gounaris
Department of Rheumatology, Evangelismos General Hospital, Ypsilanti 45-47, 10676 Athens, Greece

Charikleia Kouvidou
Department of Pathology, Evangelismos General Hospital, Ypsilanti 45-47, 10676 Athens, Greece

J. L. Barton, L. Pincus, J. Yazdany, N. Richman, T. H.McCalmont, L. Gensler, M. Dall'Era and K. H. Fye
Division of Rheumatology, Department of Medicine, University of California, San Francisco, CA 94143, USA

Cindy Mourgues, Sandrine Malochet-Guinamand and Martin Soubrier
CHU Gabriel Montpied, Service de Rhumatologie, 58 rue Montalembert, 63000 Clermont-Ferrand, France

Cherin Patrick
Department of Internal Medicine, Piti´e-Salpetrière Hospital Group, 47-83 Boulevard de l'Hôpital, 75013 Paris, France

Delain Jean-Christophe and Crave Jean-Charles
Octapharma, 92100 Boulogne-Billancourt, France

Cartry Odile
Clinique Mutualiste Catalane, 66000 Perpignan, France

Takuya Kotani, Tohru Takeuchi, Shigeki Makino and Toshiaki Hanafusa
First Department of Internal Medicine, Osaka Medical College, 2-7 Daigaku-Machi, Takatsuki, Osaka 569-8686, Japan

Helen Chioma Okoh, Sandeep Singh Lubana, Spencer Langevin, Susan Sanelli-Russo and Adriana Abrudescu
Icahn School of Medicine at Mount Sinai,QueensHospital Center, Jamaica, NY 11432, USA

Eduardo Araújo Santana Nunes
Department of Rheumatology, Santa Izabel Hospital, Praça Almeida Couto 500, 40050-410 Salvador, BA, Brazil

Mittermayer Santiago
Department of Rheumatology, Santa Izabel Hospital, Praça Almeida Couto 500, 40050-410 Salvador, BA, Brazil
Serviços Especializados em Reumatologia da Bahia, Rua Conde Filho 117, Graça, 40150-150 Salvador, BA, Brazil

Adroaldo Guimarães Rosseti Jr.
Department of Neurosurgery, Santa Izabel Hospital, Praça Almeida Couto 500, 40050-410 Salvador, BA, Brazil

Daniel Sá Ribeiro
Department of Radiology and Image Memorial Radiology Service, Santa Izabel Hospital, Praça Almeida Couto 500, 40050-410 Salvador, BA, Brazil
Serviços Especializados em Reumatologia da Bahia, Rua Conde Filho 117, Graça, 40150-150 Salvador, BA, Brazil
Sarah Norrenberg and Véronique Del Marmol
Department of Dermatology, Hôpital Erasme, Université Libre de Bruxelles, 1070 Bruxelles, Belgium

Valérie Gangji and Muhammad S. Soyfoo
Department of Rheumatology and Medical Physicine, Hôpital Erasme, Université Libre de Bruxelles, 808 Route de Lennik, 1070 Bruxelles, Belgium

Namrata Singh
Immunology, University of Iowa Hospitals and Clinics, 200 Hawkins Drive, C42 E 10, Iowa City, IA 52241, USA

Shireesh Saurabh
Mercy Iowa City, 540 E Jefferson Street, Suite 205, Iowa City, IA 52245, USA

Irene J. Tan
Section of Rheumatology, Temple University Hospital, 3200 North Broad Street, Philadelphia, PA 19140, USA

Rajaie Namas, Malini Venkatram and J. Patricia Dhar
Department of Internal Medicine, Division of Rheumatology, Wayne State University, Detroit, MI 48201, USA

Naveen Nannapaneni and Miriam Levine
Department of Internal Medicine, Wayne State University, Detroit, MI 48201, USA

Gulcin Altinok
Department of Radiology, Wayne State University, Detroit, MI 48201, USA

Marc Campos and Elena Schiopu
Division of Rheumatology, University of Michigan, Ann Arbor, MI 48109, USA

Graeme Hopper, Sanjay Gupta and Ashish Mahendra
Trauma and Orthopaedics, Glasgow Royal Infirmary, 84 Castle Street, Glasgow G4 0SF, UK

Sarath Bethapudi and David Ritchie
Radiology, Glasgow Western Infirmary, Dumbarton Road, Glasgow G11 6NT, UK

Elaine MacDuff
Pathology, Glasgow Western Infirmary, Dumbarton Road, Glasgow G11 6NT, UK

Jenny Shu
Department of Medicine, Division of Rheumatology, Western University, London, ON, Canada N6A 5W9

Lillian Barra
Department of Medicine, Division of Rheumatology, Western University, London, ON, Canada N6A 5W9
Division of Rheumatology, Arthritis Centre, Monsignor Roney Building, St. Joseph's Health Care London, 268 Grosvenor Street, London, ON, Canada N6A 4V2

Ian Ross
Department of Diagnostic Radiology, Western University, London, ON, Canada N6A 5W9

Bret Wehrli
Department of Pathology, Western University, London, ON, Canada N6A 5A5

Richard W. McCalden
Department of Orthopaedic Surgery, Western University, London, ON, Canada N6A 5A5

Takeshi Suzuki and Akiko Okamoto
Division of Rheumatology, Mitsui Memorial Hospital, Kandaizumi-cho, Chiyoda-ku, Tokyo 101-8643, Japan

Masao Sato and Katsuji Shimizu
Department of Orthopaedic Surgery, Gifu University School of Medicine, 1-1 Yanagido Gifu, Gifu 501-1194, Japan

Masao Takemura
Department of Informative Clinical Medicine, Gifu University School of Medicine, 1-1 Yanagido Gifu, Gifu 501-1194, Japan

Ryuki Shinohe
Department of Orthopadeic Surgery, Nishimino Welfare Hospital, 986 Oshikoshi Yoro, Gifu 503-1394, Japan

Eike Garbers and Falk Reuther
Klinik für Unfallchirurgie und Orthopaedie, DRK Kliniken Berlin Koepenick, Salvador-Allende-Straße 2-8, 12559 Berlin, Germany

Gunther Delling
Institut für Pathologie Hannover, Berliner Allee 48, 30175 Hannover, Germany

Meera Yogarajah, Bhradeev Sivasambu and Eric A. Jaffe
Department of Medicine, Interfaith Medical Center, Brooklyn, NY 11213, USA

Alexandra Perel-Winkler, Regina Belokovskaya and Isabelle Amigues
Department of Medicine, St. Luke's-Roosevelt Hospital Center, and Department of Medicine, Icahn School of Medicine at Mount Sinai, New York, NY 10025, USA

Melissa Larusso and Nazia Hussain
Division of Rheumatology, Department of Medicine, St. Luke's-Roosevelt Hospital Center and Department of Medicine, Icahn School of Medicine at Mount Sinai, New York, NY 10025, USA

M. Fantò, S. Salemi, R. Di Rosa and R. D'Amelio
Department of Allergy, Clinical Immunology and Rheumatology, S. Andrea Hospital, Sapienza University of Rome, Italy

F. Socciarelli and A. Bartolazzi
Department of Pathology, S. Andrea Hospital, Sapienza University of Rome, Italy

G. A. Natale, I. Casorelli, A. Pavan and S. Vaglio
Department of Immunohematology and Transfusion Unit, S. Andrea Hospital, Sapienza University of Rome, Italy

Ayesha Farooq, Vivek Choksi, Andrew Chu, Dhruti Mankodi, Sameer Shaharyar, Keith O'Brien and Uday Shankar
Aventura Hospital and Medical Center Internal Medicine Department, Aventura, FL 33180, USA

Mekdess Abebe, Nand K. Wadhwa, Mersema Abate and Edward P. Nord
Division of Nephrology, Department of Medicine, School of Medicine, State University of New York at Stony Brook, Stony Brook, NY 11794, USA

Asha Patnaik and Heidi Roppelt
Division of Rheumatology, Department of Medicine, School of Medicine, State University of New York at Stony Brook, Stony Brook, NY 11794, USA

Frederick Miller
Department of Pathology, School of Medicine, State University of New York at Stony Brook, Stony Brook, NY 11794, USA

Tomoya Miyamura and Eiichi Suematsu
Department of Internal Medicine and Rheumatology, Clinical Research Institute, National Hospital Organization, Kyushu Medical Center, Fukuoka 810-8563, Japan

Akihiro Nakamura
Department of Internal Medicine and Rheumatology, Clinical Research Institute, National Hospital Organization, Kyushu Medical Center, Fukuoka 810-8563, Japan
Department of Genetics and Development, Krembil Research Institute, University Health Network, Toronto, ON, Canada M5T 2S8

Md Abu Bakar Siddiq
Physical Medicine and Rehabilitation Department, Feni Diabetes Hospital (FDH), Feni 3900, Bangladesh
Moshiur Rahman Khasru Physical Medicine and Rehabilitation Department, BSMMU, Dhaka 1000, Bangladesh

Johannes J. Rasker
Rheumatology Department, Faculty of Behavioral Sciences, University of Twente, 7500 AE Enschede, The Netherlands

Prajwal Boddu and Abdul S. Mohammed
Department of Internal Medicine, Advocate Illinois Masonic Medical Center, 836W.Wellington Avenue, Chicago, IL 60657, USA

Chandrahasa Annem and Winston Sequeira
Department of Rheumatology, Rush University Medical Center, 1725West Harrison Street, Chicago, IL 60612, USA

Aslıhan Gürün Kaya, Aydın Çiledağ and Özlem Özdemir Kumbasar
Department of Chest Diseases, Ankara University School of Medicine, Ankara, Turkey

Orhan Küçükşahin
Department of Rheumatology, Ankara University School of Medicine, Ankara, Turkey

Çetin Atasoy
Department of Radiology, Ankara University School of Medicine, Ankara, Turkey

Christine L. Chhakchhuak and Kristine M. Lohr
Division of Rheumatology, Department of Internal Medicine, University of Kentucky, 740 South Limestone Street, Room J-515, Lexington, KY 40536, USA

Mehdi Khosravi
Division of Pulmonary and Critical Care Medicine, Department of Internal Medicine, University of Kentucky, 740 South Limestone Street, Kentucky Clinic L 543, Lexington KY 40536, USA

Carla F. Gamarra-Hilburn, Grissel Rios and Luis M. Vilá
Division of Rheumatology, Department of Medicine, University of Puerto Rico, Medical Sciences Campus, San Juan, PR 00936-5067, USA

Grigorios T. Sakellariou
Department of Rheumatology, 424 General Military Hospital, 564 03Thessaloniki, Greece

Nicoleta Kefala
Department of Internal Medicine, 424 General Military Hospital, 564 03Thessaloniki, Greece

Carlo Umberto Manzini, Michele Colaci, Amelia Spinella, Marco Sebastiani, Dilia Giuggioli and Clodoveo Ferri
Chair and Rheumatology Unit, Medical School, Azienda Ospedaliero-Universitaria, University of Modena and Reggio Emilia, Policlinico di Modena, Via del Pozzo 71, 41100 Modena, Italy

Lucio Brugioni and Maurizio Tognetti
Critical Care Unit, Azienda Ospedaliero-Universitaria Policlinico di Modena, Modena, Italy

Wafa Chebbi, Asma Fradi, Baha Zantour and Mohamed Habib Sfar
Department of Internal Medicine, University Hospital Taher Sfar, 5100 Mahdia, Tunisia

Saida Jerbi
Department of Radiology, University Hospital Taher Sfar, 5100 Mahdia, Tunisia

Wassia Kessomtini
Department of Physical Medicine, University Hospital Taher Sfar, 5100 Mahdia, Tunisia

Orhan Küçükşahin and Nurşen Düzgün
Department of Rheumatology, Ankara University Medical Faculty, Sihhiye, 06410 Ankara, Turkey

Alexis K. Okoh and Emre Kulahçioglu
Department of Internal Medicine, Ankara University Medical Faculty, Sihhiye, 06410 Ankara, Turkey

Joseph J. LaConti and Dana Ascherman
Division of Rheumatology, University of Miami Leonard Miller School of Medicine, Miami, FL 33136, USA

Jean A. Donet, Daniel A. Sussman and Amar R. Deshpande
Division of Gastroenterology, University of Miami Leonard Miller School of Medicine, Miami, FL 33136, USA

Jeong Hee Cho-Vega
Department of Pathology, University of Miami Leonard Miller School of Medicine, Miami, FL 33136, USA

Shihoko Nakajima, Keisuke Oda and Yutaka Nakiri
Department of Internal Medicine and Rheumatology, Juntendo University Nerima Hospital, Tokyo 177-8521, Japan

Satoshi Suzuki
Department of Internal Medicine and Rheumatology, Juntendo University Nerima Hospital, Tokyo 177-8521, Japan
Department of Internal Medicine Research, Sasaki Institute, Sasaki Foundation, Tokyo 101-0062, Japan

Taiki Ando and Yoshinari Takasaki
Department of Internal Medicine and Rheumatology, Juntendo University School of Medicine, Tokyo 113-8431, Japan

Manabu Sugita
Department of Emergency and Critical Care Medicine, Juntendo University Nerima Hospital, Tokyo 177-8521, Japan

Kunimi Maeda
Department of Internal Medicine and Nephrology, Juntendo University Nerima Hospital, Tokyo 177-8521, Japan

Rawhya R. El-Shereef
Rheumatology Department, Faculty of Medicine, Minia, Egypt

Zein El-Abedin
Neurology Department, Faculty of Medicine, Minia, Egypt

Rashad Abdel Aziz
Cardiology Department, Faculty of Medicine, Minia, Egypt

Ibrahim Talat, Mohammed Saleh and Hanna Abdel-Samia
ICUDepartment, Faculty of Medicine,Minia, Egypt

Amro Sameh and Mahmoud Sharha
Radiology Department, Faculty of Medicine, Minia, Egypt

Yuka Ogawa, Dai Kishida, Yasuhiro Shimojima and Yoshiki Sekijima
Department of Medicine (Neurology and Rheumatology), Shinshu University School of Medicine, 3-1-1 Asahi, Matsumoto 390-8621, Japan

Koichi Hayashi
Department of Dermatology, Shinshu University School of Medicine, 3-1-1 Asahi, Matsumoto 390-8621, Japan

B. Hodkinson and S. Botha-Scheepers
Department of Medicine, Division of Rheumatology, University of Cape Town and Groote Schuur Hospital, Cape Town 7945, South Africa

N. Osman
Division of Anatomical Pathology, National Health Laboratory Service, University of Cape Town and Groote Schuur Hospital, Cape Town 7945, South Africa

Bülent Alım
Clinic of Physical Medicine and Rehabilitation, Bayburt State Hospital, Bayburt, Turkey

Sinan Çetinel, M. Alperen Servi, Fahrettin Bostancı and Mehmet Ozan Bingöl
Clinic of Physical Medicine and Rehabilitation, Cumhuriyet University Hospital, Sivas, Turkey

Hidekazu Ikeuchi, Kana Koinuma, Masao Nakasatomi, Toru Sakairi, Yoriaki Kaneko, Akito Maeshima and Keiju Hiromura
Department of Nephrology and Rheumatology, Gunma University Graduate School of Medicine, Maebashi, Japan

Yuichi Yamazaki
Department of Medicine and Molecular Science, Gunma University Graduate School of Medicine, Maebashi, Japan

Hiroaki Okamoto
Division of Virology, Department of Infection and Immunity, Jichi Medical University School of Medicine, Shimotsuke, Japan

Toshihide Mimura
Department of Rheumatology and Applied Immunology, Faculty of Medicine, Saitama Medical University, Saitama, Japan

Satoshi Mochida
Division of Gastroenterology and Hepatology Internal Medicine, Saitama Medical University, Saitama, Japan

Yoshihisa Nojima
Department of Rheumatology and Nephrology, Japan Red Cross Maebashi Hospital, Maebashi, Japan

Tomoya Miyamura and Eiichi Suematsu
Department of Internal Medicine and Rheumatology, Clinical Research Institute, National Hospital Organization, Kyushu Medical Center, 1-8-1 Jigyohama, Chuo-ku, Fukuoka 810-8563, Japan

Akihiro Nakamura
Department of Internal Medicine and Rheumatology, Clinical Research Institute, National Hospital Organization, Kyushu Medical Center, 1-8-1 Jigyohama, Chuo-ku, Fukuoka 810-8563, Japan
Department of Genetics and Development, Krembil Research Institute, Toronto Western Hospital, 60 Leonard Avenue, Toronto, ON, Canada M5T 2S8

Brian Wu
Department of Genetics and Development, Krembil Research Institute, Toronto Western Hospital, 60 Leonard Avenue, Toronto, ON, Canada M5T 2S8

Maaman Bashir and Richard Hariman
Division of Rheumatology, Department of Medicine, Medical College of Wisconsin, Milwaukee, WI 53226, USA

Brittany Bettendorf
Division of Rheumatology, Department of Medicine, University of Iowa, Iowa City, IA 52242, USA

Shiho Iwagaitsu and Taio Naniwa
Division of Rheumatology, Department of Internal Medicine, Nagoya City University Hospital, Nagoya, Japan
Department of Respiratory Medicine, Allergy and Clinical Immunology, Nagoya City University Graduate School of Medical Sciences, Nagoya, Japan

Sara Beygi
Internal Medicine Department, Allegheny Health Network, Pittsburgh, PA, USA

Alfred Denio
Rheumatology Department, Geisinger Medical Center, Danville, PA, USA

Tarun S. Sharma
Rheumatology Department, Allegheny Health Network, Pittsburgh, PA, USA

Rebecca L. Burns
Division of Rheumatology, University of Michigan Health System, Suite 7C27, North Ingalls Building, 300 North Ingalls Street, SPC 5422, Ann Arbor, MI 48109-5422, USA

Sharukh J. Bhavnagri
Department of Diagnostic Radiology and Molecular Imaging, Oakland University William Beaumont School of Medicine, 3601 West 13 Mile Road, Royal Oak, MI 48073, USA

Zeeshan Butt and Manash K. Das
Internal Medicine Residency Program, Prince George's Hospital Center, 3001 Hospital Dr, Cheverly, MD 20785, USA

Leeza Patel
Department of Rheumatology, University of Arkansas for Medical Sciences, Little Rock, AR, USA

Christopher A. Mecoli and Alim Ramji
Division of Rheumatology, John Hopkins University School of Medicine, 733 N Broadway, Baltimore, MD 21205, USA

Myat Tun Lin Nyo
Department of Medicine, Division of Rheumatology, Sefako Makgatho Health Sciences University, Pretoria, South Africa

Mahmood M. T. M. Ally
Department of Internal Medicine, Division of Rheumatology, University of Pretoria, Pretoria, South Africa

Elsa Magreta Van Duuren
Department of Medicine, Division of Rheumatology, Sefako Makgatho Health Sciences University, Pretoria, South Africa

Regan Arendse
Division of Rheumatology, Community Rheumatology Care, University of Saskatchewan, 301-39 23rd St. East, Saskatoon, SK, Canada S7K 0H6

Sima Terebelo and Iona Chen
Maimonides Medical Center, Brooklyn, NY, USA

Fawad Aslam
Division of Rheumatology, Department of Internal Medicine, Mayo Clinic, Scottsdale, AZ, USA

Jonathan A. Flug
Department of Radiology, Mayo Clinic, Scottsdale, AZ, USA

Yousif Yonan
Department of Dermatology, Mayo Clinic, Scottsdale, AZ, USA

Shelley S. Noland
Division of Plastic Surgery, Department of Surgery, Mayo Clinic Hospital, Phoenix, AZ, USA
Department of Orthopedic Surgery, Mayo Clinic Hospital, Phoenix, AZ, USA

Index